D1145081

# ADVANCES IN PROSTAGLANDIN, THROMBOXANE, AND LEUKOTRIENE RESEARCH
## VOLUME 22

---

## Leukotrienes as Mediators of Asthma and Inflammation: Basic and Applied Research

# Advances in Prostaglandin, Thromboxane, and Leukotriene Research

## Series Editors: Bengt Samuelsson and Rodolfo Paoletti
## (Formerly *Advances in Prostaglandin and Thromboxane Research* Series)

### INTERNATIONAL ADVISORY BOARD

*Out of print

Advances in Prostaglandin, Thromboxane,
and Leukotriene Research
Volume 22

---

# Leukotrienes as Mediators of Asthma and Inflammation: Basic and Applied Research

Second International Symposium on Trends in
Eicosanoid Biology
Interlaken, Switzerland

Editors

Sven-Erik Dahlén, M.D., Ph.D.
Department of Physiology
and Pharmacology
Karolinska Institutet
Stockholm, Sweden

Per Hedqvist, M.D., Ph.D.
Department of Physiology
and Pharmacology
Karolinska Institutet
Stockholm, Sweden

Bengt Samuelsson, M.D., Ph.D.
Department of Medical Biochemistry
and Biophysics
Karolinska Institutet
Stockholm, Sweden

William A. Taylor, Ph.D.
Bayer plc
Pharmaceutical Division
Stoke Poges
Buckinghamshire, U.K.

Jürgen Fritsch, Ph.D.
Bayer AG
Scientific Relations
Leverkusen, Germany

Raven Press ☙ New York

Raven Press, Ltd., 1185 Avenue of the Americas, New York, New York 10036

Printed in Belgium

International Standard Book Number 0-7817-0247-X

Library of Congress Catalog Card Number: 94-69543

9  8  7  6  5  4  3  2  1

# Preface

This volume includes the presentations given at the Second Interlaken Symposium on *Trends in Eicosanoid Biology*. This series of symposia is organized by eicosanoid researchers at the Karolinska Institutet in Stockholm, Sweden, and made possible by an educational grant from Bayer AG. The objective of these symposia is to highlight current developments relating to the biology of arachidonic acid products, covering different aspects ranging from molecule to humans.

The title of the Interlaken Symposium in September 1992 was "*Leukotrienes as Mediators of Asthma and Inflammation: Basic and Applied Research.*" This topic was selected in view of the rapidly accumulating evidence that leukotrienes represent a group of mediators that contribute significantly to the pathobiology of asthma and perhaps to other diseases as well.

The book is organized into six sections, which correspond to the six sessions of the symposium. The first sections of this volume comprise presentations that deal with the mechanisms for synthesis of leukotrienes, how this knowledge is applied to devise strategies for inhibition of the actions or formation of leukotrienes, and presentations covering basic experimental studies with relevance to the biochemistry and physiology of leukotrienes in inflammation. Later sections of the volume, in an overview format, report on the first studies with leukotrienes and antileukotriene drugs in human volunteers and asthmatics. The chapters are written by the investigators who performed these original studies. The symposium also addressed the potential role of leukotrienes in areas other than bronchial asthma, such as rheumatoid arthritis, rhinitis, inflammatory bowel disease, and skin disorders. Furthermore, part of the symposium was devoted to closely related areas of arachidonic acid metabolism, such as the biology of the lipoxins and influences on inflammation and arachidonic acid metabolism by cytokines. In addition, each section of the book ends with a brief summary chapter written by the chairperson of that particular session, thus providing perspectives and views supplemental to the presentations.

We are convinced that this volume, which includes a collection of authoritative state-of-the-art accounts written by leading experts in the field of leukotriene and inflammation research, will be a useful reference and gateway to further investigations. The volume provides an easily accessible integration between basic and clinical findings in this important field of research.

*The Editors*

# Acknowledgments

On behalf of all participants in the International Workshop on "Leuko-trienes as Mediators of Asthma and Inflammation: Basic and Applied Research," held in Interlaken, Switzerland, September 7–12, 1992, we thank Bayer AG for making the workshop possible. We are especially grateful to Dr. Jürgen Fritsch and Mr. Klaus Gerressen for their invaluable contribution to the success of the workshop.

# Contents

*ix*

### 5. Mediators and Mechanisms in Nasal and Rheumatic Inflammation

### 6. Lipoxygenase Products and Cytokine Regulation

# Symposium Speakers and Chairmen

**William M. Abraham**   *Department of Research, Pulmonary Division, Mount Sinai Medical Center, 4300 Alton Road, Miami Beach, Florida 33140*

**Jonathan P. Arm**   *Brigham and Women's Hospital, The Seeley G. Mudd Building, 250 Longwood Avenue, Boston, Massachusetts 02115*

**K. Frank Austen**   *Department of Rheumatology and Immunology, Brigham and Women's Hospital; and Department of Medicine, Harvard Medical School, The Seeley G. Mudd Building, 250 Longwood Avenue, Boston, Massachusetts 02115*

**Neil C. Barnes**   *The London Chest Hospital, Bonner Road, London E2 9JK, England*

**Eugene R. Bleecker**   *University of Maryland, 10 South Pine Street, Baltimore, Maryland 21201*

**William W. Busse**   *Department of Medicine, University of Wisconsin-Madison, Clinical Science Center, 600 Highland Avenue, Madison, Wisconsin 53792-3244*

**John Costello**   *Kings College School of Medicine and Dentistry, Department of Thoracic Medicine, Bessemer Road, London SE5 9PJ, England*

**Clemens A. Dahinden**   *Institute for Clinical Immunology, University Hospital, Inselspital, CH-3010 Bern, Switzerland*

**Sven-Erik Dahlén**   *Department of Physiology and Pharmacology, Karolinska Institutet, S-171 77 Stockholm, Sweden*

**Edward A. Dennis**   *Department of Chemistry, University of California, San Diego, 9500 Gilman Drive, La Jolla, California 92093-0601*

**Jeffrey M. Drazen**   *Brigham and Women's Hospital, 75 Francis Street, Boston, Massachusetts 02115*

**Garret A. FitzGerald**   *Center for Experimental Therapeutics, Biomedical Research Building, University of Pennsylvania, 422 Curie Boulevard, Philadelphia, Pennsylvania 19104*

**Giancarlo Folco**   *Center for Cardiopulmonary Pharmacology, School of Pharmacy, University of Milan, Via Balzaretta 9, 20133 Milan, Italy*

**Anthony Ford-Hutchinson**   *Merck Frosst Centre for Therapeutic Research, P.O. Box 1005, Pointe Claire-Dorval, Quebec H9R 4P8, Canada*

**Phillip J. Gardiner**   *Bayer plc, Pharmaceutical Group Research Department, Stoke Court, Stoke Poges, Buckinghamshire SL2 4LY, England*

**Lawrence G. Garland**   *Department of Medicinal Chemistry, Research Division, The Wellcome Foundation Ltd., Langley Court, South Eden Park Road, Beckenham, Kent BR3 3BS, England*

**Marc E. Goldyne**   *Medicine and Dermatology Department, University of California, Veterans Affairs Medical Center, 4150 Clement Street, San Francisco, California 94121*

**Robert H. Gundel**   *Miles Preclinical Research, Miles Inc., 400 Morgan Lane, West Haven, Connecticut 06516-4175*

**Per Hedqvist**   *Department of Physiology and Pharmacology, Karolinska Institutet, S-171 77 Stockholm, Sweden*

**Joachim R. Kalden**   *University Hospital, Krankenhausstrasse 12, Erlangen 91054, Germany*

**Michael A. Kaliner**   *Institute for Asthma and Allergy, Washington Hospital Center, 106 Irving Street, N.W., Washington, D.C. 20010*

**Dietrich Keppler**   *Division of Tumor Biochemistry, Deutsches Krebsforschungszentrum, Neuenhelmer Feld 280, D-69120 Heidelberg 1, Germany*

**Howard R. Knapp**   *University of Iowa, College of Medicine, Division of Clinical Pharmacology, Iowa City, Iowa 52242-1081*

**Robert D. Krell**   *Biofor, Inc., P.O. Box 629, Waverly, Pennsylvania 18471-0629*

**Robert A. Lewis**   *Syntex Research, 3401 Hillview Avenue, P.O. Box 10850, Palo Alto, California 94304*

**Robert C. Murphy**   *Department of Pediatrics, National Jewish Center for Immunology and Respiratory Medicine, 1400 Jackson Street, Denver, Colorado 80206*

**Reiner Müller-Peddinghouse**   *Bayer AG, Business Group Pharma, Aprather Weg 18A, P.O. Box 101709, D-42096 Wuppertal, Germany*

**Paul M. O'Byrne**   *Department of Medicine, McMaster University, 1200 Main Street West, Hamilton, Ontario L8N 3Z5, Canada*

**Richard P. Phipps**   *Medical Center, University of Rochester, School of Medicine, 601 Elmwood Avenue, Rochester, New York 14642*

**Jørgen Rask-Madsen**   *Department of Medical Gastroenterology, Hvidovre Hospital, Kettegård Allé 30, DK-2650 Hvidovre, Denmark*

**Dwight R. Robinson** *Arthritis Unit, Massachusetts General Hospital, 55 Fruit Street, Boston, Massachusetts 02114*

**Bengt Samuelsson** *Department of Medical Biochemistry and Biophysics (MBB), Karolinska Institutet, S171 77 Stockholm, Sweden*

**Charles N. Serhan** *Hematology-Oncology Division, Department of Medicine, Brigham and Women's Hospital, Harvard Medical School, 221 Longwood Avenue, Boston, Massachusetts 02115*

**Elliot Sigal** *Syntex Discovery Research, 3401 Hillview Avenue, Palo Alto, California 94304*

**Andrew Szczeklik** *Department of Medicine, University School of Medicine, 8 Skawińska Street, 31-006 Cracow, Poland*

**Ian K. Taylor** *Chest and Allergy Department, Royal Infirmary Hospital, New Durland Road, Sunderland SR2 7J2, England*

**William Taylor** *Bayer plc, Pharmaceutical Group, Research Department, Stoke Court, Stoke Poges, Buckinghamshire SL2 4LY, England*

**Peter C. Weber** *Institute für Prophylaxe und Epidemiologie der Kreislaufkrankheiten, Universistät München, Pettenkofer Strasse 9, 80336 München 2, Germany*

# 1. Biosynthesis of Leukotrienes and Mode of Action of Antileukotrienes

*Advances in Prostaglandin, Thromboxane,*
*and Leukotriene Research,* Vol. 22, edited by
S.-E. Dahlén et al. Raven Press, Ltd., New York © 1994

# Novel Structural and Functional Properties of Leukotriene A$_4$ Hydrolase

## Implications for the Development of Enzyme Inhibitors

Jesper Z. Haeggström, Anders Wetterholm, Juan F. Medina, and Bengt Samuelsson

*Department of Medical Biochemistry and Biophysics, Karolinska Institutet, S-171 77 Stockholm, Sweden*

The final step in the biosynthesis of the proinflammatory substance leukotriene (LT) B$_4$ is catalyzed by a soluble monomeric enzyme, LTA$_4$ hydrolase, that is ubiquitous in mammalian tissues (1,2). The enzyme has even been detected in cells apparently devoid of 5-lipoxygenase activity, which is required for biosynthesis of LTA$_4$. Exposure of LTA$_4$ hydrolase to this natural epoxide substrate leads to enzyme inactivation and covalent modification of the protein (3,4), a phenomenon often referred to as *suicide inactivation.*

Sequence comparisons of LTA$_4$ hydrolase with certain proteases and aminopeptidases led to the identification of a zinc binding motif (Fig. 1), and further studies showed that LTA$_4$ hydrolase is indeed a zinc metalloenzyme that contains one atom of zinc (5–8). Furthermore, the enzyme was found to exhibit a second enzymatic activity that catalyzed hydrolysis of synthetic amides, i.e., a novel amidase/peptidase activity (8,9). These findings suddenly gave new insight into the structure and function of LTA$_4$ hydrolase. Here we review further work carried out to elucidate the properties of the enzyme's active center and catalytic mechanism(s) and briefly discuss the implications for the development of LTA$_4$ hydrolase inhibitors.

## REACTIVATION OF APO-LTA$_4$ HYDROLASE: CATALYTIC FUNCTION OF THE ZINC ATOM

Zinc is an essential and integral component of a broad array of enzymes involved in almost all aspects of cell metabolism (6). The metal can partic-

|  | L₁   L₂ | L₃ |
|---|---|---|
| Thermolysin | V V A Ĥ Ê L T Ĥ A V T | G A I N Ê A I S D |
|  | 142   146 | 166 |
| Leukotriene A₄ hydrolase | V I A Ĥ Ê I S Ĥ S W T | F W L N Ê G H T V |
|  | 295   299 | 318 |
| Aminopeptidase M | V I A Ĥ Ê L A Ĥ Q W F | L W L N Ê G F A S |
|  | 388   392 | 411 |
| Neutral endopeptidase | V I G Ĥ Ê I T Ĥ G F D | N T L G Ê N I A D |
|  | 583   587 | 646 |

FIG. 1. Comparison of the zinc binding regions of thermolysin and LTA₄ hydrolase, with the proposed zinc sites of neutral endopeptidase and aminopeptidase M. (Adapted from ref. 6.)

ipate either in the catalytic process or in the stabilization of protein structure. Thermolysin and related enzymes, as well as LTA$_4$ hydrolase, contain a so-called catalytic binding site at which the zinc atom is coordinated to any three of four types of residues from His, Cys, Glu, and Asp. The two primary ligands (denoted $L_1$ and $L_2$ in Fig. 1) are separated by a short spacer of about 1 to 3 amino acids, which in turn are separated from a third ligand ($L_3$) by a long spacer of about 20 to 120 amino acids. The fourth ligand is an activated water molecule that is believed to play a critical role in the catalytic reaction (10). In agreement with the single potential zinc site found in the sequence of LTA$_4$ hydrolase, analysis with atomic absorption spectrometry revealed the presence of 1.14 mol zinc per mol protein (mean value from five batches of enzyme) (7). Treatment of LTA$_4$ hydrolase with chelating agents, particularly 1,10-phenanthroline, eliminated essentially all enzymatic activity. Furthermore, zinc analysis showed that 1,10-phenanthroline had removed the zinc atom from its site of coordination and thus the apoenzyme of LTA$_4$ hydrolase had been produced. However, the loss of enzyme activities was reversible and could be regained by addition of stoichiometric amounts of $Zn^{2+}$ (and also $Co^{2+}$) to the apoenzyme (Fig. 2). Reactivation of both the epoxide hydrolase and the peptidase activity was proportional to the amount of added metal up to a molar ratio metal/protein of about 1, which suggested that a single binding site had been filled with zinc or cobalt (7,9). Apparently, removal of the intrinsic zinc atom with a chelator did not alter the protein's tertiary structure in a way such that enzyme activity was irreversibly lost. Instead, the apoenzyme could be completely reactivated, which also demonstrates the catalytic function of zinc in LTA$_4$ hydrolase.

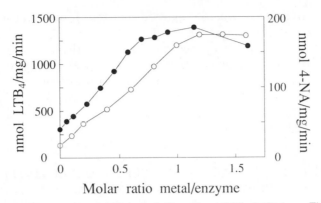

**FIG. 2.** Effects of zinc on the catalytic activities of apo-LTA₄ hydrolase. The apoenzyme was incubated with increasing amounts of ZnSO₄ and then assayed for its epoxide hydrolase (2.5 μg protein in 100 μl 25 m$M$ HEPES, pH 8) and peptidase activity (3 μg protein in 250 μl 50 m$M$ Tris-HCl, pH 8) (7,9). Activities are expressed as nmol of the respective product formed per mg and min. Filled (●) and open (○) circles denote the peptidase and epoxide hydrolase activity, respectively.

## IDENTIFICATION OF THE THREE ZINC BINDING LIGANDS

On the basis of the thermolysin/aminopeptidase sequence homology, His-295, His-299, and Glu-318 of LTA₄ hydrolase were proposed to be the ligands (L₁, L₂, and L₃) involved in zinc coordination (Fig. 1). To determine the importance of these amino acid residues in the binding of zinc to the protein and in the catalytic activities, site-directed mutagenesis was carried out on mouse LTA₄ hydrolase cDNA. In three separate mutants, codons corresponding to His-295, His-299, and Glu-318 were changed to codons encoding Tyr, Tyr, and Gln, respectively, by PCR mutagenesis on the expression plasmid pULTA4 (11).

Each mutated protein, H295Y, H299Y, and E318Q (named in single letter code to indicate the amino acid change), was expressed in *E. coli* and purified to apparent homogeneity to make zinc analyses and enzyme activity determinations possible. The zinc contents of the purified mutated proteins H295Y, H299Y, and E318Q were insignificant (0.05, 0.02, and 0.07 mol/mol, respectively). In addition, none of the three mutated enzymes displayed any significant epoxide hydrolase or peptidase activity. Nevertheless, the proteins were positively identified as mutants of LTA₄ hydrolase by their chromatographic characteristics during purification, their molecular weights, and their immunoreactivities with a polyclonal antiserum for human LTA₄ hydrolase in Western blots. Using this experimental approach, we thus obtained data which directly confirmed the predictions that His-295, His-299, and Glu-318 constitute the three zinc binding ligands of LTA₄ hydrolase. It was noteworthy that the elution profile of the mutated proteins in all chromatographic steps was almost identical to that of nonmutated recombinant mouse LTA$_4$ hydrolase, which suggested that the three-dimensional structures of the zinc-free mutants were quite similar to that of zinc containing wild-type enzyme. Therefore, the contribution of the zinc atom of LTA$_4$ hydrolase to the maintenance of its tertiary structure appears to be limited. On the other hand, the concomitant loss of both zinc content and enzyme activities in all three mutants agrees well with the properties of the apoenzyme and points out the important role of the zinc atom in the catalytic mechanism(s) of LTA$_4$ hydrolase.

## CHLORIDE ACTIVATION OF THE PEPTIDASE ACTIVITY VIA A PUTATIVE ANION BINDING SITE

The peptidase activity of LTA$_4$ hydrolase was found to be greatly stimulated by chloride ions (Table 1), an effect not observed for the conversion of LTA$_4$ into LTB$_4$ (12). This selective effect on only one catalytic activity may represent a mode of enzyme regulation. Anion activation has previously been described for several enzymes, e.g., α-amylase, cathepsin C, and angiotensin-converting enzyme (ACE). The mechanism(s) of anion activation is not fully understood and appears to vary among enzymes. In the case of LTA$_4$ hydrolase, kinetic analysis revealed that the Michaelis constant was not significantly altered by chloride ions in concentrations ranging between 12.5 and 200 m$M$, whereas the turnover number was increased almost fivefold (12). For some enzymes, experimental data have indicated that anion activation is mediated via a particular binding site in the protein. For example, binding measurements with $^{36}$Cl have shown that α-amylase possesses one binding site for Cl$^-$ per molecule of enzyme (13). Furthermore, chemical modification of α-amylase and ACE has indicated that a single lysine

**TABLE 1.** *Effects of NaCl on the peptidase activity of LTA$_4$ hydrolase*[a]

| NaCl (m$M$) | Peptidase activity (nmol/mg/min) |
|:---:|:---:|
| 1[b] | 15 |
| 10 | 80 |
| 25 | 150 |
| 50 | 250 |
| 100 | 380 |
| 200 | 510 |
| 500 | 620 |

[a] Native human LTA$_4$ hydrolase (0.5 μg) was incubated for 20 min at RT with alanine-4-nitroanilide (1 m$M$) in 250 μl 50 m$M$ phosphate buffer, pH 7.5, containing various amounts of NaCl. The reaction velocities were determined as described in ref. 12 and are expressed as nmol 4-nitroaniline/mg/min.

[b] The velocity was determined in a separate experiment using 7 μg of enzyme incubated for 60 min to reach detectable levels of product. No NaCl was used and 1 m$M$ Cl$^-$ is an estimate of the amount of anion added with the substrate.

residue may be responsible for chloride binding in their activating sites (14,15). In line with those observations, we obtained kinetic evidence suggesting that activation of the peptidase activity of LTA$_4$ hydrolase by Cl$^-$ could also be mediated by an anion binding site in the protein. Therefore, the stimulatory activity appeared to obey saturation kinetics, with a calculated affinity constant for Cl$^-$ of 100 m$M$ (Fig. 3). The concentration of Cl$^-$ is relatively high in the extracellular compartment (approximately 100 m$M$) as opposed to the intracellular (approximately 3 m$M$). Considering these differences, LTA$_4$ hydrolase may exert a possible proteolytic function only outside the cell, whereas the epoxide hydrolase activity could operate on either side of the cell membrane. However, it should be noted that the intracellular level of chloride in resting human polymorphonuclear leukocytes has been estimated to about 80 mEq/L cell water (16).

## SELECTIVE ABROGATION OF THE PEPTIDASE ACTIVITY

Several zinc proteases and mono zinc aminopeptidases, such as thermolysin, neutral endopeptidase, and aminopeptidase M, share a conserved glutamic acid located in the immediate vicinity of the first zinc binding ligand, denoted L$_1$ in Fig. 1 (cf. 6). This structural feature is also observed in LTA$_4$ hydrolase, in which a Glu residue is positioned next to the zinc binding ligand His-295. To study the role of Glu-296 for the two catalytic activities of LTA$_4$ hydrolase, we substituted this amino acid for a Gln or Ala residue by site-directed mutagenesis (17). Four to five batches of wild-type and mutated recombinant proteins were purified to apparent homogeneity and assayed for epoxide hydrolase and peptidase activity (Fig. 4).

Replacement of Glu-296 with a Gln residue in mouse LTA$_4$ hydrolase resulted in a protein E296Q with intact or even slightly increased ($\approx$150%) ability to convert LTA$_4$ into LTB$_4$, compared with unmutated wild-type enzyme (Fig. 4). In contrast, the peptidase activity toward alanine-4-ni-

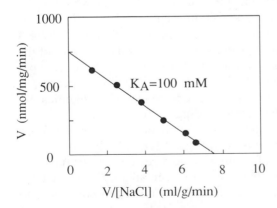

**FIG. 3.** Determination of the apparent affinity constant for NaCl. Native human LTA$_4$ hydrolase (0.5 µg) was incubated for 20 min at room temperature with alanine-4-nitroanilide (1 m$M$) in 250 µl 50 m$M$ phosphate buffer, ph 7.5 containing various amounts of NaCl (10 to 500 m$M$; cf. Table 1). The specific activities were calculated as means of triplicate samples and the kinetic data were plotted according to Eadie and Hofstee.

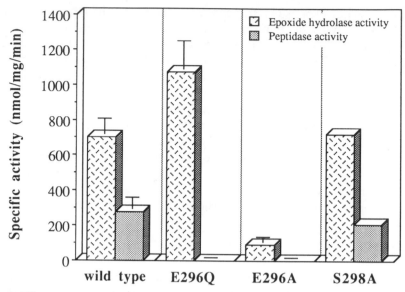

**FIG. 4.** Effects of mutagenetic replacements of Glu-296 on the epoxide hydrolase and peptidase activities of recombinant mouse LTA₄ hydrolase. Each mutant is denoted in single letter code to indicate the amino acid change. Specific activities were determined from incubations of purified enzyme with LTA₄ or alanine-4-nitroanilide, as described (17). The epoxide hydrolase and peptidase activities are expressed as nmol of product, i.e., LTB₄ and 4-nitroaniline formed per mg enzyme and min. Each bar represents a mean value, ± SD, obtained from four or five batches of enzyme, except for the mutant S298A, for which two batches were analyzed.

troanilide was practically abolished. A similar although less striking selective abrogation of the peptidase activity was observed with the mutant E296A. This enzyme displayed a substantially reduced albeit clearly detectable epoxide hydrolase activity corresponding to approximately 15% of wild-type enzyme, whereas its peptidase activity was negligible. To serve as a positive control, we also constructed the mutant S298A, in which a Ser residue located next to the second zinc binding ligand $L_2$ (cf. Fig. 1) was replaced with an Ala residue. As expected, the specific activities of S298A were quite similar to those of wild-type enzyme (Fig. 4). Zinc analyses of the purified proteins resulted in mean values of 0.97, 1.0, 0.89, 0.96 mol zinc per mol protein for wild-type enzyme, E296Q, E296A, and S298A, respectively, which confirmed that none of the mutagenetic replacements had significantly influenced the zinc content of the corresponding proteins (17).

Taken together, these results enable us to conclude that the peptidase activity, but not the epoxide hydrolase activity, of LTA₄ hydrolase is critically dependent on the presence of a glutamic acid residue at position 296. Furthermore, the fact that E296Q had intact or even slightly increased epoxide hydrolase activity suggests that Glu-296 has not been conserved to allow the biosynthesis of $LTB_4$ from $LTA_4$ but rather to maintain or develop some other biochemical function yet to be identified. Because this glutamic acid residue, as well as the binding motif of the catalytic zinc atom, is shared among a number of zinc proteases and aminopeptidases, the implications of our results may pertain to other members of these enzyme families. In fact, site-directed mutagenesis of Glu-584 in neutral endopeptidase to either an Asp or Val residue abolished its catalytic activity but not the binding of a substrate-related inhibitor (18).

## THE ROLE OF GLU-296 AS A GENERAL BASE IN THE PEPTIDASE REACTION

X-ray crystallographic analysis of thermolysin, a protease with a catalytic zinc site structurally similar to that of $LTA_4$ hydrolase, has identified Glu-143 as a putative catalytic amino acid. Two reaction mechanisms have been discussed in which Glu-143 either acts as a general base or forms an anhydride with the substrate. In the former and most favored mechanism, a water molecule is displaced from the zinc atom by the carbonyl oxygen of the substrate and is then polarized by the carboxylate of the glutamic acid to promote an attack of the carbonyl carbon of the scissile peptide bond. Simultaneously, a proton is transferred to the nitrogen of the peptide bond from an adjacent amino acid (19,20). It appears reasonable to assume that the peptidase activity of $LTA_4$ hydrolase functions according to a similar mechanism (Fig. 5).

The carboxylate of Glu-296 apparently, is not essential for the epoxide hydrolysis catalyzed by $LTA_4$ hydrolase. Therefore, replacement of the carboxyl group with an amide (E296Q) did not reduce, but rather slightly increased, the specific epoxide hydrolase activity (Fig. 4). Substitution of Glu-296 for an alanine residue (E296A) certainly reduced the epoxide hydrolase activity by more than 80%, but this effect was perhaps not unexpected, considering the chemical differences between alanine and glutamic acid, e.g., polarity and length of the side chain. Nevertheless, we cannot

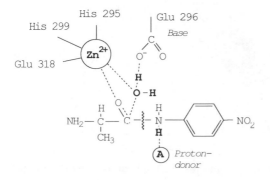

**FIG. 5.** Putative reaction mechanism for the hydrolysis of alanine-4-nitroanilide by $LTA_4$ hydrolase. (Based on the models presented in refs. 19 and 20.)

exclude that Glu-296 in some way participates in the epoxide hydrolase reaction, although this particular amino acid is not a prerequisite for catalysis.

## TWO NONIDENTICAL BUT OVERLAPPING ACTIVE SITES IN LTA₄ HYDROLASE

Several lines of evidence have indicated that the epoxide hydrolase and peptidase activities of LTA₄ hydrolase are exerted via the same active site. For example, the presence of the intrinsic zinc atom was required for both catalytic activities and they were both susceptible to inactivation by LTA₄ (7,9,21) and inhibition by the compounds bestatin and captopril (22). However, in at least two ways the activities differ, indicating that the catalytically important amino acids are not identical for the peptidase and epoxide hydrolase reactions. First, we have observed that the peptidase activity was stimulated by chloride (and other monovalent anions), in a fashion that suggested the presence of an anion binding site (12). The epoxide hydrolase activity was not stimulated by chloride but rather was slightly inhibited. Second, and more important, the results of mutagenetic replacements indicated that Glu-296, and particularly its carboxyl moiety, has a unique role in the peptidase but not in the epoxide hydrolase mechanism (17). Defined as all structural elements of the protein that participate in the catalytic reaction, the active site(s) thus appear to be overlapping rather than identical (Fig. 6).

## DEVELOPMENT OF LTA₄ HYDROLASE INHIBITORS

The strongest efforts to develop inhibitors of leukotriene biosynthesis have thus far been focused on the enzyme 5-lipoxygenase. Because 5-lipoxygenase catalyzes the formation of the key intermediate LTA₄, such inhibitors would be expected to be potent but also to block the formation of both

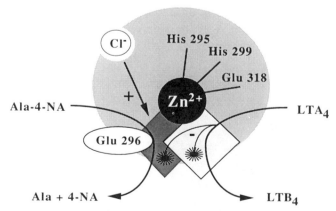

**FIG. 6.** Model for the structural and catalytic properties of LTA₄ hydrolase, a bifunctional zinc metalloenzyme.

cysteinyl-containing leukotrienes and $LTB_4$. Inhibitors aimed at more distal enzymes in the biosynthetic scheme should be more selective, and future drugs may be associated with fewer side effects. For $LTA_4$ hydrolase, which catalyzes the final and rate-limiting step in the biosynthesis of $LTB_4$ (23), not many inhibitors of significant potency and selectivity have previously been known. However, recent progress in the understanding of the enzymes structure and function has facilitated the synthesis and development of novel $LTA_4$ hydrolase inhibitors. For example, a number of known peptidase inhibitors have been tested for their effects on $LTA_4$ hydrolase (22). As mentioned above, two of the compounds, bestatin and captopril, inhibitors of aminopeptidase and ACE, respectively, were found to inhibit both catalytic activities of $LTA_4$ hydrolase. The concentrations for half-maximal inhibition varied between $10^{-5}$ and $10^{-7}$ $M$ and the peptidase activity was more susceptible than the epoxide hydrolase activity. Furthermore, a series of more than 10 peptide-based transition-state analogue inhibitors were recently synthesized (24). Those were soon followed by another class of compounds, which were based on the putative structure of a transition state between reactants and enzyme in the peptidase catalysis, as well as the hydrophobic properties of the natural epoxide substrate $LTA_4$ (25). Some of those compounds were found to be quite potent inhibitors of the peptidase activity of $LTA_4$ hydrolase with $IC_{50}$ values of less than 1 $\mu M$. In addition, Labaudinière et al. (26) have presented a new class of potent and selective inhibitors of $LTA_4$ hydrolase, one of which appeared metabolically stable after oral administration to rats. Interestingly, some of these compounds also displayed $LTB_4$ receptor binding activity (27).

## SUMMARY

Recent work in our laboratory, some of which is described in this report, has established that $LTA_4$ hydrolase is a bifunctional metalloenzyme that contains one zinc atom, essential for both catalytic activities. The well-characterized epoxide hydrolase activity, i.e., the conversion of $LTA_4$ into $LTB_4$ is inhibited by exposure to $LTA_4$, and this irreversible enzyme inactivation also affects the peptidase activity. In contrast, the peptide hydrolysis proceeds without any signs of enzyme inactivation, can be stimulated by physiologic concentrations of chloride ions, and is critically dependent on the presence of a Glu residue in position 296 of the protein. A model of the active center, which summarizes these novel structural and functional properties of $LTA_4$ hydrolase, is presented in Fig. 6.

## ACKNOWLEDGMENT

This work was financially supported by the Swedish Medical Research Council (03X-217, 03X-10350), Stiftelsen Lars Hiertas minne, Magnus Bergvalls Foundation, and O.E. & Edla Johanssons Foundations.

## REFERENCES

1. Samuelsson B. *Science* 1983;220:568–75.
2. Samuelsson B, Funk CD. *J Biol Chem* 1989;264:19469–72.
3. Evans JF, Nathaniel DJ, Zamboni RJ, Ford-Hutchinson AW. *J Biol Chem* 1985;260:10966–70.
4. Örning L, Jones DA, Fitzpatrick FA. *J Biol Chem* 1990;265:14911–6.
5. Malfroy B, Kado-Fong H, Gros C, Giros B, Schwartz JC, Hellmiss R. *Biochem Biophys Res Commun* 1989;161:236–41.
6. Vallee BL, Auld DS. *Biochemistry* 1990;29:5647–59.
7. Haeggström, JZ, Wetterholm A, Shapiro R, Vallee BL, Samuelsson B. *Biochem Biophys Res Commun* 1990;172:965–70.
8. Minami M, Ohishi N, Mutoh H, et al. *Biochem Biophys Res Commun* 1990;173:620–6.
9. Haeggström JZ, Wetterholm A, Vallee BL, Samuelsson B. *Biochem Biophys Res Commun* 1990;173:431–7.
10. Vallee BL, Auld DS. *Proc Natl Acad Sci USA* 1990;87:220–4.
11. Medina JF, Wetterholm A, Rådmark O, et al. *Proc Natl Acad Sci USA* 1991;88:7620–4.
12. Wetterholm A, Haeggström, JZ. *Biochim Biophys Acta* 1992;1123:275–81.
13. Levitzki A, Steer ML. *Eur J Biochem* 1974;41:171–80.
14. Lifshitz R, Levitzki A. *Biochemistry* 1976;15:1987–93.
15. Shapiro R, Riordan JF. *Biochemistry* 1983;22:5315–21.
16. Simchowitz L, De Weer P. *J Gen Physiol* 1986;88:167–94.
17. Wetterholm A, Medina JF, Rådmark O, et al. *Proc Natl Acad Sci USA* 1992;89:9141–5.
18. Devault A, Nault C, Zollinger M, et al. *J Biol Chem* 1988;263:4033–40.
19. Pangburn MK, Walsh KA. *Biochemistry* 1975;14:4050–4.
20. Kester WR, Matthews BW. *Biochemistry* 1977;16:2506–16.
21. Wetterholm A, Medina JF, Rådmark O, et al. *Biochim Biophys Acta* 1991;1080:96–102.
22. Örning L, Krivi G, Fitzpatrick FA. *J Biol Chem* 1991;266:1375–8.
23. Sun FF, McGuire JC. *Biochim Biophys Acta* 1984;794:56–64.
24. Yuan W, Zhong Z, Wong CH, Haeggström JZ, Wetterholm A, Samuelsson B. *Bioorg Med Chem Lett* 1991;1:551–6.
25. Yuan W, Wong CH, Haeggström JZ, Wetterholm A, Samuelsson B. *J Am Chem Soc* 1992;114:6552–3.
26. Labaudinière R, Hilboll G, Leon-Lomeli A, et al. *J Med Chem* 1992;35:3156–69.
27. Labaudinière R, Hilboll G, Leon-Lomeli A, et al. *J Med Chem* 1992;35:3170–9.

*Advances in Prostaglandin, Thromboxane, and Leukotriene Research*, Vol. 22, edited by S.-E. Dahlén et al. Raven Press, Ltd., New York © 1994

# 5-Lipoxygenase Activating Protein and Leukotriene C$_4$ Synthase: Therapeutic Targets for Inhibiting the Leukotriene Cascade

## A. W. Ford-Hutchinson

*Merck Frosst Centre for Therapeutic Research, Pointe Claire–Dorval, Quebec H9R 4P8, Canada*

Leukotrienes are products of arachidonic acid metabolism derived through the 5-lipoxygenase enzyme pathway and have been implicated as mediators of inflammatory and allergic reactions, including human bronchial asthma (Fig. 1). Various therapeutic approaches have been used to modulate either the production or the action of leukotrienes, and a number of drugs have entered clinical trials (1,2). The most advanced of these agents are the leukotriene D$_4$–receptor antagonists, such as MK-571, MK-679, and ICI 204,219 (1). In addition, various classes of inhibitors of leukotriene biosynthesis have been described (2). These include either direct 5-lipoxygenase inhibitors, such as zileuton and ICI D2318, which directly inhibit the enzyme through a variety of mechanisms, or a second class of agents, termed leukotriene biosynthesis inhibitors, which have no effect on the 5-lipoxygenase enzyme itself. These inhibitors, which include structures of the indole, quinoline, and quindole classes, bind with high affinity to a 5-lipoxygenase activating protein (FLAP), the expression of which is required for cellular leukotriene biosynthesis. Because leukotriene D$_4$–receptor activation has been shown to be an important event in diseases such as human bronchial asthma, an alternative approach would be to inhibit the enzyme leukotriene C$_4$ synthase. Evidence presented below indicates that this enzyme is a unique enzyme distinct from other more generalized glutathione S-transferase enzyme systems.

## 5-LIPOXYGENASE ACTIVATING PROTEIN

Leukotriene synthesis occurs only in intact cells after exposure to defined stimuli that can induce a considerable elevation in intracellular calcium. This

*13*

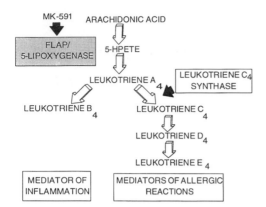

**FIG. 1.** Pathways of leukotriene biosynthesis.

is consistent with the suggestion that there is a regulatory process for the activation of 5-lipoxygenase. Further evidence for this is that the synthesis of leukotrienes by various cell types after stimulation with either calcium ionophore (3,4), thapsigargin (5), f-Met-Leu-Phe (6), or antigen (7) is associated with translocation of 5-lipoxygenase from the cytosol to a membrane fraction. In polymorphonuclear leukocytes this translocation was shown to be inhibited by leukotriene biosynthesis inhibitors such as the indole structure MK-886 (8). Compounds such as MK-886 block leukotriene biosynthesis in intact cells under all physiologic conditions studied to date but have no effect on the 5-lipoxygenase enzyme and are not inhibitors of phospholipase $A_2$ (9). Further studies with MK-886 have led to the isolation and identification of a novel 18-kDa membrane protein which has been termed 5-lipoxygenase activating protein (FLAP) (10). This protein was first identified using photoaffinity probes based around the structure of MK-886 and was purified to homogeneity on affinity columns to which the drug was coupled (10). In a series of dual transfection studies, it was demonstrated that the presence of FLAP was required for the cellular activation of 5-lipoxygenase and for cellular leukotriene biosynthesis in response to relevant stimuli (11). A series of studies utilizing photoaffinity analogs of various leukotriene biosynthesis inhibitors and a radioligand binding assay have demonstrated that leukotriene biosynthesis inhibitors, such as MK-886, bind to FLAP with high affinity and that this binding is correlated with the ability of different structures to inhibit leukotriene biosynthesis (12). In addition to the indoles, two other classes of inhibitors, i.e., quinolines and hybrid indole–quinoline structures, which have been termed quindoles and which are exemplified by MK-0591, have also been shown to bind with high affinity to FLAP (12–15). Therefore, FLAP binding assays (12) represent an important screening approach to searching for new leukotriene biosynthesis inhibitors.

The current hypothesis of how FLAP is involved in the activation of 5-lipoxygenase is illustrated in Fig. 2. After activation of the cell a rise in

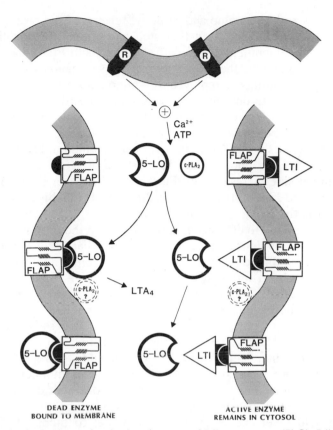

**FIG. 2.** Hypothetical scheme for the involvement of 5-lipoxygenase (5LO), 5-lipoxygenase activating protein (FLAP), and high molecular weight cytosolic phospholipase $A_2$ ($cPLA_2$) in cellular leukotriene biosynthesis and inhibition of leukotriene biosynthesis by inhibitors (LTI) such as MK-886 or MK-0591.

intracellular calcium occurs, which causes activation of both 5-lipoxygenase and high molecular weight cytosolic phospholipase $A_2$ (16). Both enzymes undergo a translocation to a membrane site at which 5-lipoxygenase, in cooperation with FLAP, metabolizes liberated arachidonic acid to leukotrienes. Leukotriene biosynthesis inhibitors bind to FLAP and may either directly compete with 5-lipoxygenase for binding to the protein or may cause a conformational change in FLAP, leading to a decreased affinity of 5-lipoxygenase for its membrane binding site.

The development of high-affinity ligands for FLAP has allowed analysis of the drug binding site. On the basis of hydropathic analysis of the amino acid sequences of FLAP, it has been proposed that the protein contains three transmembrane domains corresponding to residues 5-28, 63-93, and 118-141. This model suggests that two short hydrophilic loops link the transmem-

brane domains with the amino and carboxyl termini of the protein on oppo-
site sides of a membrane. As a first step to defining the location of the
binding site, the attachment of photoaffinity ligands to FLAP has been studied (17). Unfortunately, the attachment of these ligands to FLAP is not
stable under the conditions employed for amino acid sequencing, and therefore it is impossible to determine the exact amino acid to which the ligand
covalently attaches. However, reagents that cleave polypeptides at specific
amino acids have been used to localize peptide fragments to which these
photoaffinity ligands bind (17). Using cynogen bromide, it has been possible
to determine that the photoaffinity ligands are attached to FLAP on the
amino terminal side of residue 89. Further studies after digestion with io-
dozobenzoic acid have further defined the site of attachment to a peptide
fraction that is the amino terminal of [72]Trp.

A second approach to defining important areas in the protein is to look for
amino acid residues conserved among species. Therefore, the amino acid
sequences and binding characteristics of FLAP from a number of mammalian species have been determined (18). As observed in a radioligand binding
assay, FLAP from 10 different mammalian species specifically bound leukotriene biosynthesis inhibitors with $IC_{50}$ values for MK-886 ranging from 12
to 120 n$M$. This is consistent with the fact that drugs such as MK-886
effectively inhibit leukotriene biosynthesis both in vitro and in vivo in a
variety of mammalian species (9). cDNA molecules for FLAP from six of
these species were isolated and sequenced (Rhesus monkey, horse, pig,
sheep, rabbit, and mouse). All species displayed a high degree of overall
homology, with each species being at least 92% identical to human FLAP at
the amino acid level and at least 85% identical to human FLAP at the
nucleotide level. No insertions or deletions were observed, and many of the
amino acid differences among species were conservative substitutions. Positions at which amino acids do occur among species tend to be clustered in
specific regions of the protein, such as residues 127–138 and 35–38. A number of stretches of FLAP are highly conserved and, in particular, two regions
of FLAP (residues 39–68 and 74–123) are completely conserved among all
eight species (18).

The above two approaches suggest that the residues 39–68 within FLAP
might be important for inhibitor binding. Therefore, a series of site-directed
mutagenesis studies on human FLAP were carried out, the site-directed
mutants being expressed in COS-7 cells where FLAP is localized to the
100,000 × g membrane fraction and where binding studies can be carried out
(16). These studies have suggested that the amino acids in the region of
residues 42–61 play a critical role in inhibitor binding. In particular, an
aspartate residue at position 62 seems to be required for inhibitor binding,
because when [62]Asp in human FLAP is substituted with an asparagine residue extremely low levels of inhibitor binding were observed, although with
a glutamate substitution at this position full inhibitor binding was retained (17).

## CLINICAL EVALUATION OF LEUKOTRIENE
## BIOSYNTHESIS INHIBITORS

Leukotriene biosynthesis inhibitors that bind to FLAP have undergone limited clinical evaluation in human subjects. The first compound to be studied was the indole derivative MK-886 (9). This drug has been shown to be biochemically effective in humans through inhibition of ionophore A23187-induced leukotriene $B_4$ synthesis in human blood ex vivo (19). Functionally, MK-886 was shown to cause a modest inhibition of the early- and late-phase asthmatic response to antigen challenge, which was associated with a partial inhibition of the excretion of urinary leukotriene $E_4$ (20). The inhibition of the antigen response was less than that observed with potent leukotriene $D_4$-receptor antagonists such as MK-571 (21). This observation, together with the fact that only partial inhibition of urinary leukotriene $E_4$ excretion was observed at the maximal tolerated dose, suggested that a more potent derivative of MK-886 was needed for clinical evaluation in human subjects. Such a compound has since been developed, belongs to the quindole class of compounds, and is known as MK-0591 (15) (Fig. 3). This compound has a high affinity for FLAP, as evidenced by an $IC_{50}$ value of 1.6 n$M$ in the FLAP binding assay, and also inhibits the photoaffinity labeling of FLAP by two different photoaffinity ligands. It is a potent inhibitor of leukotriene biosynthesis in a variety of intact leukocyte preparations. In vivo, MK-0591 is a potent inhibitor of leukotriene biosynthesis, as is evidenced in ex vivo challenge of blood obtained from treated dogs, rats, and squirrel monkeys, in a rat pleurisy model and as monitored by the inhibition of the urinary excretion of leukotriene $E_4$ in normal dogs and antigen-challenged allergic dogs and sheep (15). In humans, MK-0591 has been tested at single doses ranging from 25 to 500 mg, and at doses of 250 mg or greater complete inhibition of leukotriene production for up to 24 hr after the dose, as measured by ex vivo inhibition of leukotriene $B_4$ in whole blood and the urinary excretion of leukotriene $E_4$, was observed (22). The use of compounds such as MK-0591 will allow definitive studies to be carried out on the role of leukotrienes in various diseases and will also be of value in determining whether leukotriene biosynthesis inhibitors will show superior activity to leukotriene $D_4$-receptor antagonists in diseases such as human bronchial asthma.

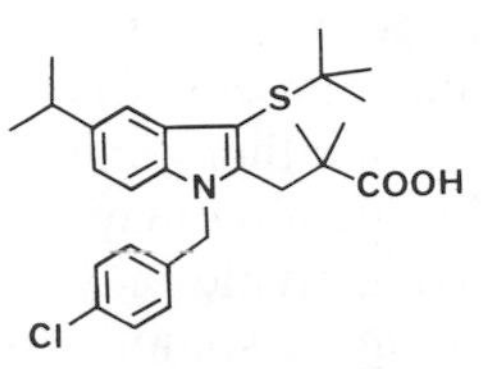

*MK-886* 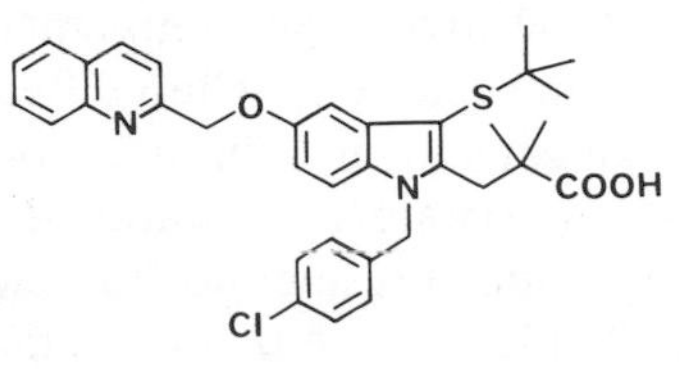          *MK-0591*

**FIG. 3.** Structures of MK-886 and MK-0591.

## LEUKOTRIENE $C_4$ SYNTHASE

Leukotriene $C_4$ synthase is a glutathione S-transferase–like enzyme that catalyzes the conjugation of leukotriene $A_4$ with glutathione. If this enzyme were a unique enzyme distinct from the more generalized glutathione S-transferase enzyme systems, it could represent an appropriate therapeutic target for regulation of production of the peptidolipid leukotrienes. The enzyme-catalyzed, stereospecific opening of the epoxide leukotriene $A_4$ occurs through sn-2 attack of glutathione at C6. Early studies have produced partial purifications of leukotriene $C_4$ synthase from various sources, including mouse mastocytoma cells (fourfold purification) (23), RBL-1 cells (10-fold purification) (24), and guinea pig lung (91-fold purification) (25–27). In addition, the enzyme has been characterized in human platelets (28), human endothelial cells (29), and vascular smooth-muscle cells (30). The above studies indicate that the dominant enzymic activity is associated with a membrane-bound enzyme rather than a soluble enzyme, which distinguishes the enzyme from the abundant cytosolic glutathione S-transferases found, for example, in the liver. However, the situation is somewhat complicated in that the more generalized glutathione S-transferases can catalyze the formation of leukotriene $C_4$ from leukotriene $A_4$. Therefore, in rat liver various glutathione S-transferase isozymes catalyze this reaction, the highest specific activity being observed with a homodimer of the Yb subunit, and isozymes containing the Yb subunit in general showed better activity than isozymes containing either the Ya and/or the Yc subunits (31). However, these enzymes did not show the regiospecificity that should be a characteristic of this enzyme. Glutathione S-transferase isozymes isolated from rat brain have also been examined for leukotriene $C_4$ synthase activity, the highest activity being observed with an acidic glutathione S-transferase, GST-$Yn_1Yn_1$ (32).

More recently, we have carried out an extensive purification and characterization of human leukotriene $C_4$ synthase from human monocyte cell lines, such as differentiated U937 cells. A substantial increase in leukotriene $C_4$ synthase activity in U937 cells was observed after differentiation with 1.3% dimethylsulfoxide for 3 days, whereas differentiation with phorbol-12-myristate-13-acetate produced no increase in specific activity compared with undifferentiated cells (31). The level of enzymic activity in undifferentiated U937 cells was similar to that found in freshly isolated human blood monocytes. In addition, the HL-60 myeloblast leukemia cell line was shown to express leukotriene $C_4$ synthase activity when differentiated into either neutrophil- or macrophage-like cells by growth in the presence of either dimethylsulfoxide or phorbol-12-myristate-13-acetate, respectively, although the levels of enzymic activity under these conditions were comparable only to undifferentiated U937 cells (32). The enzymic activity could be solubilized from microsomal pellets by the anion detergent taurocholate. Under these conditions, microsomal glutathione S-transferase remained in the membrane. The enzyme could also be distinguished from $\alpha$, $\mu$, $\pi$, and $\theta$ glutathione S-transferases through chromatographic separation, substrate specificity, and Western blot analysis (32). A purification scheme for LTC$_4$ synthase from either differentiated U937 cells or the human monocytic leukemia cell line THP-1 is shown in Fig. 4 (33). The steps include solubilization of membrane-bound leukotriene C$_4$ synthase from microsomal membranes by the anionic detergent taurocholate; successive anion-exchange chromatography steps in the presence of the taurocholate plus Triton X-100, followed by a similar separation but in the presence of taurocholate plus *n*-octyl glucoside; and leukotriene C$_2$ affinity chromatography on a matrix that was constructed by first biotinylating synthetic leukotriene C$_2$ and then immobilizing the biotinylated leukotriene on streptavidin–agarose. A number of key factors allowed this purification, including the finding that the enzymic activity in preparations enriched more than 500-fold was absolutely dependent on the presence of divalent cations (specifically Mg$^{2+}$) and phospho-

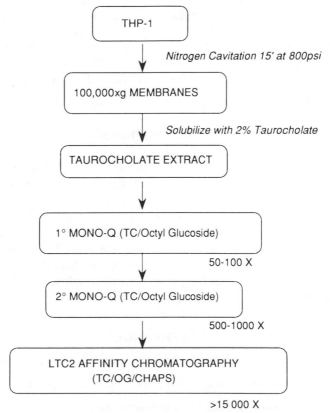

**FIG. 4.** Purification scheme for leukotriene C$_4$ synthase activity in human monocyte preparations.

lipids (specifically phosphatidylcholine) in the enzymic incubation mixtures and that reduced glutathione, which is required at 2 to 4 m$M$ for stabilization of the enzyme, irreversibly inactivated the enzyme when present at 5 m$M$ or greater during cycles of freezing and thawing. The final fractions contained an enzyme preparation that was more than 10,000-fold purified and contained three polypeptides with molecular masses of 37.1, 24.5, and 18.0 kDa. The 18-kDa polypeptide is thought to be associated with the enzymic activity, as it could be specifically labeled by a radioionated leukotriene $C_4$ photoaffinity probe (azido[$^{125}$I]leukotriene $C_4$). To determine if this specifically labeled protein was unique and distinct from microsomal glutathione S-transferase, the rank order of potencies of glutathione, various leukotrienes, and their analogues for competition of the photolabeling of the 18-kDa polypeptide and inhibition of leukotriene $C_4$ synthase and microsomal glutathione S-transferase activities was determined (34). The rank order of potencies for competition of photolabeling with azido[$^{125}$I]-leukotriene $C_4$ of the 18-kDa protein was found to be leukotriene $C_2$ $\geqslant$ azido[$^{127}$I]-leukotriene $C_4$ $\approx$ leukotriene $C_4$ > leukotriene $D_4$ > leukotriene $E_4$ > leukotriene $A_4$ $\approx$ leukotriene $B_4$ > S-hexyl glutathione $\geqslant$ glutathione. This rank order of potencies corresponded exactly with the rank order of inhibition of leukotriene $C_4$ synthase biosynthetic activity but showed no correlation with inhibition of microsomal glutathione S-transferase activity. It is therefore concluded that leukotriene $C_4$ synthase either is composed of 18-kDa polypeptides or contains an 18-kDa subunit.

## CONCLUSIONS

Regulation of either the production or the action of leukotrienes is potentially an important therapeutic approach for the treatment of allergic and inflammatory diseases. This regulation can be achieved at several levels. In particular, compounds that bind with high affinity to FLAP have shown therapeutic promise and may represent an important way to inhibit production of all leukotrienes. In addition, the studies described above suggest that leukotriene $C_4$ synthase is a unique enzyme and therefore is an important potential therapeutic target for prevention of synthesis of the peptidolipid leukotrienes.

## REFERENCES

1. Kouitert L, Barnes NC. In: Barnes PJ, ed. *New drugs for asthma*. London: IBC; 1992;2: 78–93.
2. Ford-Hutchinson AW. In: Barnes PJ, ed. *New drugs for asthma*. London: IBC; 1992;2: 94–102.
3. Rouzer CA, Kargman S. *J Biol Chem* 1988;263:10980–8.
4. Wong A, Hwang SM, Cook MN, Hogaboom GK, Crooke ST. *Biochemistry* 1988;27: 6763–9.

5. Wong A, Cook MN, Foley JJ, Sarau HM, Marshall P, Hwang SM. *Biochemistry* 1991;30: 9346–4.
6. Kargman S, Prasit P, Evans JF. *J Biol Chem* 1991;266:23745–52.
7. Wong A, Cook MN, Hwang SM, Sarau HM, Foley JJ, Crooke ST. *Biochemistry* 1992;31: 4046–53.
8. Rouzer CA, Ford-Hutchinson AW, Morton HE, Gillard JW. *J Biol Chem* 1990;265:1436–42.
9. Gillard JW, Ford-Hutchinson AW, Chan C, et al. *Can J Physiol Pharmacol* 1989;67:456–64.
10. Miller DK, Gillard JW, Vickers PJ, et al. *Nature* 1990;343:278–81.
11. Dixon RAF, Diehl RE, Opas E, et al. *Nature* 1990;343:282–4.
12. Charleson S, Prasit P, Leger S, et al. *Mol Pharmacol* 1992;41:873–9.
13. Evans JR, Léveillé C, Mancini JA, et al. *Mol Pharmacol* 1991;40:22–7.
14. Mancini JA, Prasit P, Coppolino MG, et al. *Mol Pharmacol* 1992;41:267–72.
15. Brideau C, Chan C, Charleson S, et al. *Can J Physiol Pharmacol* 1992;70:799–807.
16. Clark JD, Lin L-L, Kriz RW, et al. *Cell* 1991;65:1043–51.
17. Vickers PJ, Adam M, Charleson S, Coppolino MG, Evans JF, Mancini JA. *Mol Pharmacol* 1992;42:94–102.
18. Vickers PJ, O'Neill GP, Mancini JA, Charleson S, Abramovitz M. *Mol Pharmacol* 1992;42:1014–5.
19. Tanaka W, Dallob A, Winchell G, et al. *Am Rev Respir Dis* 1990;141:A32 [Abstract].
20. Friedman BS, Bel EH, Buntinx A, et al. *Am Rev Respir Dis* 1993;147:839–44.
21. Rasmussen JB, Margolskee DJ, Eriksson LO, Williams VC, Andersson KE. *Ann NY Acad Sci* 1991;629:436.
22. Tanaka W, Dallob A, Friedman BS, Brecher EB, Seibold JR. *Proceedings 8th International Conference on Prostaglandins and Related Compounds.* Montreal, 1992;643 [Abstract].
23. Söderström M, Mannervik B, Hammarström S, *Methods Enzymol* 1990;187:306–12.
24. Yoshimoto T, Soberman RJ, Lewis RA, Austen KF. *Proc Natl Acad Sci USA* 1985;82: 8399–8403.
25. Yoshimoto T, Soberman RJ, Spur B, Austen KF. *J Clin Invest* 1988;81:866–71.
26. Izumi T, Honda Z, Ohishi N, et al. *Biochim Biophys Acta* 1988;959:305–15.
27. Izumi T, Honda Z, Ohishi N, Kitamura S, Seyama Y, Shimizu T. In: Samuelsson B, Wong PY-K, Sun FF, eds. *Advances in prostaglandin, thromboxane, and leukotriene research,* Vol. 19. New York: Raven Press; 1989:90–3.
28. Söderström M, Mannervik B, Garkov V, Hammarström S. *Arch Biochem Biophys* 1992; 294:70–4.
29. Claesson H-E, Haeggström J. *Eur J Biochem* 1988;173:93–100.
30. Feinmark SJ, Cannon PJ. *Biochim Biophys Acta* 1987;922:125–35.
31. Chang M, Rao MK, Reddanna P, et al. *Arch Biochem Biophys* 1987;259:536–47.
32. Nicholson DW, Ali A, Klemba MW, Munday NA, Zamboni RJ, Ford-Hutchinson AW. *J Biol Chem* 1992;267:17849–57.
33. Nicholson DN, Klemba MW, Rasper DM, Zamboni RJ, Ford-Hutchinson AW. *Eur J Biochem* 1992;209:725–34.
34. Ali A, Zamboni RJ, Ford-Hutchinson AW, Nicholson DW. *FEBS Lett* 1993;317:195–201.

*Advances in Prostaglandin, Thromboxane, and Leukotriene Research*, Vol. 22, edited by S.-E. Dahlén et al. Raven Press, Ltd., New York 1994

# Mode of Action of the Leukotriene Synthesis (FLAP) Inhibitor BAY X1005

## Implications for Biological Regulation of 5-Lipoxygenase

A. Hatzelmann, R. Fruchtmann, *K. H. Mohrs, *S. Raddatz, M. Matzke, †U. Pleiss, ‡J. Keldenich, and R. Müller-Peddinghaus

*Institute for Cardiovascular and Arteriosclerosis Research, *Chemistry Science Laboratories, †Institute of Pharmacokinetics, and ‡Biophysical Research, Bayer AG, D-42096 Wuppertal, Germany*

In the early 1980s, Vanderhoek et al. (1) demonstrated that the 15-LOX (15-lipoxygenase) metabolite 15-HETE (15-hydroxyeicosatetraenoic acid) is an endogenous inhibitor of 5-LOX that served as a lead for the prototypic quinoline-based 5-LOX inhibitor Rev-5901, which lacked bioavailability (2). Based on the chemical structure of Rev-5901, we started a program aimed at enhancing the potency of Rev-5901 and gaining oral activity. This synthetic program led to the identification of BAY X1005 [(R)-2-[4-(quinolin-2-yl-methoxy)phenyl]-2-cyclopentyl acetic acid] (Fig. 1), which in preclinical studies proved to be effective in models of acute inflammation and asthma after oral application (3–6). These in vivo effects were expected to be due to the selective inhibition of leukotriene biosynthesis as BAY X1005 is a selective inhibitor of both 5-HETE and leukotriene (LTB$_4$, LTC$_4$) synthesis in various in vitro systems (7). There is virtually no inhibition of the cyclooxygenase pathway or any antioxidant effect (7).

This article summarizes our present knowledge about the mode of action of BAY X1005 and also discusses some biological implications with respect to BAY X1005 target protein(s).

Although the major part of this chapter was presented at the Second International Symposium on Trends in Eicosanoid Biology, this article is reprinted with permission from *Agents and Actions* 1994, vol. 43, © 1994 Birkhäuser Publishers, Basel, Switzerland.

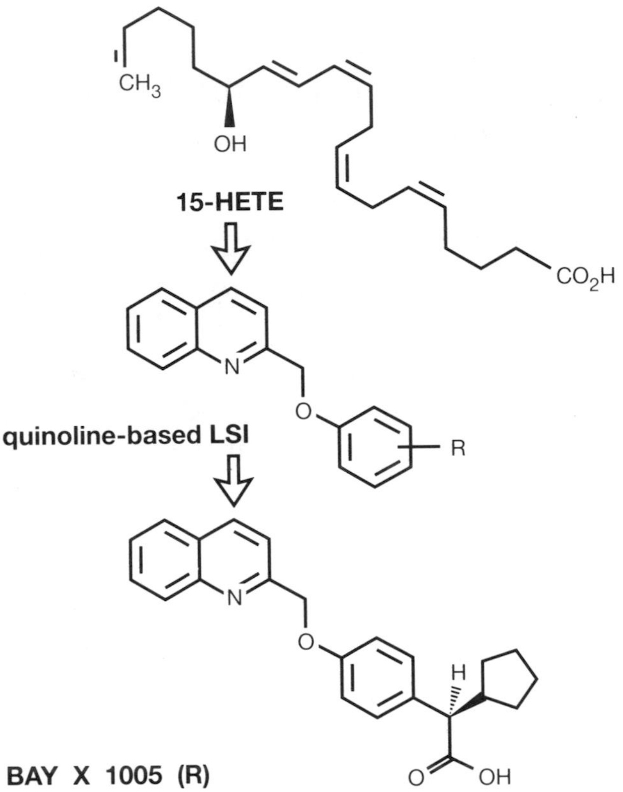

**FIG. 1.** 15-HETE hypothesis (i.e., 15-HETE as endogenous 5-lipoxygenase inhibitor) leading via prototypic quinoline-based leukotriene synthesis inhibitors to the synthesis of the enantiomeric quinoline BAY X1005.

## MOLECULAR SITE OF ACTION OF BAY X1005

Using $Ca^{2+}$ ionophore A23187-stimulated human PMNL (polymorphonuclear leukocytes) we found that BAY X1005 neither significantly affected arachidonic acid release nor the synthesis of platelet activating factor at concentrations that totally inhibited 5-LOX activity. Thus, the inhibition of 5-LOX activity by BAY X1005 was not a consequence of inhibition of phospholipase $A_2$ activity (8). In addition, compared with the inhibition of leukotriene synthesis in intact human PMNL, about 800-fold higher concentrations of BAY X1005 were required to inhibit leukotriene formation in a corresponding cell-free system (PMNL supernatant), suggesting that the inhibitory action of BAY X1005 cannot be explained by a direct effect of this compound on 5-LOX (8).

In an attempt to identify possible other target proteins of BAY X1005 [$^{14}$C]BAY X1005 was used for binding studies in human PMNL (8). The quantitative analysis of specific binding revealed two binding sites for BAY X1005. After subcellular fractionation of sonicated cells, a BAY X1005 high-affinity binding site was localized in the microsomal fraction ($280,000 \times g$ pellet) whereas a low-affinity binding site was present in the granule fraction ($10,000 \times g$ pellet).

The localization of the low-affinity binding site led us to speculate whether the putative target protein might be involved in the regulation of granule release. However, although this possibility could be excluded (9), recent experiments have pointed to an involvement of the low-affinity binding site in the regulation of NADPH-oxidase activity (7). The biological significance of the low-affinity binding site has to be elucidated.

With respect to the BAY X1005 high-affinity binding site, it was observed that the $K_d$ values of this BAY X1005 binding site ($K_d$, 0.165 μmol/L) was almost identical to the $IC_{50}$ value for inhibition of $LTB_4$ synthesis ($IC_{50}$, 0.22 μmol/L). Moreover, the $IC_{50}$ values for inhibition of BAY X1005 binding at the high-affinity binding site (range $IC_{50}$, 0.04–3.5 μmol/L) were almost identical to the $IC_{50}$ values for inhibition of $LTB_4$ synthesis for a series of other quinoline derivatives, including the reference compounds Rev-5901 and WY-50,295, but not for the direct 5-LOI, A-64077, and AA-861 (8). These results suggested a possible causal relationship between the binding of quinoline derivatives to the BAY X1005 high-affinity binding site and the inhibition of leukotriene synthesis in human and rat PMNL (8). The leukotriene synthesis inhibitor (LSI) MK-886, an indole derivative (10), was reported to bind with high affinity to a membrane-bound 18-kDa protein termed FLAP (5-lipoxygenase activating protein) (10,11). This protein was shown to be essential for leukotriene synthesis in intact cells (12), and therefore appeared to be a likely candidate for the BAY X1005 high-affinity binding site, although MK-886 and BAY X1005 share no obvious common structural features. Indeed, MK-886 inhibited $LTB_4$ synthesis as well as BAY X1005 binding to the high-affinity binding site with almost identical $IC_{50}$ values in human PMNL (8). This finding, in addition to the same subcellular localization, strongly suggested that the target protein of BAY X1005 mediating leukotriene synthesis inhibition is identical to FLAP. Additional indirect evidence supporting this notion came from a recent report showing that another series of quinolines compete with MK-886 for photoaffinity labeling of human FLAP (13). To test the interaction of the quinoline derivatives with FLAP directly, we synthesized a [³H]-labeled analogue carrying an azido group to perform photoaffinity labeling experiments (14). Taking the microsomal fraction of human PMNL, one of these compounds specifically labeled a protein with a molecular weight of about 19 kDa. The labeling of this protein was inhibited by MK-886, and was recognized by a polyclonal rabbit anti-FLAP antiserum (14). These experiments showed that, similar to the indol-derivative MK-886, the target protein of quinoline derivatives mediating inhibition of leukotriene synthesis is identical to FLAP.

Originally, FLAP was thought to have a unique structure (11,12) and to serve as a 5-LOX docking protein (15). Recent findings show structural similarities between FLAP and LTC$_4$ synthase (29). FLAP is now viewed as an arachidonic acid or 5-LOX substrate binding protein (19), which might share its structure and related functions with other free fatty acid binding proteins. Interestingly, using another photoaffinity label, the major specifically labeled protein in the microsomal fraction was not a 19-kDa species but had an estimated molecular weight of about 30 kDa (Hatzelmann, unpublished results). Similar to FLAP, the labeling of this protein was inhibited by MK-886. Experiments to identify this protein are in progress.

## COMPETITIVE BINDING OF INHIBITORS AND SUBSTRATES TO FLAP AND 5-LOX

The physiological function of FLAP has not been fully elucidated up to now. However, it was first proposed that FLAP might serve as a 5-LOX anchoring protein at the membrane site [15]. This hypothesis was based on the fact that 5-LOX Ca$^{2+}$ dependently translocates from the cytosol to a membrane site on stimulation (16) and that MK-886 both prevents and reverses this translocation process in human PMNL (17). In principle, the same results were reported for a quinoline derivative using HL-60 cells (18). Our group was able to confirm the inhibition of 5-LOX translocation by MK-886 using BAY X1005 in A23187-stimulated human PMNL, implying that 5-LOX translocation is tightly linked to leukotriene synthesis (Fig. 2). Yet, still some questions remain as to the direct FLAP/5-LOX interaction, the 5-LOX translocation to cellular membranes, even in the absence of FLAP as shown in osteosarcoma cells (20), and why the stable 5-LOX translocation in certain cells is irreversibly inhibited by the FLAP binding compound MK-886, which, in most circumstances, reverts 5-LOX translocation (21).

Novel aspects concerning the role of FLAP in cellular leukotriene biosynthesis were revealed from structure/function studies performed with different quinoline derivatives. As mentioned above, about 800-fold higher concentrations of BAY X1005 were necessary to inhibit 5-LOX activity in a cell-free system (10,000 $\times$ $g$ supernatant) compared to intact cells. The inhibition of 5-LOX activity by BAY X1005 in the cell-free system was likely to represent a direct effect of the compound on 5-LOX. Indeed, preliminary results indicated that BAY X1005 inhibited 5-LOX competitively. To determine whether the large difference in potency mentioned above for BAY X1005 could be demonstrated for other quinoline derivatives, we extended these studies to additional compounds. With respect to the substance class of phenyl-substituted (quinolin-2-yl-methoxy) compounds, the ratios of the IC$_{50}$ values for inhibition of leukotriene synthesis in the cell-free system and

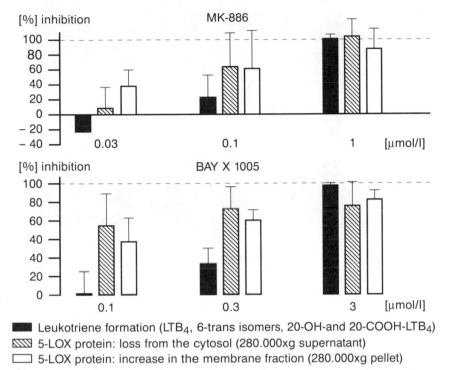

**FIG. 2.** Leukotriene synthesis inhibitor (MK-886 and BAY X1005) effects on leukotriene synthesis and 5-LOX translocation in A23187-stimulated human PMNL. (Methods are indicated in refs. 8 and 14.)

in intact cells, respectively, were calculated and found to range from 1 to 2,000 (19). Plotting of the two values resulted in a random distribution suggesting that no relationship existed between the inhibition of leukotriene synthesis in the cell-free system and in intact cells. This apparent discrepancy could be explained by the fact that the potency of the LSI in intact cells increased with higher lipophilicity, expressed as $K$ value (partition coefficient). The $K$ value is a parameter for the ability of a substance to accumulate in a lipid (hydrophobic) phase (19). The positive influence of a high $K$ value on the potency of the compounds suggested that the binding site of the target protein (FLAP) was located within the membrane. Consequently, the compound at the binding site would be in equilibrium with the drug in the lipid phase of the membrane (Fig. 3). The most important biochemical consequence was that the real affinity of the compounds to FLAP was lower than the apparent affinity as represented by the $IC_{50}$ value for leukotriene synthesis inhibition in intact cells. Therefore, $IC_{50}$ values generated using intact cells could only be compared at equal $K$ values. If one plotted the real affinity of various compounds stratified by their $K$ value, an inverse rela-

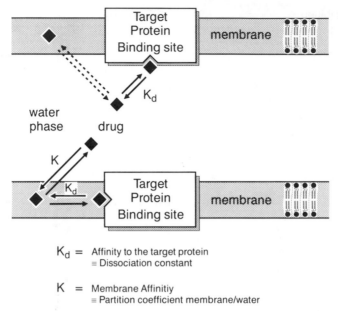

$K_d$ =  Affinity to the target protein
         ≡ Dissociation constant

$K$  =  Membrane Affinitiy
        ≡ Partition coefficient membrane/water

**FIG. 3.** Drug potency related to membrane and target protein affinity. (For methodological details see ref. 19.)

tionship between the compound affinity for 5-LOX or FLAP became evident (19).

Our interpretation of this finding was twofold: (i) Compounds with a high affinity for 5-LOX were predicted to have a low affinity for FLAP, and therefore such compounds represent direct 5-LOI (Fig. 4). To the contrary, compounds with a high affinity for FLAP would have a low affinity for 5-LOX, and therefore such compounds represent LSI (Fig. 4). In addition, compounds should be detectable with an intermediate affinity for both 5-LOX and FLAP, which should be able to bind to both proteins with equal affinity (Fig. 4). Such a situation may be exemplified by NDGA (nordihydroguaiaretic acid). This compound is the only 5-LOI identified that is able to interact with FLAP in addition to 5-LOX, which might be explained by the symmetric nature of this molecule resulting in an intermediate affinity for either protein. (ii) Considering the latter possibility, we thought that 5-LOX versus FLAP inhibition might reflect a physiological condition, and proposed a model in which FLAP would be able to bind 5-LOX arachidonic acid released from membrane phospholipids by the action of phospholipases. After effective translocation of 5-LOX from the cytosol to a membrane, FLAP would direct arachidonic acid to the 5-LOX enzyme (Fig. 4). According to this model, 5-LOX would have a high affinity and FLAP a low affinity for arachidonic acid to allow 5-LOX to pick up arachidonic acid from FLAP. The consequence of this model would be that FLAP specifically regulates

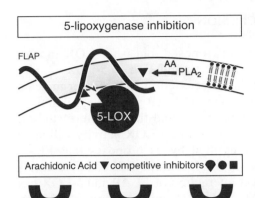

**FIG. 4.** Hypothesis on 5-lipoxygenase inhibitors as false substrates in place of arachidonic acid (AA), which is postulated to be transferred from FLAP (5-lipoxygenase activating protein) to 5-LOX. LSI (BAY X1005) are bound to FLAP and are postulated to compete with AA. LOI inhibits 5-LOX directly, probably by competition with AA. Equal binding of 5-LOX inhibitory compounds to FLAP and 5-LOX would result in mixed LOI/LSI.

the access of 5-LOX to its substrate. In support of this model, BAY X1005 binding at the high-affinity binding site (FLAP) can be inhibited by *cis*-unsaturated but not by *trans*-unsaturated or saturated fatty acids (19,22,23). Since our proposition that FLAP functions as an arachidonic acid transfer protein for 5-LOX (Fig. 4), presented at the 1992 Interlaken Workshop, two articles have been published that provide additional support. By applying a novel photoaffinity analogue of arachidonic acid, Mancini et al. (24) demonstrated the labeling of FLAP expressed to high levels in Sf9 insect cells. In addition, using the same cellular system, Abramovitz et al. (25) showed that FLAP stimulated the utilization of arachidonic acid by 5-LOX.

In this context, it is important to note that the intracelluar site at which 5-LOX and FLAP act to metabolize arachidonic acid has recently been identified to be the nuclear envelope. This has been shown for human neutrophils and monocytes (26), as well as for rat peritoneal macrophages (27). This finding was surprising because there was general consensus at that time that 5-LOX was catalytically active at or close to the plasma membrane. Yet the fact that these proteins, required for the initial step of leukotriene synthesis, were localized along the nuclear envelope appeared analogous to arachidonic acid metabolism via the cyclooxygenase pathway, as both the cyclooxygenases 1 and 2 have been located to the nuclear envelope and endoplasmatic reticulum in mouse 3T3 fibroblasts (28). It remains to be clarified whether arachidonic acid metabolism preferentially takes place at the nuclear membrane due to the fact that these membranes are known to be rich in arachidonyl-phospholipids, or whether leukotrienes and arachidonic acid metabolites of the cyclooxygenase pathway function not only as extracellularly released mediators but also as intracellular messengers.

## CONCLUSION

With the identification of FLAP and its proposed role as a 5-LOX anchoring protein at membrane sites (11,12,15), the regulation of 5-LOX activity seemed to be well understood. The data discussed in this chapter indicate that our present concept of the importance of FLAP and the regulation of 5-LOX activity may be even more complicated and that in future studies, additional protein(s) involved in the regulation of 5-LOX activity will most probably be identified. The model presented by us proposes that FLAP binds and transfers arachidonic acid to 5-LOX and the LSI compete at this arachidonic acid binding site. A direct interaction of FLAP and 5-LOX has not yet been demonstrated. As FLAP does not simply function as a 5-LOX anchoring protein, it remains to be shown how LSI interfere with the 5-LOX translocation process and with 5-LOX activity. To answer these questions, specific compounds are now available to serve as biochemical tools. In addition, there is hope that 5-LOX inhibitors, represented by BAY X1005, as future drugs will provide substantial benefit to patients suffering from inflammatory and/or allergic disease.

## REFERENCES

1. Vanderhoek JY, Bryant RW, Bailey JM. *J Biol Chem* 1980;255:10061–6.
2. Coutts SM, Khandwala A, van Inwegen R, et al. In: Bailey JM, ed. *Prostaglandins, leukotrienes and lipoxins, biochemistry, mechanism of action, and clinical applications.* New York: Plenum Press, 1985.
3. Müller-Peddinghaus R, Fruchtmann R, Ahr H-J, et al. *J Lipid Mediat* 1993;6:245–8.
4. Müller-Peddinghaus R, Kohlsdorfer C, Theisen-Popp P, et al. *J Pharmacol Exp Ther* 1993:267:51–7.
5. Gorenne T, Labat C, Gascard JP, et al. *J Pharmacol Exp Ther* 1993;268:868–72.
6. Gardiner PJ, Cuthbert NJ, Francis HP, et al. *Eur J Pharmacol* 1994;258:95–102.
7. Fruchtmann R, Mohrs K-H, Hatzelmann A, et al. *Agents Actions* 1993;38:188–95.
8. Hatzelmann A, Fruchtmann R, Mohrs KH, Raddatz S, Müller-Peddinghaus R. *Biochem Pharmacol* 1993;45:101–11.
9. Hatzelmann A, Fruchtmann R, Mohrs K-H, Raddatz S, Müller-Peddinghaus R. *Biochem Pharmacol* 1994;48:31–9.
10. Gillard J, Ford-Hutchinson AW, Chan C, et al. *Can J Physiol Pharmacol* 1989;67:456–64.
11. Miller DK, Gillard JW, Vickers PJ, et al. *Nature* 1990;343:278–81.
12. Dixon RAF, Diehl RE, Opas E, et al. *Nature* 1990;343:282–4.
13. Evans JF, Leveillé C, Mancini JA, et al. *Mol Pharmacol* 1991;40:22–7.
14. Müller-Peddinghaus R, Kast R, Hatzelmann A, Fruchtmann R, Gardiner PJ. Advances in understanding and treatment of asthma and COPD. Workshop held December 1–2, 1993, Key West, Florida, U.S.A. In press (1995).
15. Ford-Hutchinson AW. *Trends Pharmacol Sci* 1991;12:68–70.
16. Rouzer CA, Kargman S. *J Biol Chem* 1988;263:10980–8.
17. Rouzer CA, Ford-Hutchinson AW, Morton HE, Gillard JW. *J Biol Chem* 1990;265:1436–42.
18. Kargmann S, Prasit P, Evans JF. *J Biol Chem* 1991;266:23745–52.
19. Hatzelmann A, Goossens J, Fruchtmann R, Mohrs KH, Raddatz S, Müller-Peddinghaus R. *Biochem Pharmacol* 1994;47:2259–68.
20. Kargmann S, Vickers PJ, Evans JF. *J Cell Biol* 1992;119:1701–9.
21. Coffey M, Peters-Golden M, Fantono JC III, Sporn PHS. *J Biol Chem* 1992;267:570–6.

22. Kast R, Fruchtmann R, Kupferschmidt R, et al. *Agents Actions* 1994;41:C166–8.
23. Charleson S, Evans JF, Leger S, et al. *Eur J Pharmacol Mol Pharmacol* 1994;267:275–80.
24. Mancini JA, Abramovitz M, Cox ME, et al. *FEBS Lett* 1992;318:277–81.
25. Abramovitz M, Wong E, Cox ME, Richardson CD, Li C, Vickers PJ. *Eur J Biochem* 1993;215:105–11.
26. Woods JW, Evans JF, Ethier D, et al. *J Exp Med* 1993;178:1935–46.
27. Peters-Golden M, McNish RW. *Biochem Biophys Res Commun* 1993;196:147–53.
28. Regier MK, DeWill DL, Schindler MS, Smith WL. *Arch Biochem Biophys* 1993;301:439–44.
29. Lam BK, Penrose JF, Freeman GJ, Austen KF. *Proc Natl Acad Sci* 1994;91:7663–7.

*Advances in Prostaglandin, Thromboxane, and Leukotriene Research*, Vol. 22, edited by S.-E. Dahlén et al. Raven Press, Ltd., New York © 1994

# Inhibition of Leukotriene Production by Inhibitors of Lipoxygenation

*Lawrence G. Garland and †Simon T. Hodgson

*Research Directorate, and *†Department of Medicinal Chemistry, Research Division, The Wellcome Foundation, Ltd., Beckenham, Kent BR3 3BS, England

The enzyme 5-lipoxygenase (arachidonate: oxygen 5-oxidoreductase, EC 1.13.11.34) catalyzes the oxygenation of arachidonic acid to 5-HPETE and its subsequent dehydration to form $LTA_4$. This is the substrate for synthesis of $LTB_4$ and the peptidoleukotrienes ($LTC_4$, $LTD_4$, $LTE_4$) (1,2), which have a range of biologic activities consistent with their putative roles as mediators of allergy and inflammation in the asthmatic airway (see ref. 3 for recent summary). 5-Lipoxygenase is believed to be a cytoplasmic enzyme that undergoes calcium-dependent translocation to the plasma membrane on cell activation, probably due to association with the membrane protein 5-lipoxygenase activating protein (FLAP) (4,5). Human 5-lipoxygenase has been purified to virtual homogeneity (6), and the recombinant enzyme has been expressed using several different expression systems (7–11), yielding a monomeric 78-kDa protein. In keeping with other lipoxygenase enzymes (e.g., 15-lipoxygenases from soybeans or rabbit reticulocytes and 12-lipoxygenase from porcine leukocytes), purified recombinant human 5-lipoxygenase has been shown to contain non-heme iron (at least one atom of iron per molecule), which is essential for activity (12). cDNA sequences have been determined for at least 10 different lipoxygenases from plant and animal sources, and comparison of the equivalent amino acid sequences for the different enzymes has highlighted five or six conserved histidine residues. From site-directed mutagenesis studies it appears that three histidine residues (at positions 367, 372, and 551), glutamine 558, and glutamate 376 are essential for activity (13–15), and it is speculated that these residues are responsible for coordinating with iron in the active site.

## MECHANISM OF CATALYSIS

Because it has been available in pure form and is a fairly stable enzyme, soybean lipoxygenase has often been used as a model for the mechanism of catalysis brought about by mammalian 5-lipoxygenase. Now that it is known that the two enzymes share certain critical amino acid residues and that both contain non-heme iron, the analogy is even more reasonable. In the native state, the iron in soybean lipoxygenase is in the ferrous ($Fe^{2+}$) form, but in the catalytically active enzyme the iron is in the ferric ($Fe^{3+}$) form. The mechanism of catalysis proposed by Gibian and Galaway (16) involves transfer of an electron from the pentadienyl unit of the substrate to $Fe^{3+}$ in the catalytic site of the enzyme to generate a radical cation. A basic amino acid residue abstracts a proton from the radical cation, yielding the pentadienyl radical, which is then oxygenated by molecular oxygen. This is depicted as

Free radicals have been detected by ESR in anaerobic solutions of soybean lipoxygenase and substrate, consistent with pentadienyl radicals being intermediates in the lipoxygenase reaction (17). Recently, Chamulitrat and Mason (18) used a rapid-mixing, continuous-flow ESR technique to investigate further the peroxidation of fatty acids by soybean lipoxygenase under aerobic conditions. All fatty acids tested with two or more double bonds gave fatty acid peroxyl radicals. The direct detection of peroxyl radicals as well as carbon-centered radicals supports the mechanism of catalysis shown in Fig. 1. Hydroperoxide produced by the soybean lipoxygenase is capable of converting the enzyme from its native $Fe^{2+}$ form to the active $Fe^{3+}$ form. This probably explains the characteristic progress curve for the lipoxygenase reaction, which exhibits an initial lag before the linear rate is achieved. The enzyme also catalyzes its own inactivation before substrate becomes limiting, possibly due to protein denaturation by high local concentrations of radicals.

It is likely that a similar catalytic mechanism occurs in mammalian 5-lipoxygenase but thus far the evidence is indirect. For thiol-stabilized preparations of isolated 5-lipoxygenase, addition of fatty acid hydroperoxides (e.g., 5-HPETE) promotes activity, whereas high concentrations of thiol inhibit activity. An inverse relationship exists between the amount of hydroperoxide required to activate the enzyme and the concentration of thiol present (19). The inhibition of 5-lipoxygenase by thiols could be due to either reductive inactivation of the enzyme or elimination of endogenous fatty acid peroxides. Experiments with soybean lipoxygenase show that dithiothreitol (DTT) and other antioxidants act by reducing the non-heme iron from the

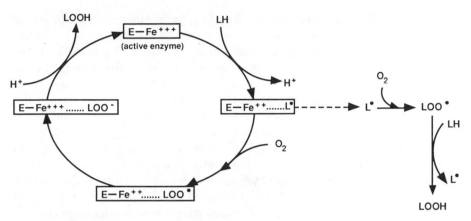

**FIG. 1.** Mechanism for lipoxygenation under aerobic conditions. E-Fe$^{3+}$, active oxidized enzyme: LH, fatty acid: L$^\bullet$, fatty acid carbon-centered (pentadienyl) radical: LOO$^\bullet$, fatty acid peroxyl radical: LOOH, fatty acid hydroperoxide. (Modified from ref. 18.)

Fe$^{3+}$ to the Fe$^{2+}$ form (20). This mechanism could also explain inhibition of mammalian 5-lipoxygenase and the requirement for hydroperoxide to regenerate the Fe$^{3+}$ form of the enzyme in the presence of thiols. Among the thiols tested, glutathione is an effective inhibitor of 5-lipoxygenase (19) and the concentrations required (0.1 to 1 m$M$) are within the range found in tissues (21). In the recent ESR study of soybean lipoxygenase (18), antioxidants such as vitamin E and Trolox C decreased the intensity of arachidonate peroxyl radical that could be detected. This decrease was accompanied by an increase in phenoxyl radical, consistent with scavenging of the peroxyl radical by the antioxidant. Antioxidant reactivity was related to the oil/water partitioning of the scavengers, vitamin E being more effective than Trolox C. Therefore, in intact mammalian leukocytes the activity of 5-lipoxygenase may be limited by endogenous antioxidants that act by reductively inactivating the enzyme (e.g., glutathione) and scavenging fatty acid hydroperoxide (e.g., vitamin E). However, stimulation of leukocytes by a variety of agents not only activates 5-lipoxygenase but also promotes generation of $O_2^-$ and, by dismutation, $H_2O_2$. Therefore, at an inflammatory focus lipid peroxidation by the $H_2O_2$, together with lipoxygenase-derived peroxyl radicals, will tend to surmount the control of 5-lipoxygenase by endogenous antioxidants.

## MECHANISMS OF ACTION OF INHIBITORS

From model experiments such as those described above, it is evident that the mechanisms whereby the 5-lipoxygenase reaction might be inhibited include the following: competition with fatty acid substrate; chelation of non-heme iron; reduction of the non-heme iron to the inactive $Fe^{2+}$ form; and scavenging of fatty acid peroxyl radical intermediate. It is also likely that inhibitors will be found that possess several if not all of these properties in the same molecule.

Of the many different inhibitors of 5-lipoxygenase that have been described, only a few examples will be used to illustrate features of the mechanism of action. For many compounds, potency as lipoxygenase inhibitors agrees with the strength of antioxidant activity (22). Studies using soybean lipoxygenase as a model enzyme have shown that catechols such as nordihydroguiaretic acid (20) and $N$-alkylhydroxylamines (23) inhibit the enzyme by reducing the $Fe^{3+}$ form of the enzyme to the $Fe^{2+}$ state. Such model experiments also show that the hydroperoxy fatty acid product can convert the $Fe^{2+}$ form of the enzyme back to the $Fe^{3+}$ form through a pseudoperoxidase activity of the enzyme (24). Therefore, in the presence of some reducing inhibitors and hydroperoxy fatty acid, the enzyme cycles between the $Fe^{3+}$ and $Fe^{2+}$ forms with the consumption of hydroperoxide and also possibly the inhibitor (Fig. 2). The fundamental ability of mammalian 5-lipoxygenase to undergo a similar reaction is illustrated when lipid hydroperoxides activate thiol-stabilized purified enzyme (19,25). Furthermore, purified 5-lipoxygenase from mammalian leukocytes catalyzes the degradation of lipid hydroperoxide (e.g., 13-HPOD) when certain potent inhibitors are added to the reaction (26,27). Inhibitors of various chemical classes have this effect, including hydroxamates, $N$-hydroxyureas, and hydroxybenzofurans. The pseudoperoxidase activity of purified mammalian 5-lipoxygenase requires the enzyme to be fully catalytically active and is particularly stimulated by potent inhibitors of the lipoxygenation reaction. These observations suggest that the model of reductive inactivation described for soybean lipoxygenase also applies to mammalian 5-lipoxygenase.

Among the most widely used inhibitors of lipoxygenase enzymes are the pyrazoline derivatives phenidone and BW 755C (28). A detailed study of the mechanism of inhibition of mammalian 5-lipoxygenase by these compounds has not been made, but such a study using plant lipoxygenase shows that

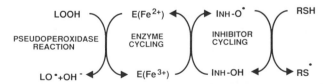

**FIG. 2.** Proposed scheme for lipoxygenase-catalyzed pseudoperoxidase reaction stimulated by a reducing inhibitor. LOOH, lipid hydroperoxide: LO•, unstable alkoxide radical: E-$Fe^{2+}$, reduced enzyme: INH-OH, inhibitor: INH-O•, oxide radical: R-SH, thiol-reducing agent. (Modified from ref. 27.)

these compounds are not in themselves able to inhibit the reaction (29). The active inhibitors are oxidation products generated either by molecular oxygen (when the compounds are allowed to stand in oxygenated buffers) or by the pseudoperoxidase activity of the enzyme in the presence of a fatty acid hydroperoxide. The active species is not the ultimate oxidation product but rather is radical intermediates obtained by a one-electron oxidation of the compound. The importance of this oxidation of phenidone to the radical intermediate is illustrated by the observation that ascorbic acid, by reducing the radical back to phenidone, prevents the inhibition of soybean lipoxygenase. The oxidation of phenidone by the pseudoperoxidase activity of lipoxygenase will tend to inhibit the enzyme reversibly through reduction of the iron in the catalytic site to the inactive $Fe^{2+}$ form. In addition, incubation of the enzyme with phenidone and lipid hydroperoxide causes the inhibitor to become covalently bound to the enzyme, presumably owing to the interaction between a phenidone radical and a nucleophilic amino acid residue in the enzyme. This covalent interaction results in the irreversible inactivation of the enzyme.

Hydroxybenzofuran derivatives (e.g., L-656,224) also probably inhibit 5-lipoxygenase by reducing iron at the catalytic site of the enzyme, in this case by donation of an electron from the hydroxyl group. The reaction product formed from such compounds is probably the phenoxyl radical. This radical interacts readily with the enzyme and, indeed, with other proteins outside of the catalytic site, suggesting that the radical is rather stable (30). Like the pyrazolines, the hydroxybenzofurans may therefore inhibit 5-lipoxygenase irreversibly by covalently binding to the enzyme, as well as reversibly through a reductive mechanism.

Analogues of arachidonic acid containing a hydroxamic acid moiety were synthesized originally as inhibitors of 5-lipoxygenase, with the rationale that they would bind strongly to iron at the active site of the enzyme (31). Subsequently, several series of 5-lipoxygenase inhibitors have been described that contain either hydroxamic acid or N-hydroxyurea groups linked to a lipophilic aryl unit. Examples of such inhibitors include the so-called acetohydroxamate BW A4C and the N-hydroxyureas BW B70C and zileuton (A-64077) (32–36). There is no doubt that such compounds bind strongly to iron in solution. For example, the binding constant for BW A4C has been measured to be in the order of $10^{12}$/mol. However, the potency for 5-lipoxygenase inhibition among a range of analogues is not related to this property (unpublished observations), and it is probable that their mechanism of action is more complex. Electrochemical evidence shows that BW A4C and BW B70C have relatively high electrode potentials ($E_0$ c. 2 V against a normal hydrogen electrode) and are not powerful redox compounds. However, both compounds inhibit lipid peroxidation in a model system based on the oxidation of linoleic acid by a thermolabile azo compound (37), and this property is clearly separate from the iron-chelating property of the compounds. These observations led to the suggestion that such compounds inhibit 5-lipoxygenase by scavenging lipid peroxides at the active site of the enzyme. However, the ability of hydroxamates and $N$-hydroxyureas to stimulate a pseudoperoxidase activity of mammalian 5-lipoxygenase strongly suggests that these compounds are also reductive inhibitors of the enzyme (26,27). This has been illustrated clearly by experiments with the $N$-hydroxyurea CPHU, which is quite a potent inhibitor of mammalian 5-lipoxygenase in vitro ($IC_{50}$ = 0.1 $\mu M$) and also stimulates the pseudoperoxidase activity of the enzyme, as monitored by consumption of lipid hydroperoxide (27). The results were consistent with CPHU undergoing a single electron oxidation to form the nitroxide radical and at the same time reducing the iron in the catalytic site of the enzyme to the inactive $Fe^{2+}$ form. The presence of a reducing agent such as DTT protected the CPHU from degradation by the pseudoperoxidase activity by converting the nitroxide radical back to CPHU. Depending on the reactivity of the nitroxide radical, it cannot be ruled out that this class of inhibitor also becomes covalently bound to the enzyme.

The mechanism of action of hydroxamates and $N$-hydroxyureas therefore involves up to four separate properties: iron chelation (a minor component), lipid peroxyl radical scavenging, reduction of non-heme iron and, under certain circumstances, possibly covalent binding. The lipophilic aryl moiety clearly locates the inhibitors in the phase of the cell membrane at which the enzyme is active, but it is unclear whether a more detailed analogy with the fatty acid substrate (as suggested in ref. 34) is appropriate.

A number of substrate analogues are inhibitors of 5-lipoxygenase in vitro. This includes acetylenic analogues of arachidonic acid, analogues of $LTA_4$, and metabolites of arachidonic acid such as 15-HPETE and 15-HETE (see ref. 38 for details). None of these has sufficient selectivity or activity in vivo to be considered important inhibitors. Historically, compounds such as Rev-5901 were considered to have structural similarity to 15-HETE, which is a moderately potent inhibitor of 5-lipoxygenase. This series of quinolines has led to compounds that are now recognized as having further properties that include inhibition of 5-lipoxygenase activation by FLAP and $LTD_4$-receptor antagonism.

Two series of compounds have been reported that are neither redox agents nor iron chelators but appear to be active-site inhibitors of 5-lipoxygenase (39–42). In one series, the methoxyalkyl thiazoles, certain analogues that contain chiral centers (e.g., ICI 216800) show a marked difference in potency between enantiomers (39). Because this difference was observed using high-speed supernatant from RBL-1 cells as the enzyme source, it is likely that it reflects a potency difference at the active site of the enzyme. The class of compounds has very great selectivity for inhibition of 5-lipoxygenase rather than cyclooxygenase, but activities against either 12- or 15-lipoxygenase have not been reported. These compounds lose potency in whole blood, probably as the result of plasma protein binding, which limits their activity in vivo. However, some of the series (e.g., ICI 211965) have moderate oral activity.

Further development led to a second series of potent orally active non-redox inhibitors exemplified by ZD 2138 (42). This compound is active at low concentrations against 5-lipoxygenase in vitro ($IC_{50}$ values 3 to 25 n$M$), has high selectivity for lipoxygenase with respect to cyclooxygenase (25,000-fold), and is not greatly affected by plasma protein binding. Details about selectivity among different lipoxygenase enzymes and mechanism of action have not yet been reported. However, it is not a powerful iron chelator or redox agent, nor is it a FLAP inhibitor. Therefore, ZD 2138 possibly acts by binding tightly to the active site of the enzymes and competing with the fatty acid substrate. If so, it is the most powerful inhibitor to act only through this mechanism.

## RANGE OF INHIBITOR TYPES

From the above it is clear that many different molecular species might inhibit 5-lipoxygenase in vitro, especially due to antioxidant properties. As testimony to this, during the last 10 years more than 600 patent applications have been filed by at least 38 different pharmaceutical companies claiming 5-lipoxygenase inhibitors with various degrees of selectivity.

### Antioxidants

A wide range of compounds with antioxidant activity have been identified as 5-lipoxygenase inhibitors. Most reasonably, lipophilic phenols block the enzyme but hindered phenols, analogues of BHT, have attracted much attention, as many examples are inhibitors of both cyclooxygenase and lipoxygenase and have oral activity. One of the earliest examples was prifelone from Riker (43), and further developments led to KME-4 from Kanagafuchi, which has undergone clinical evaluation.

Merck has progressed 4-oxy-phenols related to vitamin E. The benzofura-nols such as L-656,224 were mentioned earlier. Many structural variants of this series have been evaluated for potency, bioavailability, and toxicity. Early work on the 4-benzofuranols (44) has been extended to the 2,3-dihy-drobenzofuranols, among which at least two compounds have been selected for development: L-651,896, which lacks systemic activity, is a potent top-ical anti-inflammatory agent, and L-670,630 is orally active (45,46). L-670,630 has high potency and selectivity for 5-lipoxygenase in vitro and does not generate methaemoglobinemia in vivo which is frequently a prob-lem with redox-active 5-lipoxygenase inhibitors (see below).

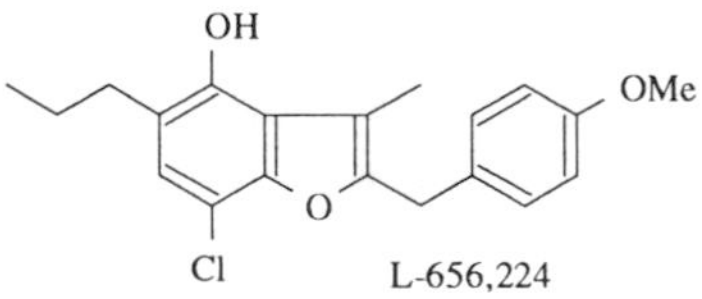

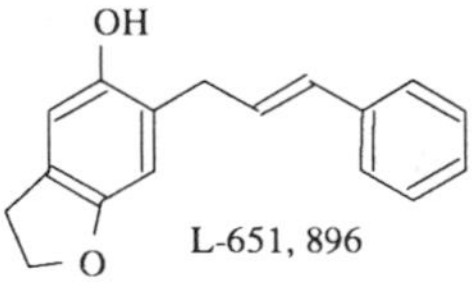

Perhaps related to phenols are the extensive series of hydroxysubstituted heterocycles from Merck and Abbott. As examples, one class of compound from each company is shown below. Hydroxythiazole (2) is selective for 5-rather than 12- or 15-lipoxygenase but is not active after oral dosing (47).

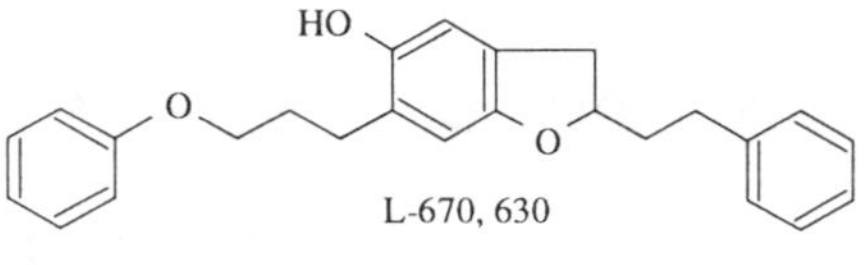

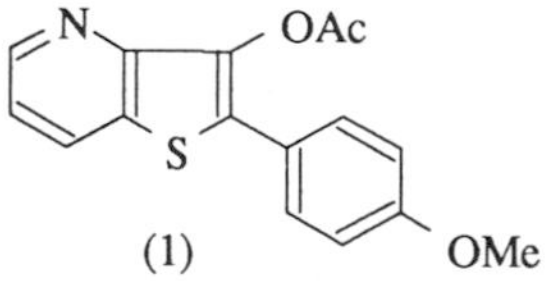

Another extensive range of antioxidant lipoxygenase inhibitors contains two adjacent heteroatoms in a ring usually conjugated with a third hetero-atom. The original compound of this type was phenidone, which was fol-lowed by a series of compounds exemplified by BW 755C and nafazatrom and, more recently, by indazolinones (e.g., ICI 207968). These compounds suffer from short duration of action in vivo (nafazatrom) or toxicity (BW 755C), and attempts to achieve compounds of this type that were both orally active and nontoxic were largely unsuccessful.

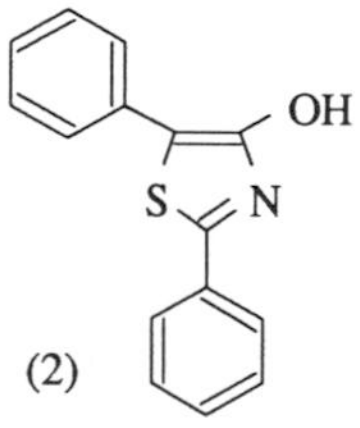

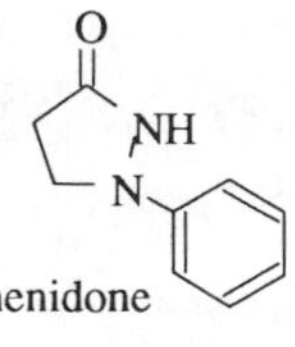

Phenidone

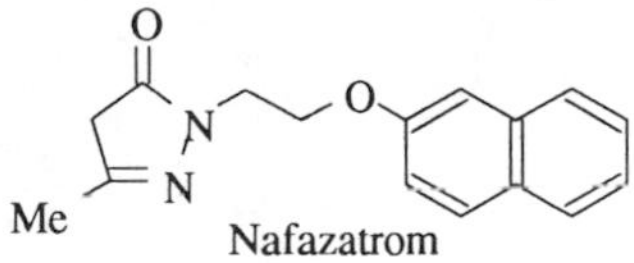

Nafazatrom

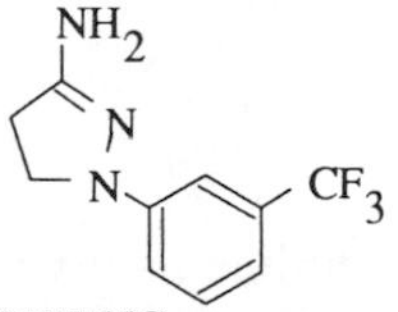

BW755C

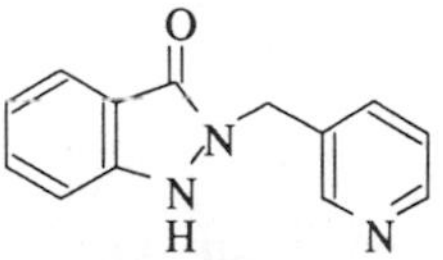

ICI 207968

A large family of conjugated heterocycles exemplified by Merck's phenothiazines (e.g., L-651,392) and Bayer's benzothiazines (3) are potent inhibitors of 5-lipoxygenase in vitro; some have oral activity, but no development candidates have been identified.

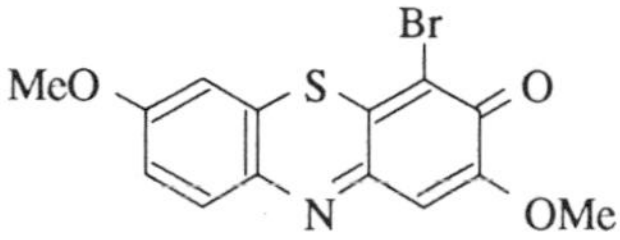

L-651,392

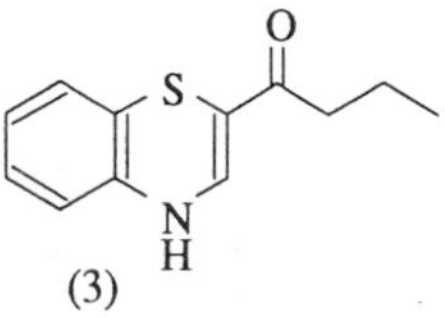

(3)

Certain piroxicam analogues containing the "enol-amide" structure shown below are described as "dual" inhibitors of cyclooxygenase and lipoxygenase, although the cyclooxygenase activity is usually dominant. An example of this type of compound is tenidap from Pfizer.

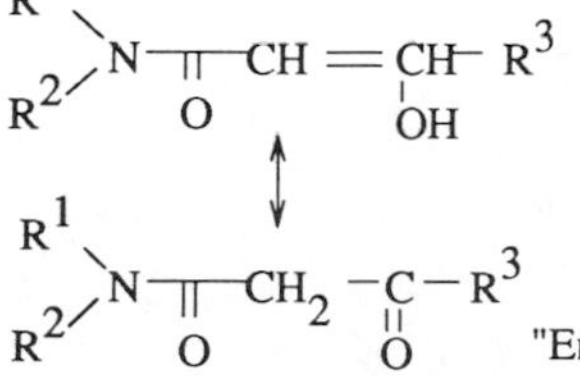

"Enol-amide"

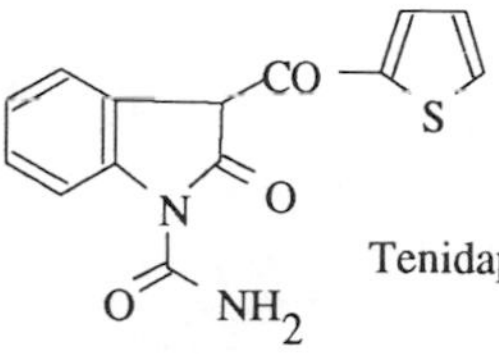

Tenidap

A range of quinone/quinol-based antioxidants with lipoxygenase-inhibitory activity includes the prototype compound AA-861 from Takeda and lonapolene from Syntex. The Takeda compound has been evaluated clinically, but its therapeutic potential is not well documented. Lonapolene was evaluated topically for psoriasis but was withdrawn as it provoked dermatitis.

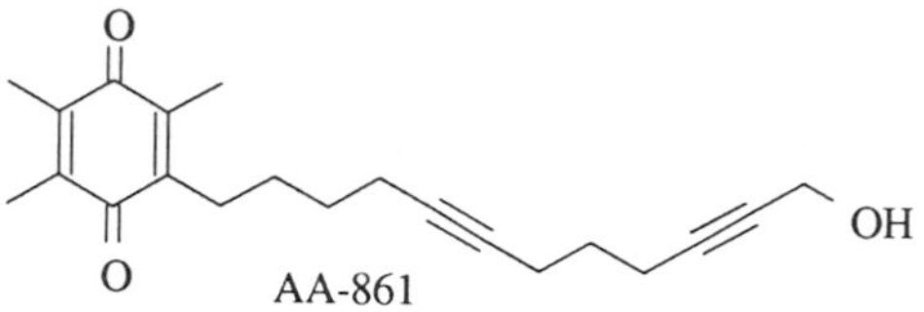

AA-861

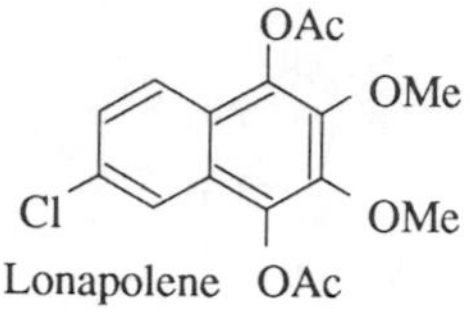

Lonapolene OAc

## Iron Chelators

The rationale for synthesis of this type of molecule is outlined above. The original (so-called "straight") hydroxamates are very potent inhibitors in vitro but have poor activity in vivo because of their rapid metabolism to the corresponding carboxylic acid. This metabolism of the hydroxamic acid moiety is blocked when it is incorporated into a "reversed" hydroxamate.

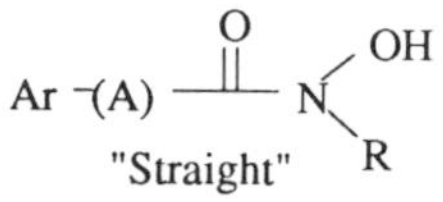

"Straight"

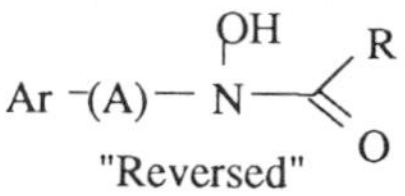

"Reversed"

For this reason, very few "straight" hydroxamates have been pursued. However, tepoxalin, which is a dual inhibitor, falls into this class and, perhaps surprisingly, the effect of this compound appears to persist for many hours after oral dosing (48).

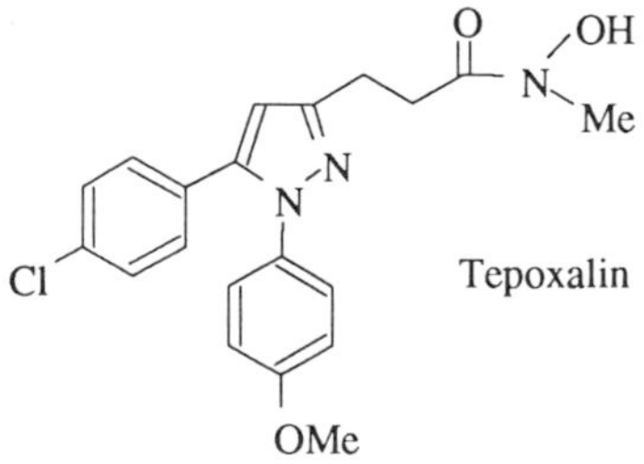

Tepoxalin

The reversed hydroxamates, exemplified by BW A4C, and the *N*-hydroxyureas, exemplified by zileuton, were the first 5-lipoxygenase inhibitors with reasonable selectivity (especially against cyclooxygenase) that are not toxic and have moderate persistence after oral dosing. Analogues with greater metabolic stability and longer duration of action are now known (e.g., BW B70C, A-78773) (49,50).

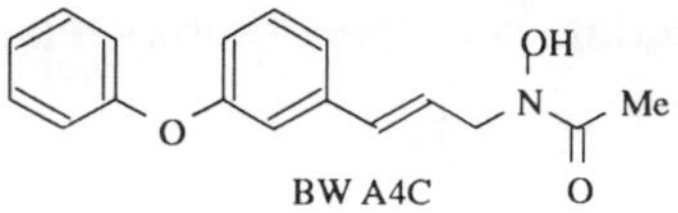

BW A4C

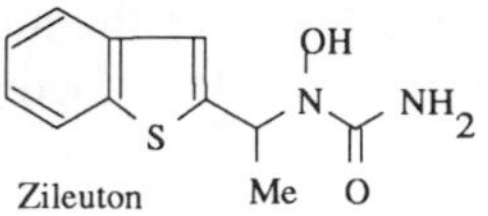

Zileuton

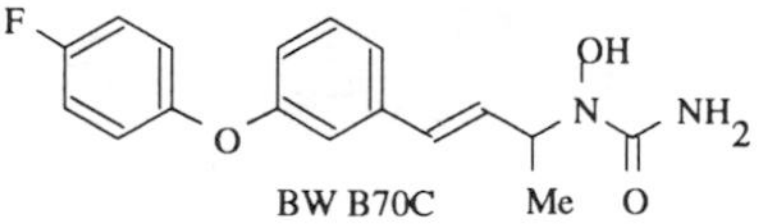

BW B70C

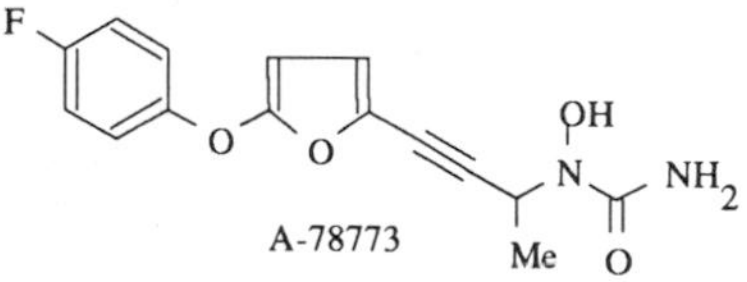

A-78773

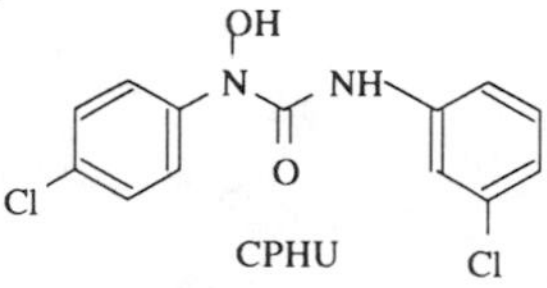

CPHU

At least five other companies have filed patent applications on 5-lipoxy-genase inhibitors based on hydroxamates and *N*-hydroxyureas, including molecules with aryl moieties derived from a variety of nonsteroidal anti-inflammatory drugs (e.g., 4). In addition, a range of heterocyclic and car-bocyclic compounds incorporating the *N*-hydroxyurea concept have been described, including the compounds shown below (5–7). The development status of these molecules is not generally known.

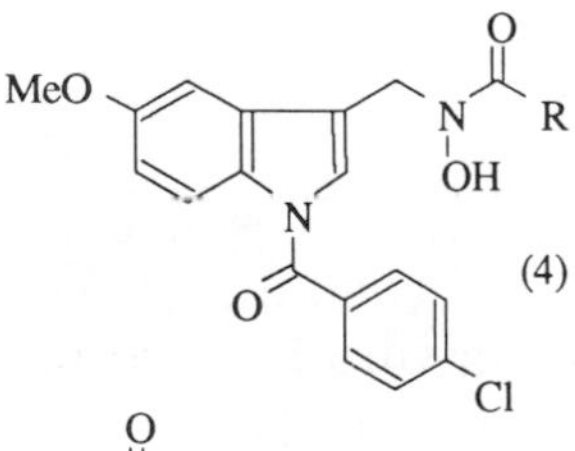

(4)

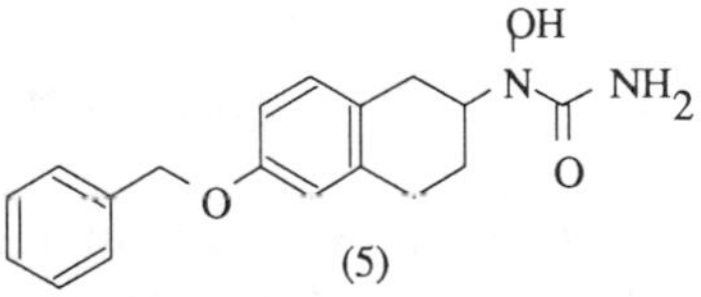

(5)

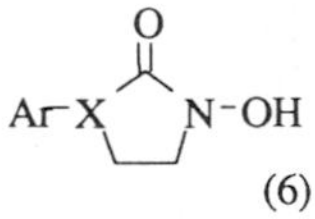

(6)

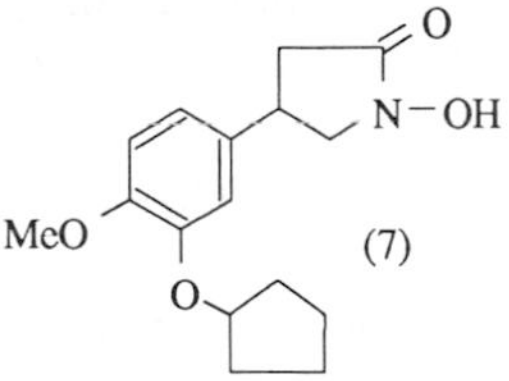

(7)

## Substrate-Based Inhibitors

The proposed relationship between the structure of Rev-5901 and 15-HETE shown below illustrates why this compound might be considered as an active-site inhibitor of 5-lipoxygenase. However, Rev-5901 is now thought to block 5-lipoxygenase through interaction with FLAP. This com-pound does not have good oral activity but is being evaluated in asthma by the inhalation route. The methoxythiazoles (e.g., ICI 211965, ICI 216800) and the methoxypyrans (e.g., ZD 2138) shown below are believed to act by binding tightly to the catalytic site of the enzyme. As mentioned earlier,

ZD 2138 is one of the most potent and long-acting, selective 5-lipoxygenase inhibitors yet described and is in phase II trials.

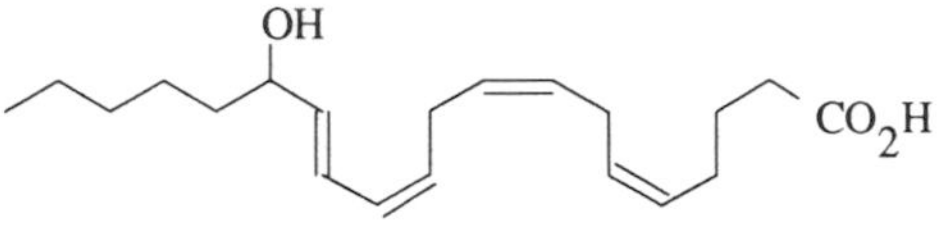

15-HETE

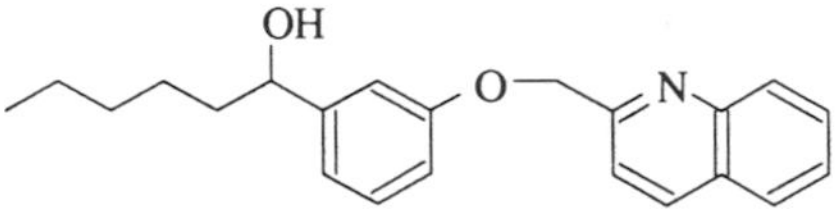

Rev-5901

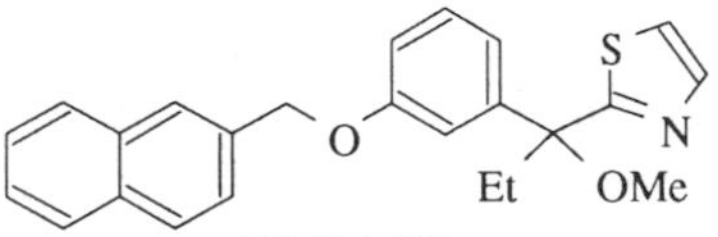

ICI-211,965

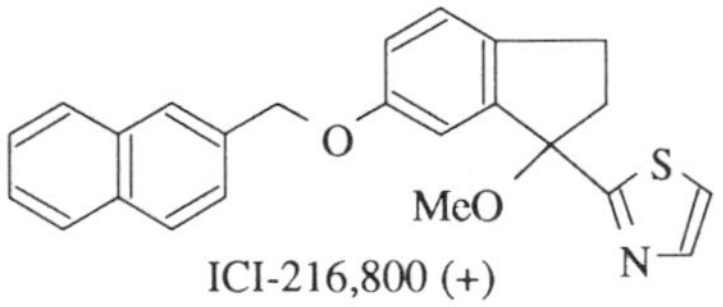

ICI-216,800 (+)

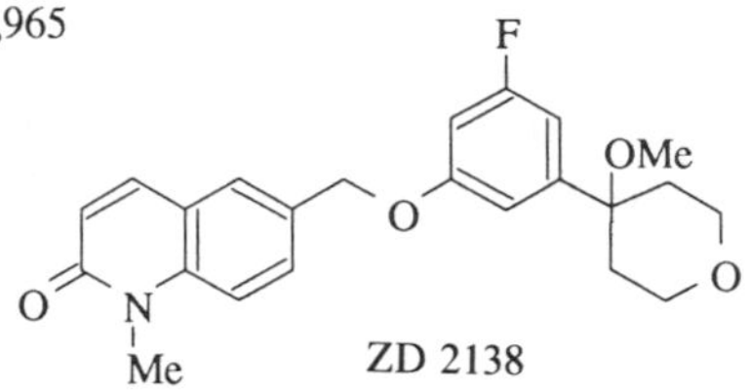

ZD 2138

## BIOAVAILABILITY AND TOXICITY

Despite the wealth of inhibitors of 5-lipoxygenase that have been identified, it is pertinent to note that very few have reached clinical trial. This reflects the problems of achieving not only potency in vitro but also bioavailability (particularly metabolic stability) and lack of toxicity.

Many inhibitors are short acting in vivo. For some molecules this might be due to their degradation by the pseudoperoxidase activity of the enzyme itself. For others, such as hydroxamates and *N*-hydroxyureas, for which this is not a problem, duration of action in vivo is limited by more conventional metabolic transformations before excretion. The measurement of LTB$_4$ generation in ionophore-stimulated blood ex vivo, taken from predosed animals or humans, has been a useful way of monitoring the persistence of 5-lipoxygenase inhibition after oral dosing (see refs. 33 and 38 for details). This technique illustrates the short duration of action in vivo of several standard inhibitors (e.g., NDGA, nafazatrom), which limits their value as experimental probes (33). It has also provided a way of monitoring improvement in duration of action gained by systematically blocking sites of metabolism. This was done with the hydroxamates and *N*-hydroxyureas, where the relative metabolic instability of prototype compounds such as BW A4C and zileuton (each of which has a t$_{1/2}$ in humans of 2 to 3 hr) has been significantly improved in later members of the series, such as BW B70C and A-78773. Other recently described inhibitors have long durations of action after oral dosing; for example, ZD 2138 at a single dose of 5 mg/kg p.o. in dogs inhibited blood $LTB_4$ synthesis ex vivo for at least 32 hr, and in rats the $ED_{50}$ was 4 mg/kg p.o. measured 10 hr after dosing (42).

This ex vivo technique for measuring persistence of 5-lipoxygenase inhibition has the potential to be misleading when lipophilic compounds are distributed beyond the plasma compartment. This appears to happen with the dihydrobenzofuranol L-670,630, which is effective at low doses against antigen-induced bronchospasm in several species when plasma levels of the free drug are barely detectable (46). This finding is a reminder that 5-lipoxygenase inhibition in the plasma compartment may not always translate to equivalent inhibition in the lungs, and compound testing regimens should include measurements in both.

Many 5-lipoxygenase inhibitors whose activity is based on a redox mechanism have systemic toxicity that results from the redox activity rather than from 5-lipoxygenase inhibition. Characteristically, such compounds reduce hemoglobin to methemoglobin (which diminishes the oxygen-carrying capacity of the blood) and, in addition, hepatotoxicity is a common occurrence. Such toxicity has limited the value of several different series of inhibitors, including the early pyrazolines (e.g., BW 755C), the indazolinones (e.g., ICI 207968) and certain of the dihydrobenzofuranols. Structural modification to avoid toxicity often results in loss of potency and oral activity. An exception is L-670,630, in which inclusion of bulky substituents that abolish the ability to form methemoglobin does not diminish potency or oral activity (46).

The hydroxamate and *N*-hydroxyurea series of compounds are not powerful reducing agents and do not induce methemoglobinemia. Simple aryl *N*-hydroxyureas are known to be mutagens through their ability to form hydroxylamine; this illustrates one reason why the potent 5-lipoxygenase inhibitor CPHU could not be considered a therapeutically useful compound. The problem is avoided by separating the nitrogen atom of the *N*-hydroxyurea from the resonance system associated with the aryl moiety by at least one carbon atom. No class-specific toxicology has been identified among 5-lipoxygenase inhibitors. The prototype compound zileuton has low toxicity in animals and has, by now, been evaluated safely at high dosage in a large number of subjects (more than 1,500), some for up to 2 years. This clinical experience shows that sustained inhibition of 5-lipoxygenase is not per se associated with undesirable side effects that may limit the therapeutic utility of this class of drugs.

## CLINICAL EFFICACY

Before evaluating the efficacy of 5-lipoxygenase inhibitors in chronic conditions such as asthma, it is first necessary to show that the compound is capable of inhibiting the enzyme in the target organ for prolonged periods of time. The blockade of ionophore-induced $LTB_4$ release in blood taken from treated individuals (33,38) illustrates activity of compounds in the blood compartment, and inhibition of the rise in urinary $LTE_4$ provoked by airway challenge, for example, by allergen inhalation in atopics (51), provides some measure of activity in the lungs.

Early clinical trials with 5-lipoxygenase inhibitors were carried out without first making these fundamental pharmacologic assessments, and it is likely that compounds such as AA-861 and nafazatrom, which brought about no relief in asthma, were cleared rapidly and blocked lung 5-lipoxygenase for only a short time if at all. Prototype compounds with adequate duration of action in humans include BW A4C and zileuton. In volunteers, BW A4C was well tolerated and achieved almost complete blockade of 5-lipoxygenase in blood for 24 hr with a dose of 400 mg t.i.d. (52). This compound was not pursued further, but zileuton has been evaluated clinically, high doses being used to compensate for its relatively short half-life. At 3 hr after a single oral dose of 800 mg to asthmatics, zileuton decreased the ionophore-induced production of $LTB_4$ by 74% and significantly decreased airway responses provoked by inhalation of cold, dry air (53). In a double-blind, placebo-controlled study, a single dose of 600 mg brought about a modest increase in $FEV_1$ (0.4 L above a mean basal level of 2.3 L) (54), similar to that seen with an $LTD_4$ receptor antagonist (55). Because zileuton has no direct relaxant effect on airway smooth muscle, this bronchodilatation must be due to blockade of a sustained, leukotriene-mediated constrictor tone on the airways. Treatment for 28 days with zileuton 600 mg four times per day significantly improved airway function in mild-to-moderate asthmatics (56). It is not yet clear whether oral zileuton has an anti-inflammatory effect in asthmatic airways, with a possible steroid-sparing effect, but these studies are apparently in hand.

The early clinical results with zileuton in asthma and other inflammatory conditions, especially ulcerative colitis (57), are encouraging, but the obvious shortcoming of the compound is its relatively short duration of action. Compounds that are intrinsically more potent and are cleared less rapidly, such as ZD 2138 and A-78773, are likely to be more useful drugs. Both of these compounds have been evaluated by the oral route in volunteers; they are apparently well absorbed, well tolerated, and achieve prolonged inhibition of 5-lipoxygenase in blood stimulated ex vivo (58–60). Such compounds are likely to be effective in asthma, with modest doses being required only once or twice per day. Clinical studies with both compounds are either about to start or are already in progress, and the results will be awaited with great interest.

### REFERENCES

1. Samuelsson B, Funk CD. *J Biol Chem* 1989;264:19469–72.
2. Samuelsson B, Haeggstrom JZ, Wetterholm A. *Ann NY Acad Sci* 1991;629:89–99.

3. Placentini GL, Kaliner MA. *Am Rev Respir Dis* 1991;143:596–9.
4. Miller DK, Gillard JW, Vickers PJ et al. *Nature* 1990;343:278–81.
5. Dixon RAF, Diehl RE, Opas E, et al. *Nature* 1990;343:282–4.
6. Rouzer CA, Samuelsson B. *Proc Natl Acad Sci USA* 1985;82:6040–4.
7. Matsumoto T, Funk CD, Radmark O, Hoog J-O, Jornvall H, Samuelsson B. *Proc Natl Acad Sci USA* 1988;85:26–30.
8. Dixon RAF, Jones RE, Diehl RE, Bennett CD, Kargman S, Rouzer CA. *Proc Natl Acad Sci USA* 1988;85:416–20.
9. Rouzer CA, Rands E, Kargman S, Jones RE, Register RB, Dixon RAF. *J Biol Chem* 1988;263:10135–40.
10. Noguchi M, Matsumoto T, Nakamura M, Noma M. *FEBS Lett* 1989;249:267–70.
11. Denis D, Falgueyret J-P, Riendeau D, Abramovitz M. *J Biol Chem* 1991;266:5072–9.
12. Percival MD. *J Biol Chem* 1991;266:10058–61.
13. Nguyen T, Falgueyret J-P, Abramovitz M, Riendeau D. *J Biol Chem* 1991;266:22057–62.
14. Zhang YY, Rådmark O, Samuelsson B. *Proc Natl Acad Sci USA* 1992;89:485–9.
15. Ishii S, Noguchi M. Miyano M, Matsumoto T, Noma M. *Biochem Biophys Res Commun* 1992;182:1482–90.
16. Gibian MJ, Galaway RA. In: Van Tammelin EE, ed. *Bio-organic chemistry*, Vol. 1. New York: Academic Press; 1977;117–30.
17. de Groot JJMC, Veldink GA, Vliegenthart JFG, Boldingh J, Wever R, van Gelder BF. *Biochim Biophys Acta* 1975;377:71–9.
18. Chamulitrat W, Mason RP. *J Biol Chem* 1989;264:20968–73.
19. Riendeau D, Denis D, Choo LY, Nathaniel DJ. *Biochem J* 1989;263:565–72.
20. Kemal C, Louis-Flamberg P, Krupiriski-Olsen R, Shorter AL. *Biochemistry* 1987;26:7064–72.
21. Meister A. *J Biol Chem* 1988;263:17205–8.
22. Thody VE, Buckle DR, Foster KA. *Biochem Soc Trans* 1987;15:416–7.
23. Clapp CH, Banerjee A, Rotenberg SA. *Biochemistry* 1985;24:1826–30.
24. Streckert G, Starr H-J. *Lipids* 1975;10:847–54.
25. Rouzer CA, Samuelsson B. *FEBS Lett* 1986;204:293–6.
26. Riendeau D, Falgueyret J-P, Guay J, Ueda N, Yamamoto S. *Biochem J* 1991;274:287–92.
27. Falgueyret J-P, Desmarais S, Roy PJ, Riendeau D. *Biochem Cell Biol* 1992;70:228–36.
28. Randall RW, Eakins KE, Higgs GA, Salmon JA, Tateson JE. *Agents Actions* 1980;10:553–5.
29. Cucurou C, Battioni JP, Thang DC, Nam NH, Mansuy D. *Biochemistry* 1991;30:8964–70.
30. Rouzer CA, Riendeau D, Falgueyret J-P, Lau CK, Gresser MJ. *Biochem Pharmacol* 1991;41:1365–73.
31. Corey JE, Cashman JR, Kantner SS, Wright SW. *J Am Chem Soc* 1984;106:1503–4.
32. Jackson WP, Islip PJ, Kneen G, Pugh A, Wates PJ. *J Med Chem* 1988;31:499–500.
33. Tateson JE, Randall RW, Reynolds CH, et al. *Br J Pharmacol* 1988;94:528–39.
34. Summers JB, Mazdiyasni H, Holms JH, Ratajczyk JD, Dyer RD, Carter GW. *J Med Chem* 1987;30:574–80.
35. Summers JB, Kim KH, Mazdiyasni H, et al. *J Med Chem* 1990;33:992–8.
36. Carter GW, Young PR, Albert DH, et al. *J Pharmacol Exp Ther* 1991;256:929–37.
37. Darley-Usmar VM, Hersey A, Garland LG. *Biochem Pharmacol* 1989;38:1465–9.
38. Salmon JA, Garland LG. In: Jucker E, ed. *Progress in drug research*, Vol. 37. Basel: Birkhäuser Verlag; 1991:9–90.
39. McMillan RM, Girodeau J-M, Foster SJ. *Br J Pharmacol* 1990;101:501–3.
40. McMillan RM, Bird TGC, Crawley GC, et al. *Agents Action* 1991;34:110–2.
41. Bird TGC, Bruneau P, Crawley GC, et al. *J Med Chem* 1991;34:2176–86.
42. Foster SJ, Crawley GC, Walker ERH, McMillan RM. *Br J Pharmacol* 1992;106:71P.
43. Moore GGI, Swingle KF. *Agents Actions* 1982;12:674–83.
44. Lau CK, Bélanger PC, Scheigetz J et al. *J Med Chem* 1989;32:1190–7.
45. Hammond ML, Zambias RA, Chang MN, et al. *J Med Chem* 1990;33:908–18.
46. Lau CK, Bélanger PC, Dufresne C, et al. *J Med Chem* 1992;35:1299–1318.
47. Kerdesky FA, Holmes JA, Moore JL, et al. *J Med Chem* 1991;34:2158–65.
48. Robinson CP. *Drugs Future* 1990;15:902–4.
49. Salmon JA, Jackson WP, Garland LG. In: Samuelsson B, Ramwell PW, Paoletti R, Folco

G, Granström E, eds. *Advances in prostaglandin, thromboxane, and leukotriene research,* Vol. 21. New York: Raven Press; 1991:109–12.
50. Brooks DW, Stewart AO, Kerkman DJ, et al. *Patent* WO92/01682, 1992.
51. Taylor GW, Taylor I, Black P, et al. *Lancet* 1989;1:584–8.
52. Nicholls A, Posner J. *Br J Clin Pharm* 1991;31:577P.
53. Israel E, Dermarkarian R, Rosenberg M, et al. *N Engl J Med* 1990;323:1740–4.
54. Israel E, Rubin P, Pearlman H, Cohn J, Drazen J. *Am Rev Respir Dis* 1992;145: A16(Abstract).
55. Hui KP, Barnes NC. *Lancet* 1991;337:1062–3.
56. Israel E, Drazen J, Pearlman H, Cohn J, Rubin P. *J Allergy Clin Immunol* 1992;89:236.
57. Collawn C, Rubin P, Perez N, et al. *Am J Gastroenterol* 1992;87:342–6.
58. McMillan RM, Crawley GC, Walker ERH, Williams AJ, Yates RA, Foster SJ. *Eighth International Conference on Prostaglandins and Related Compounds* 1992; Abstract 152.
59. Bell RL, Young P, Malo PE, et al. *Eighth International Congress on Prostaglandins and Related Compounds* 1992; Abstract 154.
60. Rubin PD, Dubé LM, Winkelman LG, Cohn J, Brandwein SR. *Eighth International Congress on Prostaglandins and Related Compounds* 1992; Abstract 638.

*Advances in Prostaglandin, Thromboxane,
and Leukotriene Research*, Vol. 22, edited by
S.-E. Dahlén et al. Raven Press, Ltd., New York © 1994

# Leukotriene Receptors and Their Selective Antagonists

P. J. Gardiner, T. S. Abram, S. R. Tudhope, N. J. Cuthbert,
P. Norman, and *C. Brink

*Research Department, Bayer plc, Stoke Poges, Buckinghamshire SL2 4LY
England; and *Centre Chirurgical Marie Lannelongue, Departement de
Physiologie Humaine, F-92350 Paris, France*

## PATHOPHYSIOLOGIC ROLE

The discovery of the structure of and the subsequent synthesis of the leukotrienes (LTs) led to many studies demonstrating their many biologic actions. The cysteinyl LTs, $LTC_4$, $LTD_4$, and $LTE_4$ were shown to be potent
smooth-muscle contractile agonists; they also increased vascular permeability and mucous production (1). The putative mediator of asthma, SRS-A,
was shown to be a mixture of LTs. As a consequence, most of the studies
that attempted to identify the pathophysiologic role of LTs centered around
asthma. Asthmatics have higher basal plasma levels of cysteinyl LTs compared with normal subjects, and the level of cysteinyl LTs increases further
during an asthma attack (2). The fact that inhalation of $LTC_4$ or $LTD_4$
induces asthma-like symptoms was also demonstrated (2). These findings
indirectly implicated the cysteinyl LTs in the pathogenesis of asthma.

## LT RECEPTORS

Early studies of the cysteinyl LTs demonstrated that they act via specific
membrane receptors; this was done using three different techniques: ste-
reoisomers of $LTC_4$ or $LTD_4$, a selective LT antagonist (FPL 55712), and
ligand binding studies (3–6). These studies suggested that multiple cysteinyl
LT receptors exist on guinea pig tissues. However initial studies with human
bronchial muscle suggested that only one LT receptor type (provisionally
called the $LTD_4$ or LT1 receptor) was present on this tissue (7). As a consequence, many groups attempted to identify and develop new, highly potent, and selective $LTD_4$/LT1 antagonists in the hope that they would provide a valuable new treatment for asthma. Almost 15 years after the
identification of the LTs, our knowledge of the receptor(s) through which
cysteinyl LTs act has increased considerably. This new information means

that we should reexamine the receptor targets for those LT antagonists that are being developed for the treatment of asthma.

Only the cysteinyl LTs and not the proinflammatory mediator $LTB_4$ will be discussed at length in this chapter.

## CYSTEINYL LEUKOTRIENE RECEPTOR TYPES

### $LTD_4$/LT1 Receptors and Their Antagonists

#### Functional Studies

Shortly after the discovery of the structure and subsequent synthesis of cysteinyl LTs, preclinical studies showed that the chromone FPL 55712 (which was known to antagonize SRS-A) was a weak but selective LT antagonist (5,7). FPL 55712 given orally was inactive in both animals and humans and had only a very short duration of action when given intravenously. However, this antagonist selectively blocked the contractile effects of both $LTC_4$ and $LTD_4$ on human bronchial muscle. This suggested that new drugs with LT receptor profiles similar to that of FPL 55712 but with higher potency, selectivity, and better pharmacokinetics may well provide a valuable new therapy for asthma. Various groups, over a relatively short period, identified a plethora of structurally distinct drugs, all with the required LT antagonist profile; some of these have subsequently progressed to clinical trials for evaluation in asthmatics.

The most studied cysteinyl LT antagonists are probably SK & F 104353, ICI 204219, ONO 1078, RO 245913, and MK 571 (8–12). Functional and ligand binding studies, using a range of tissues taken predominantly from the guinea pig, have shown these drugs to be effective antagonists of $LTD_4$. However, the situation is complicated by the fact that $LTC_4$ (in the presence of L-serine borate, an inhibitor of $LTC_4$ metabolism) has a similar potency to that of $LTD_4$ on many guinea pig tissues, yet none of these second-generation LT antagonists was able to block many of the actions of $LTC_4$. The most notable demonstrations of this selective antagonism were performed with guinea pig trachea and ileum (13,14). These results led to the suggestion that different types of cysteinyl LT receptors exist, one type being designated as the $LTD_4$/LT1 receptor.

This $LTD_4$/LT1 receptor could not be functionally characterized as predominantly activated by $LTD_4$ because $LTC_4$ (even in the presence of inhibitors of its metabolism) was generally equipotent and equally effective compared with $LTD_4$. Instead, characterization of the $LTD_4$/LT1 receptor initially relied on studies using the selective LT antagonists, as they were purported to antagonize only $LTD_4$ on guinea pig tissues. However, it soon became apparent that nomenclature based on $LTD_4$ being the most potent agonist for this receptor type was confusing, because these putative $LTD_4$/LT1-receptor antagonists also antagonized $LTC_4$ (in the absence or presence of inhibitors of $LTC_4$ metabolism) on human bronchial muscle. These results indicated that $LTD_4$ was not the only agonist selective for the $LTD_4$/LT1 receptor. Irrespective of receptor nomenclature, using LT antagonists provided evidence for the existence of at least two cysteinyl LT receptor types, one sensitive to a range of LT antagonists and another insensitive to such antagonists.

## Ligand Binding Studies

After reports indicating the existence of an $LTD_4$/LT1 receptor, many radioligand binding studies were performed using $[^3H]LTD_4$. Plasma membranes from a range of species and tissues (predominantly lung) were shown to have G-protein–coupled, saturable, and reversible binding sites for $LTD_4$ (15–21). The characteristics of these $LTD_4$ binding sites were similar among species, in that $LTD_4$ had $K_D$ and $\beta_{max}$ values in the range of 0.1 to 3.4 n$M$ and 42 to 1,100 fmol/mg protein, respectively (Table 1). Although $LTC_4$ displayed a relatively low affinity for the $LTD_4$/LT1 site, the selective LT antagonists all inhibited $LTD_4$ binding with potencies similar to those seen in functional studies. More recently, a number of attempts have been made to solubilize and purify the binding site as the first stage in cloning and sequencing the $LTD_4$/LT1 receptor (22). Initial studies suggest that the site is located in the plasma membrane and that this site is a glycoprotein with an apparent molecular weight of 70 kDa.

## Signal Transduction

Some of the complex pathways of signal transduction have been partially dissected by Crooke and colleagues (23), using DMSO-differentiated U937

**TABLE 1.** *Characteristics and species distribution of the $[^3H]LTD_4$ binding site*

| Species | Tissue/cells | Binding data | |
|---------|--------------|--------------|---|
| | | $K_D$ (nM) | $\beta_{max}$ (fmol/mg protein) |
| Guinea pig | Lung | 0.2 | 1,100 |
| | Ventricular myocardium | 3.4 | 850 |
| Rat | Lung | 0.12 | 42 |
| | Basophils | 0.9 | 800 |
| Sheep | Trachea | 0.4 | 268 |
| Human | Lung | 0.15 | 68 |
| | PMN | 1.1–2.3 | 116–275 (per PMN) |

From refs. 15–21.

cells. In brief, $LTD_4$ interacts with a plasma membrane receptor and then the LT receptor interacts with at least two G-proteins; 5 to 20 sec later $Ca^{2+}$ is mobilized from at least three sources. During the next 4 to 7 min, activation of topoisomerase I occurs, producing enhanced transcription of the phospholipase activating protein (PLAP) and, subsequently, increased phospholipase $A_2$ ($PLA_2$) activity. This increased $PLA_2$ activity results in the release of arachidonic acid and its metabolism to produce or release cyclooxygenase and/or lipoxygenase products.

## $LTC_4$/LT2 Receptors and Their Antagonists

### Function

As mentioned in the previous section, the cysteinyl LT antagonists in many tissues do not block $LTC_4$ responses; this implies the existence of a second LT-receptor type. The initial suggestion that this second receptor was selectively activated by $LTC_4$ was soon disputed when it was demonstrated that $LTD_4$ antagonists had limited activity in some tissues and failed to block high doses of $LTD_4$ (14,24). This fact provided evidence of an antagonist-resistant component in the $LTD_4$ response.

If different LT receptor types exist, then tissues or cells with homogeneous populations of such receptor types should also exist. Such systems would be invaluable in characterizing the cysteinyl LT receptors as opposed to working on tissues with multiple receptor types. Using $LTC_4$, $LTD_4$, and $LTE_4$ and the putative $LTD_4$/LT1 antagonists, we have identified two different groups of tissues.

The first group comprises two tissues: rat lung strip and guinea pig gallbladder. $LTC_4$ (in the absence and presence of L-serine borate) and $LTD_4$ were approximately equipotent and equally effective contractile agonists on both of these tissues, and both $LTC_4$ and $LTD_4$ were antagonized by the LT antagonists with a similar rank order of potency (Fig. 1). Unlike in the guinea pig trachea and ileum, there was no evidence of a LT antagonist-resistant component to the $LTC_4$ or $LTD_4$ contractile responses. This suggests the presence of only one receptor type.

The second group comprises two tissues: sheep bronchial muscle and ferret spleen strip. $LTC_4$ and $LTD_4$ were approximately equipotent and equally effective contractile agonists on both of these tissues, but none of the LT antagonists blocked $LTC_4$- or $LTD_4$-induced contractions (Fig. 2). $LTE_4$ was a partial agonist on these two tissues, with a similar $pK_p$ against $LTC_4$ (in the absence and presence of L-serine borate) as against $LTD_4$. This adds strength to the argument that both LTs are acting through the same receptor.

Using these two groups of tissues, we sought to identify selective agonists and/or antagonists of the two cysteinyl LT receptor types.

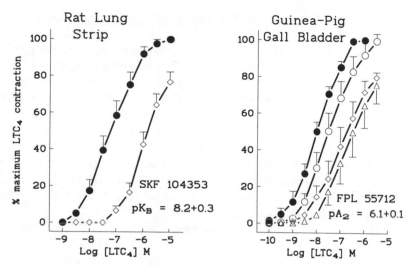

**FIG. 1.** Antagonism of $LTC_4$-induced contractions of isolated rat lung strip and guinea pig gallbladder in the presence of L-serine borate. Rat lung strips were treated with either vehicle (●) or $10^{-7}$ M SKF 104353 (◇). Guinea pig gallbladder was treated with either vehicle (●), $1.6 \times 10^{-6}$ M FPL 55712 (○), $1.6 \times 10^{-5}$ M FPL 55712 (◇), or $4.7 \times 10^{-5}$ M FPL 55712 (△). Each point is the mean ± SEM of four observations. $LTD_4$-induced contractions of these two tissues were also antagonized by SKF 104353 and FPL 55712. Other $LTD_4$/LT1 antagonists, i.e., ICI 198615 and MK 571, also antagonized $LTC_4$- and $LTD_4$-induced contractions of these two tissues.

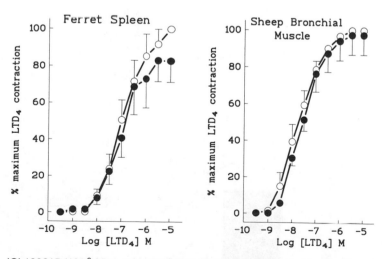

**FIG. 2.** ICI 198615 ($10^{-6}$ M): lack of LT antagonism on the isolated ferret spleen strip and sheep bronchial muscle. Each point is the mean ± SEM of four observations. $LTC_4$- (± L-serine borate) induced contractions of both tissues were also unaffected by ICI 198615 (●$10^{-6}$ M). SKF 104353 ($10^{-6}$ M) and MK 571 ($10^{-6}$ M) were also ineffective against $LTC_4$ and $LTD_4$ on these two tissues.

### BAY u9773

This compound is a cysteinyl leukotriene analogue; the cysteinyl group of the LT molecule has been replaced by $p$-mercaptobenzoic acid (Fig. 3). BAY u9773 blocked both $LTC_4$- and $LTD_4$-induced contractions of sheep bronchial muscle and of ferret spleen (Fig. 4). BAY u9773 was also an effective antagonist against $LTC_4$- and $LTD_4$-induced contractions of rat lung strip and guinea pig gallbladder, suggesting that BAY u9773 is not selective with respect to the type of LT receptor (Fig. 5). However, we did demonstrate that BAY u9773 is a selective cysteinyl LT antagonist as this compound was ineffective against contractions induced by non-LTs on the four tissues tested; BAY u9773 was also inactive against $LTB_4$-induced $Ca^{2+}$ influx in human PMNs (Poll, personal communication).

When BAY u9773 was tested on heterogeneous LT receptor systems such as the guinea pig trachea or ileum, in contrast to the existing LT antagonists, BAY u9773 was effective against both $LTD_4$-induced (no antagonist-resistant component was evident) and $LTC_4$-induced (in the absence and presence of L-serine borate) contractions (25).

BAY u9773, when used alone or in conjunction with $LTD_4/LT1$ antago-

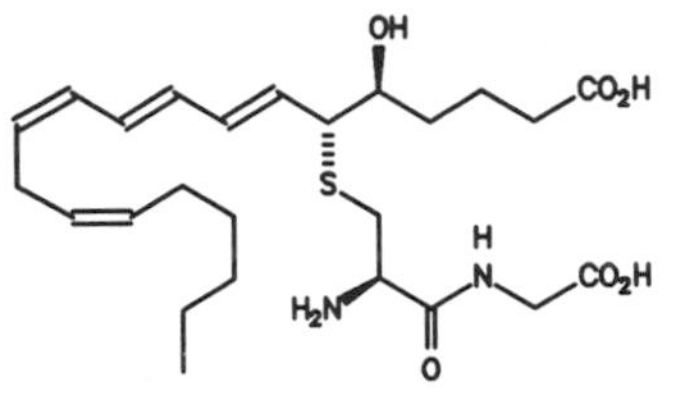

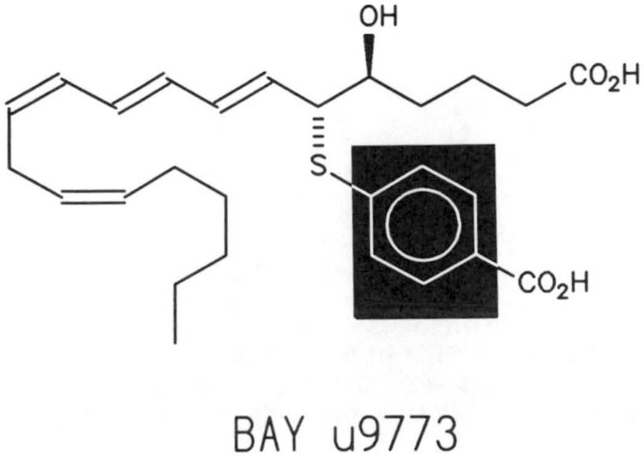

**FIG. 3.** Structure of the LT analogue BAY u9773.

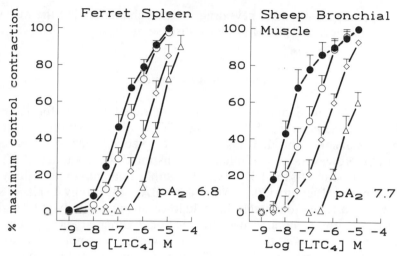

**FIG. 4.** BAY u9773 antagonism of $LTC_4/LT2$ receptor-mediated responses on the ferret spleen and sheep bronchial muscle. Each point is the mean ± SEM of five observations. $LTC_4$ alone (●), BAY u9773 $10^{-7}$ $M$ (○), BAY u9773 $10^{-6}$ $M$ (◇), BAY u9773 $10^{-5}$ $M$ (△). BAY u9773 was equally effective against $LTC_4$ in the presence of L-serine borate and had similar $pA_2$ values against $LTD_4$ on both tissues.

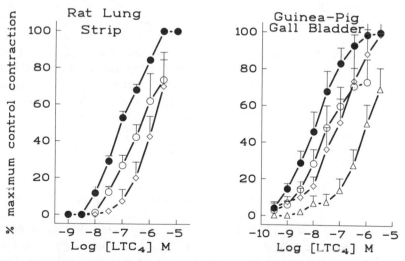

**FIG. 5.** BAY u9773 antagonism of $LTD_4/LT1$ receptor-mediated responses. $LTC_4$ concentration–response curves were obtained after incubation with either vehicle (●), $10^{-7}$ $M$ BAY u9773 (○), $10^{-6}$ $M$ BAY u9773 (◇), or $3 × 10^{-5}$ $M$ BAY u9773 (△). All tissues were bathed in Tyrode's solution containing indomethacin ($3 × 10^{-6}$ $M$) and L-serine borate ($4.5 × 10^{-2}$ $M$). Each point is the mean ± SEM of four observations on rat lung strip and six observations on gallbladder. $LTD_4$-induced contractions of these two tissues were also antagonized by BAY u9773 with a similar potency.

nists, represents a valuable new drug tool for characterizing the cysteinyl LT-receptor types in pathophysiologic disease models.

### Ligand Binding Studies

Many studies, predominantly on lung membranes, were performed using [$^3$H]LTC$_4$. It had been suggested that an LTC$_4$ binding site insensitive to LT antagonists existed, and that this site was the second type of LT receptor (15,26–29). However, we and others demonstrated the existence of LT analogues that bound to the [$^3$H]LTC$_4$ site with a relatively high affinity but had no functional activity (30). Furthermore, BAY u9773 only displaces such binding with a K$_i$ approximately 100-fold lower than its affinity at LTC$_4$/LT2 receptors (Norman, unpublished observation). Other studies around the same time demonstrated that this LTC$_4$ binding site was not a receptor but a glutathione S-transferase (31). LTC$_4$ binds extremely well to the glutathione S-transferase, probably masking LTC$_4$ binding to the true receptor sites. This nonreceptor binding by LTC$_4$ may also help to explain why it has a much lower affinity for LTD$_4$ binding sties than would be expected in the light of functional studies. LTC$_4$ is probably binding to glutathione S-transferase(s), leaving little or no LTC$_4$ available for competition at the [$^3$H]LTD$_4$ site.

A better strategy for ligand binding studies aimed at characterizing the LTC$_4$/LT2-receptor type would be to use tissues with homogeneous populations of receptors, e.g., ferret spleen. [$^3$H]LTD$_4$ could be used as the ligand for this receptor, as it is functionally active and has a low affinity for glutathione S-transferase. Further confirmation of a homogeneous population of this receptor type might come from the use of radiolabeled LT antagonists (e.g., [$^3$H]ICI 198615). If a homogeneous population of the LTC$_4$/LT2 receptors is present, then ICI 198615 should not bind to these sites. However, ICI 198615 seems to bind to more than just the LTD$_4$/LT1 site, which may produce false-positives on some tissues (32).

### Signal Transduction

In contrast to the LTD$_4$/LT1 receptor, relatively little is known of the mechanisms involved in the LTC$_4$/LT2-receptor–signal transduction pathway. We have shown that the voltage-operated calcium-channel antagonist nifedipine partially blocks both LTC$_4$- and LTD$_4$-induced contractions of ferret spleen to the same degree (Cuthbert, personal communication). This adds strength to the argument that both LTs are acting through the same receptor and implies that extracellular Ca$^{2+}$ is involved in the early stages of signal transduction.

## LT3 Receptor

### *Functional Studies*

When BAY u9773 was tested on tissues with mixed LT-receptor populations, as might be expected from a dual LT1/LT2 antagonist, BAY u9773 generally antagonized both $LTD_4$ and $LTC_4$ responses. However, on one tissue, guinea pig lung strip (GPLS), a significant discrepancy became evident. $LTC_4$ and $LTD_4$ both induced contractions in GPLS, and $LTD_4$/LT1 antagonists were partially effective against such responses, as was indomethacin. However, a significant component of both the $LTC_4$ and $LTD_4$ responses was resistant to both the LT antagonists and to indomethacin.

If an $LTC_4$/LT2 receptor was present in GPLS (as in guinea pig trachea), BAY u9773 should antagonize both $LTC_4$- and $LTD_4$-induced contractions, but BAY u9773 was only partially effective. This suggests that either a further LT-receptor type exists that is resistant to BAY u9773 or that subtypes of the $LTC_4$/LT2 receptor exist, with BAY u9773 acting only at one subtype.

Although the identification of BAY u9773 represents a significant advance in the characterization of LT receptors, by itself it cannot provide conclusive evidence for the existence of two separate LT receptors. If such receptors do exist, then selective agonists and antagonists for each receptor type should exist. The identification of such compounds is critical in extending our knowledge of LT receptors. It is possible that the difference between the LT receptors is small, especially as both $LTC_4$ and $LTD_4$ seem to act at both receptors and as BAY u9773 antagonizes both receptors. Perhaps the two receptors are not distinct types but merely subdivisions of one type. If this is the case, identifying selective antagonists for the $LTC_4$/LT2 receptors may be difficult, although it has been achieved for the $LTD_4$/LT1 receptor.

## PRELIMINARY CLASSIFICATION OF LT RECEPTORS

A number of proposals have already been made with respect to the nomenclature of LT receptors. These include, for example, "$LTD_4$/LT1," "$LTC_4$/LT2," "$pLT_1$," "$LTB_4$" receptors. However, such suggestions are either misleading, e.g., $LTD_4$/LT1 or $LTC_4$/LT2, or do not take into account the $LTB_4$ receptors, e.g., LT1, LT2, or pLT1. To overcome such problems, we suggest that the best strategy would be to use a compromise hybrid of novelty and previous nomenclatures; the nomenclature we are proposing is illustrated in Table 2.

In brief, the LT receptor class is identified by the letter "L," which covers both the cysteinyl and noncysteinyl LTs. The significant differences between cysteinyl and $LTB_4$-receptor types is dealt with by the nomenclature

**TABLE 2.** *Preliminary classification of LT receptors*

| Tissue/cells with homogeneous LT | Rank order agonist potency | Antagonist(s) | Receptor nomenclature |
|---|---|---|---|
| Rat lung strip Guinea pig gallbladder | $D_4 = C_4 > E_4 > B_4 = 0$ | ICI 198,615 SK&F 104,353 BAY u9773 | PL1 |
| Sheep bronchus Ferret trachea/spleen | $C_4 = D_4 > E_4 > B_4 = 0$ | | PL2 |
| Guinea pig lung strip[a] | $C_4 = D_4 > E_4 > B_4$ | None | PL3 |
| PMNs, eosinophils[b] | $B_4 \gg D_4 = C_4 = E_4 = 0$ | LY 223982 | BL |

[a] This is not a homogeneous population. The PL1 is also present, but in the presence of indomethacin neither PL1 nor PL2 antagonists are effective.

[b] Recent studies suggest that PL receptors are present on such cells, but PL antagonists are ineffective against $LTB_4$ and BL antagonists are ineffective against $LTD_4$ or $LTC_4$.

"PL" (as $LTC_4$ and $LTD_4$ are the predominant agonists at one L receptor class; "P" represents "peptido") and "BL" ("B" represents $LTB_4$, which is the predominant agonist at the other L class). Further subdivisions or subtypes of the PL receptor type are defined by antagonist-sensitive or antagonist-insensitive responses and are incorporated as "PL1" and "PL2." PL1 receptors are sensitive to all existing LT antagonists and PL2 are insensitive to all known LT antagonists, except for BAY u9773. Further subtypes can be identified numerically, e.g., PL3; this subtype responds equally to $LTC_4$ and to $LTD_4$. However, these responses are resistant to all existing LT antagonists, including BAY u9773.

This nomenclature is a working hypothesis and as new data emerge from working with selective LT agonists and antagonists and as the cloning and sequencing of receptors advance, the need for modification may well arise.

## LEUKOTRIENE RECEPTORS ON HUMAN PULMONARY TISSUES

Although of academic interest, the main aim of characterizing LT receptors is to help identify an ideal pharmacologic profile for new LT agonists or antagonists as potential therapeutics for a range of pathologic states. Asthma is the most studied disease with respect to the application of LT antagonists. Early studies demonstrated that $LTC_4$ and $LTD_4$ equipotently and equally effectively contracted human bronchial muscle (HBM) and that LT antagonists were effective against the contractions induced by either of these LTs. These results have never been disputed, and despite the lower potency (approximately one order of magnitude compared with most animal tissues) shown by LT antagonists on this tissue, HBM seems to contain a homogeneous PL1-receptor population.

Early reports from experiments with LTs suggested that the predominant site of action was the small airways. We therefore evaluated LTs and their antagonists on human parenchymal lung strip (HLS). We repeatedly found that the potencies of the LT antagonists against both $LTC_4$ and $LTD_4$ on HLS were markedly less than the already low values seen with HBM. In an attempt to investigate the discrepancy between LT antagonist potency on HBM and HLS, and because lung strips contain both airway and vascular tissue, we evaluated LT agonists and antagonists on human pulmonary veins (HPV) (33). $LTC_4$ and $LTD_4$ had comparable contractile activity on HPV, but the PL1 antagonists were ineffective against these responses (Fig. 6). In contrast, BAY u9773 ($10^{-6}$ $M$) antagonized both $LTC_4$ and $LTD_4$ responses in HPV. However, BAY u9773 also showed some agonist activity, suggesting that this compound was a partial agonist on this tissue. These results indicate the presence of PL2 receptors on HPV. This may help to explain the poor activity of PL1 antagonists on HLS, i.e., part of the LT contractile response is probably due to activation of PL2 receptors on the vascular tissue present. The overall conclusion from these studies is that more than one PL receptor exists in humans.

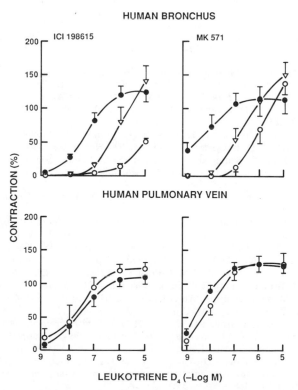

**FIG. 6.** Activity of ICI 198615 and MK 571 on human pulmonary tissues. $LTD_4$ was added alone (●) or in the presence of $10^{-7}$ $M$ (▽) or $10^{-6}$ $M$ (○) of the LT antagonist. Contractions are expressed as percent of histamine (50 $\mu M$) in bronchus and percent of 5-HT (10 $\mu M$) in pulmonary veins. Each point is the mean ± SEM of three to six observations.

As mentioned previously, asthma is presently the therapeutic area most strongly associated with LTs. Current clinical findings suggest that PL1 antagonists could be highly beneficial in the treatment of this disease. It will be intriguing to discover whether or not PL2 antagonists or mixed PL1/PL2 antagonists will show similar or even better pharmacologic profiles than the PL1 antagonists. Alternatively, the PL2 receptor (sub)type has pathophysiologic significance in other areas, e.g., the cardiovascular field.

## ACKNOWLEDGMENT

We thank Ms. K. Francis and Ms. L. Bovington for the preparation of this manuscript, and Ms. S. Fitch for invaluable comments on its content.

## REFERENCES

1. Wasserman MA. In: Hollinger MA, ed. *Reviews in pulmonary pharmacology and toxicology*. New York: Elsevier Science Publishing; 1986;1:1–22.
2. Drazen JM, Maguire W, Israel E, Pichurko B. In: Kaliner M, Barnes PJ, Persson C, eds. *Lung biology in health and disease*. New York: Marcel Dekker; 1991;49:301–25.
3. Baker SR, Boot JR, Jamieson WB, Osborne DJ, Sweatman WJF. *Biochem Biophys Res Commun* 1981;103:1258–64.
4. Tsai B, Bernstein PR, Macia RA, Conaty J, Krell RD. *Prostaglandins* 1982;23:489–506.
5. Krell RD, Osborn R, Wickery L, et al. *Prostaglandins* 1981;22:387–409.
6. Pong SS, DeHaven RN. *Proc Natl Acad Sci USA* 1983;80:7415–9.
7. Buckner CK, Krell RD, Laravuso DB, Coursin DB, Bernstein PR, Will JA. *J Pharmacol Exp Ther* 1986;237;558–62.
8. Hay DWP, Newton JF, Torphy TJ, Gleason JG. *Drugs Future* 1990;15:240–4.
9. Krell RD, Aharony D, Buckner CK, et al. *Am Rev Respir Dis* 1990;141:978–87.
10. Adaikan PG, Lau LC, Kottegoda SR, Ratnam SS. In: Samuelsson B, Paoletti R; Ramwell PW; eds. *Advances in prostaglandins, thromboxane and leukotrienes research*, Vol. 17. New York: Raven Press; 1987:549–53.
11. O'Donnell M, Crowley MJ, Yaremko B, O'Neill N, Welton AF. *J Pharmacol Exp Ther* 1991;259:751–8.
12. Jones TR, Zamboni R, Belley M, et al. *Can J Physiol Pharmacol* 1989;67:17–28.
13. Synder DW, Krell RD. *J Pharmacol Exp Ther* 1984;231:616–22.
14. Gardiner PJ, Abram TS, Cuthbert NJ. *Eur J Pharmacol* 1990;182:291–9.
15. Mong S, Wu H-L, Scott MO, et al. *J Pharmacol Exp Ther* 1985;234:316–25.
16. Hogaboom GK, Mong S, Stadel DM, Crooke ST. *J Pharmacol Exp Ther* 1985;233:686–93.
17. Metters KM, Frey EA, Ford-Hutchinson AW. *Eur J Pharmacol* 1991;194:51–61.
18. Scerau HM, Mong S, Foley JJ, Wu H-L, Crooke ST. *J Biol Chem* 1987;262:4034–41.
19. Mong S, Chi-Rosso G, Hay DM, Crooke ST. *J Pharmacol Exp Ther* 1988;34:590–6.
20. Lewis MA, Mong S, Vessella RL, Crooke ST. *Biochem Pharmacol* 1985;34:4311–7.
21. Bouchelouche PN, Berild D. *Second J Clin Lab Invest* 1991;51:Suppl 204:47–55.
22. Watanabe T, Shimizu T, Miki I, et al. *J Biol Chem* 1990;265:21237–41.
23. Crooke ST, Sarau H, Saussy D, Winkler J, Foley J. In: Samuelsson B, Dahlén SE, Fritsch J, Hedquist P, eds. *Advances in prostaglandin, thromboxane, and leukotriene research*, Vol. 20. New York: Raven Press; 1990:127–37.
24. Hand JM, Schwalm SF, Engelbach IM, Aven MA, Musser JH, Kreff AF. *Prostaglandins* 1989;37:181–91.
25. Cuthbert NJ, Tudhope SR, Gardiner PJ, et al. *Ann NY Acad Sci* 1991;629:402–4.
26. Bruns RF, Thomsen WJ, Paysley TA. *Life Sci* 1983;33:645–53.

27. Lewis MA, Mong S, Vesilla RL, Hoogaboom GK, Wu H-L, Crooke ST. *Prostaglandins* 1984;27:961–74.
28. Rovati GE, Oliva D, Sautebin L, Folco GC, Welton AF, Nicosia S. *Biochem Pharmacol* 1985;34:2831–7.
29. Pong SS, Dehaven RN, Kuehl FA Jr, Egan RW. *J Biol Chem* 1983;258:9616–9.
30. Norman P, Abram TS, Kluender HC, Gardiner PJ, Cuthbert NJ. *Eur J Pharmacol* 1987; 143:323–34.
31. Sun FF, Chau LY, Spur B, Corey EJ, Lewis RA, Austen KF. *J Biol Chem* 1986;261: 8540–6.
32. Mong S. *Methods Enzymol* 1990;187:421–33.
33. Labat C, Ortiz L, Norel X, et al. *J Pharmacol Exp Ther* [*in press*].

*Advances in Prostaglandin, Thromboxane,
and Leukotriene Research,* Vol. 22, edited by
S.-E. Dahlén et al. Raven Press, Ltd., New York © 1994

# Summary: The Enzymes, Accessory Proteins, and Receptors of Leukotriene Metabolism and Their Inhibition and Antagonism

Edward A. Dennis and *Robert D. Krell

*Department of Chemistry, University of California, San Diego, La Jolla,
California 92093-0601; and *Biofor, Inc., Wavery, Pennsylvania 18471-0629*

Many important inflammatory mediators are derived from arachidonic acid. Of major interest are the prostaglandins, including the thromboxanes and prostacyclins, produced by the cyclooxygenase pathway, and the leukotrienes as well as the lipoxins and HETES, produced by the lipoxygenase pathway. The production of all of these mediators depends critically on the availability of free arachidonic acid. The control point for the production of that free arachidonic acid potentially involves many different membrane receptor events and signal transduction pathways (1,2). Presumably, they all involve the activation of a phospholipase, either directly or through secondary mediators, as indicated in Fig. 1. This phospholipase is believed to act in or on membranes because that is where substrate is localized, although other subcellular localizations are also possible. The most reasonable candidate for the type of phospholipase would be a phospholipase $A_2$, because the bulk of the arachidonic acid is found esterified in the *sn*-2 position of membrane phospholipids.

When phospholipase $A_2$ acts on a phospholipid to release arachidonic acid, the other product is a lysophospholipid, which is itself a biologic detergent quite lytic to membranes and which must be hydrolyzed further by a lysophospholipase to water-soluble products or be reacylated. When the phospholipids contain ether linkages in the *sn*-1 position and are acted on by phospholipase $A_2$, the lysophospholipid product is actually lyso PAF which, on acylation, forms platelet-activating factor or PAF, which is also a potent proinflammatory lipid mediator implicated in many disease processes. The inhibition of cyclooxygenase by aspirin and other nonsteroidal anti-inflammatory drugs (NSAIDs) is very well known. There has been a great deal of interest in inhibiting the lipoxygenase pathway or developing receptor an-

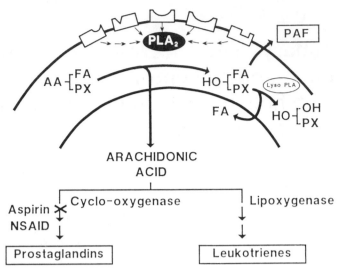

**FIG. 1.** Role of phospholipase $A_2$ in arachidonic acid production. From Dennis (1).

tagonists to the various products of this pathway, which is the focus of this report. It is important also to acknowledge that if one could inhibit the phospholipase $A_2$ (3), one should be able to block production of the substrate for both the cyclooxygenase and the lipoxygenase pathways as well as for the production of PAF.

## LEUKOTRIENE INHIBITION AND ANTAGONISM

The question of whether there is a single pool of arachidonic acid or whether the cyclooxygenase and lipoxygenase utilize different pools is still unresolved, and the possibility must therefore be considered of inhibiting phospholipase $A_2$ specifically for the leukotrienes. If we focus specifically on the leukotriene products, one could potentially interfere with either the biosynthetic enzymes via specific inhibitors or the leukotriene products via receptor antagonists. There are several potential points of intervention to be considered, as indicated in Fig. 2.

Free arachidonic acid is the substrate of the 5-lipoxygenase (5-LO) with the aid of its accessory protein, 5-lipoxygenase activating protein (FLAP), and the resulting leukotriene $A_4$ (LTA$_4$) can be converted to leukotriene $B_4$ (LTB$_4$) by the LTA$_4$ hydrolase. Alternatively, the LTA$_4$ can be transformed with glutathione to form leukotriene $C_4$ (LTC$_4$) with the enzyme LTC$_4$ synthase, which has also been referred to as glutathione S-transferase.

There is in this way a key bifurcation of the biosynthetic pathway between the nonpeptidyl-containing LTB$_4$ and the peptidyl-containing LTC$_4$. The

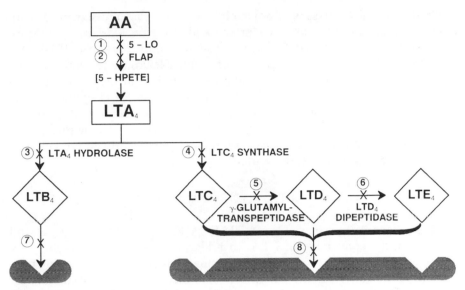

**FIG. 2.** Potential inhibitor and antagonist sites specific for leukotriene biosynthesis and receptor action.

$LTC_4$ can undergo further metabolism to leukotriene $D_4$ ($LTD_4$) and leuko-triene $E_4$ ($LTE_4$). The question of whether the formation of $LTD_4$ and $LTE_4$ should be considered as part of the anabolic or biosynthetic pathway or as a catabolic pathway is a matter that has not been sufficiently addressed. Because receptors with selectivity for $LTD_4$ have been identified and an-tagonists to them have been made, it has been assumed that the γ-glutamyl transpeptidase is anabolic and that the $LTD_4$ dipeptidase is catabolic. How-ever, this requires further clarification.

Potential points of inhibition include the 5-lipoxygenase itself or its acces-sory protein (FLAP), $LTA_4$ hydrolase for the nonpeptidyl leukotrienes or $LTC_4$ synthase for the peptidyl leukotrienes. Of course, development of potent and selective receptor antagonists for $LTB_4$, $LTC_4$, $LTD_4$, and $LTE_4$ constitutes the other main approach to inhibition, and this approach has met with considerable success.

We consider here the underlying biochemistry of the 5-lipoxygenase, FLAP, $LTA_4$ hydrolase, $LTC_4$ synthase, and the receptors for the $LTB_4$ and the peptidyl leukotrienes, as well as their potential as inhibitory targets.

### 5-LO AND FLAP

5-Lipoxygenase has been extensively explored as a potential target for pharmacologic control of the production of proinflammatory leukotrienes.

Several mechanistic classes of novel chemicals have been discovered, with a few entering clinical trials (see Garland and Hodgson, *this volume*). More recently, a protein termed 5-lipoxygenase-activating protein (FLAP) has been discovered, which is obligatory for cellular leukotriene synthesis (see Ford-Hutchinson, *this volume*). Evidence suggests that membrane-associated FLAP serves as an intracellular "receptor" for the 5-LO enzyme during activation, placing it in proximity to the substrate arachidonic acid, provided by phospholipase $A_2$. Compounds capable of interfering with the interaction of 5-LO with FLAP have been discovered and have recently entered clinical trials. The results are eagerly awaited.

## LTA$_4$ HYDROLASE

Leukotriene $A_4$ hydrolase (4) is a 70 kDa enzyme that contains $Zn^{2+}$ and carries out the conversion of $LTA_4$ to $LTB_4$, the major pharmacologically active nonpeptidyl leukotriene. $LTB_4$ stimulates adhesion of circulating neutrophils to vascular endothelium and directs them to sites of inflammation. The substrate and related analogues, such as $LTA_3$ and $LTA_5$, are irreversible inhibitors of the enzyme.

Interestingly, the enzyme also has aminopeptidase activity, and although this reaction may use the $Zn^{2+}$ and a carbonyl side chain in the catalytic site differently, inhibitors based on the peptidase activity work well as $LTA_4$ hydrolase inhibitors. However, the question of the physiologic function of the enzyme remains to be addressed, i.e., whether the potential peptidase activity and/or the $LTA_4$ hydrolase dominates under normal and pathologic conditions. Interesting inhibitors of the enzyme have been developed, based in part on its aminopeptidase activity (5).

## LTC$_4$ SYNTHASE

Leukotriene $C_4$ synthase catalyzes the conversion of $LTA_4$ to the first of the cysteinyl leukotrienes, $LTC_4$, by virtue of its glutathione S-transferase-like activity. Ford-Hutchinson (*this volume*) described the first successful purification and characterization of membrane-bound $LTC_4$ synthase from differentiated U937 cells or THP-1 cells. It was concluded that $LTC_4$ synthase is either an 18-kDa polypeptide or that this peptide may be one subunit of a homodimer. Purification of the enzyme offers yet another potential target for pharmacologic control of cysteinyl leukotrienes.

## LTB$_4$ RECEPTORS

Antagonists of the receptor for the nonpeptide leukotriene $LTB_4$ have been discovered (6). Because $LTB_4$ exerts profound effects on the polymorphonuclear leukocyte (PMN) as well as on other white cells (e.g., chemotaxis, chemokinesis, activation, and degranulation), these types of compounds may well prove to be anti-inflammatory. As yet, none of these compounds has proceeded to clinical trials.

## $LTC_4$, $LTD_4$, AND $LTE_4$ RECEPTORS

Not surprisingly, cysteinyl leukotriene receptors have been clearly demonstrated to be highly heterogeneous (see Gardiner et al., *this volume*; 7). In human intrapulmonary conducting airway smooth muscle, a single type of cysteinyl leukotriene receptor has been identified that interacts with all three cysteinyl leukotrienes (8). Several distinct chemical classes of potent and selective antagonists, including SKF 104,353 (9), ICI 204,219 (10), MK 571 (11), and its single enantiomer, MK 679, have been developed and have been shown to be capable of blocking exogenous aerosol $LTD_4$ in healthy volunteers, as well as in antigen- and exercise-induced provocation in allergic asthmatics. There is justification for the high level of enthusiasm for the early clinical data that have been obtained with these compounds to date.

## ACKNOWLEDGMENT

Support for preparation of this manuscript (to EAD) was provided by NIH grants GM 20,501 and HD 26171.

## REFERENCES

1. Dennis EA. *Bio/Technology* 1987;5:1294–1300.
2. Dennis EA, Rhee SG, Bilah MM, Hannun YA. *FASEB J* 1991;5:2068–77.
3. Dennis EA. *Advances in prostaglandin, thromboxane and leukotriene research.* New York: Raven Press; 1990:217–23.
4. Samuelsson B, Funk CD. *J Biol Chem* 1989;264:19469–72.
5. Yuan W, Wong C-H, Haeggstrom JZ, Wetterholm A, Samuelsson B. *J Am Chem Soc* 1992;114:6552–3.
6. Boyd RJ, Jackson WT. *Fourth International Conference of the Inflammation Research Association.* White Haven, PA; Oct 23–27, 1988.
7. Synder DW, Krell RD. *J Pharmacol Exp Ther* 1984;231:616–22.
8. Buckner CK, Krell RD, Laravuso, RB Coursin, DB, Bernstein PR, Will JA. *J Pharmacol Exp Ther* 1986;237:558–62.
9. Hay DWP, Muccitelli RM, Tucker SS, et al. *J Pharmacol Exp Ther* 1987;243:474–81.
10. Krell RD, Aharony D, Buckner CK, et al. *Am Rev Respir Dis* 1990;141:978–87.
11. Jones TR, Zamboni R, Belley M, et al. *Can J Physiol Pharmacol* 1989;67:17–28.

# 2. Basic Mechanisms in Inflammation

Advances in Prostaglandin, Thromboxane,
and Leukotriene Research, Vol. 22, edited by
S.-E. Dahlén et al. Raven Press, Ltd., New York © 1994

# Cytokine Regulation of Mouse Mast-Cell–Specific Protease Genes

## H. Patrick McNeil and K. Frank Austen

*Department of Rheumatology and Immunology, Brigham and Women's Hospital,
and Department of Medicine, Harvard Medical School,
Boston, Massachusetts 02115*

Mast cells are heterogeneous, comprising at least two major subtypes in human, mouse, and rat tissues. Histochemical staining, sensitivity to fixatives, and morphologic criteria distinguish perivascular connective tissue mast cells (CTMC) from intestinal mucosal mast cells (MMC) in rats and mice. The serosal mast cell (SMC) that lines the peritoneal cavities of these animals has been considered to be an example of the CTMC, as SMC are morphologically and histochemically similar to CTMC. However, as discussed below, the composition of neutral proteases in the microvascular CTMC differs from those present in SMC, indicating that there are at least three subtypes of mouse mast cells. A second important difference between the subtypes is that proliferation of MMC in response to helminth infection is dependent on T-lymphocyte–derived cytokines [1,2], whereas it has been considered that maintenance of CTMC is relatively T-lymphocyte–independent, as their numbers are normal in T-cell–deficient animals. Differences between human mast cells at different locations in their sensitivity to formalin fixation, together with a selective deficiency of mast cells in the intestinal mucosa of patients with T-cell immunodeficiency [3], indicates that division of human mast cells into subtypes may also be generally applicable [4]. Human mast cells are not distinguishable by histochemistry, but ultrastructural analysis of secretory granule morphology is consistent with a division into two general subtypes [5–9]. Secretory granules of human mast cells display a variety of structures by electron microscopy, which include lattice or grating-like structures, scrolls, and mixed patterns. Mast cells located in the skin, breast parenchyma, lymph node, and bowel submucosa reveal few closed scrolls and are predominantly "scroll-poor," whereas "scroll-rich" morphology is found in mast cells in intestinal mucosa and lung parenchyma. These morphologic features are not a characteristic of rat or mouse mast cell granules, which are usually amorphous and homogeneous in structure.

Apart from granule morphology and dependence on T-cell factors, the expression of mast-cell–specific secretory granule proteases is considered to be the most definitive marker yet employed for discrimination among subtypes of human mast cells. Immunohistochemistry has been used to divide human mast cells into those staining positive with antitryptase antibodies alone, designated $MC_T$, and those staining with antibodies to tryptase and chymase, designated $MC_{TC}$ (10). $MC_{TC}$ cells also contain mast cell carboxypeptidase-A (MC-CPA) (11) and a cathepsin G-like enzyme activity (12). Scroll-rich cells are predominantly $MC_T$, whereas scroll-poor cells are predominantly $MC_{TC}$ cells (8,13). Because approximately 8% of mast cells from all human tissues display mixed morphologic granule patterns, and some in bowel submucosa stain positive for chymase only ($MC_C$) (13), both overlap and additional phenotypes are probable. Furthermore, antitryptase antibodies are reactive with the products of at least two distinct tryptase cDNAs (14). Whereas only one human mast cell chymase and two tryptases have been identified, the granules of murine mast cells have been resolved into at least six proteases by sodium dodecyl sulfate polyacrylamide gel electrophoresis and N-terminal amino acid sequencing (15). The molecular weights of these proteases are 26, 28, 29, 29, 30–31, and 32 kDa. They have been termed mouse mast cell protease (MMCP)-1 through -6, respectively, and a seventh has been defined by genomic cloning and identification of mRNA in mast cells (16). MC-CPA has an $M_r$ of 36 kDa (17). The recognition of multiple mouse protease genes afforded the opportunity to study their cytokine-induced differential transcription during mast cell differentiation from bone marrow progenitors and their expression in in vivo mast cells to define mast cell heterogeneity. These studies provide a basis for the selective expression of protease genes by various mast cell subsets, and illustrate a close association between mast cell phenotype and exposure to tissue-specific cytokines.

## CLONING OF MULTIPLE MOUSE MAST CELL PROTEASE GENES

Oligonucleotides were designed that contained sequences encoding portions of the N-terminal region of the protease molecules which had been defined by resolution of granule proteins (15). These oligonucleotides were used to screen cDNA libraries prepared from Kirsten sarcoma virus-transformed mast cells and nontransformed bone marrow-derived mast cell (BMMC) mRNA to isolate cDNAs encoding MMCP-4 (18), MMCP-5 (19), MMCP-6 (20), and MC-CPA (17). cDNAs encoding MMCP-2 were cloned by cross-hybridization using the homologous rat mast cell protease (RMCP)-II cDNA as a probe (21). The cDNAs were then used as probes to isolate from genomic libraries their respective genes, and by cross-hybridization the genes encoding MMCP-1 (22), a mouse mast-cell–like serine protease

(MMCP-L) (18), and MMCP-7 (16). cDNAs corresponding to these three latter genes were subsequently isolated (16,23,24) from mast cell libraries.

The mast cell serine protease genes exhibit similar genomic structures. The MMCP-1, -2, -4, and -5 (MMCP-3 has not been cloned) and MMCP-L genes possess five exons and contain conserved exon/intron junctions. Exon 1 contains the 5′-untranslated region and the protein coding portion for the signal and activation peptides. The regions encoding the three components of the catalytic triad present in all serine proteases are located on exons 2, 3, and 5. The genes span from 2.3 to 3.1 kb, the variation being due to variable intron length. The MMCP-6 and MMCP-7 genes are smaller (1.8 and 2.3 kb, respectively) and differ slightly from the MMCP-1 to -5 genes. In the MMCP-6 gene, an additional intron separates the 5′-untranslated region from the N-terminal protein coding portion, resulting in an extra exon. The remaining exon/intron junctions of MMCP-6 and MMCP-7 are in similar locations to the MMCP-1 to -5 genes. The MMCP-7 gene contains a further variation at its 5′ end. The region corresponding to intron 1 in the MMCP-6 gene is incorporated into a large exon 1, owing to the absence of an intron splice sequence at the 3′ end of this region. Therefore, the MMCP-7 gene contains only five exons, but its structure remains more similar to the MMCP-6 gene than to the MMCP-1 to -5 genes. The chromosomal location of the MMCP genes has recently been defined using the inheritance pattern of recombinant inbred mouse strains (25). The MMCP-1, -2, -4, and -5 genes are clustered together on chromosome 14 adjacent to the genes encoding the mouse lymphocyte granule proteases, granzymes B, C, E, and F (26). The MMCP-6 gene is located on chromosome 17, whereas the murine MC-CPA gene is on chromosome 3.

Structural analysis of the MMCP cDNAs indicates that they encode serine protease molecules that are initially translated as preproenzymes. The zymogens contain 18 to 21 amino acid hydrophobic signal peptides and activation peptides of two (MMCP-1 to -5 plus MMCP-L) or 10 (MMCP-6 and -7) amino acids. Based on homology to the pancreatic enzymes and from an examination of the substrates lining the putative substrate binding pockets, MMCP-1 to -5 plus MMCP-L are predicted to function as chymases, whereas MMCP-6 and MMCP-7 are tryptases. MMCP-2, MMCP-4, and MMCP-L contain a $Ser^{176}$ residue at the base of the substrate binding region, analogous to the $Ser^{189}$ in chymotrypsin, which confers specificity for cleavage of amino acids with aromatic side chains. MMCP-1 and MMCP-5 possess a Thr and Asn, respectively, at this site. MMCP-5 also contains a novel $Val^{199}$ in an otherwise highly conserved substrate binding region, and MMCP-2 and MMCP-L contain a $Glu^{199}$ and $Ser^{198}$, respectively, in this region (Table 1). In addition to these unique residues around the active site, MMCP-5 exhibits a number of novel structural features, including a Gly-Glu activation peptide (Table 1), which indicate that it represents a distinct subset from the other mouse mast cell chymases (19). These variations and the

**TABLE 1.** *Activation peptides and amino acid residues forming the substrate binding cleft of mast cell chymases*

| Chymase | Activation peptide | Amino acid residues forming the substrate binding cleft | | |
|---|---|---|---|---|
| | | [176] | [197–199] | [207] |
| MMCP-1 | Glu-Glu | Thr | Ser-Tyr-Gly | Ala |
| MMCP-2 | Glu-Glu | Ser | Ser-Tyr-Glu | Ala |
| MMCP-4 | Glu-Glu | Ser | Ser-Tyr-Gly | Ala |
| MMCP-L | Glu-Glu | Ser | Ser-Ser-Gly | Ala |
| MMCP-5 | Gly-Glu | Asn | Ser-Tyr-Val | Ala |
| RMCP-1 | ND | Ser | Ser-Tyr-Gly | Ala |
| RMCP-II | Glu-Glu | Ala | Ser-Tyr-Gly | Ala |
| Dog chymase | Glu-Glu | Ser | Ser-Tyr-Gly | Ala |
| Human chymase | Gly-Glu | Ser | Ser-Tyr-Gly | Ala |

Adapted from ref. 19.
ND, not determined.

common gene locus argue that the chymases have highly restricted functions dictated by their participation in the efferent limb of the immune response. MMCP-6 and MMCP-7 possess an Asp[188] analogous to Asp[189] in trypsin, which is the critical substrate-binding residue for cleavage of peptide bonds at basic amino acid residues. The division of the MMCPs into chymases and tryptases is also supported by the chromosomal organization of all the chymases at one locus, separate from MMCP-6. The MC-CPA cDNAs encode an exopeptidase with a 15-residue signal peptide, a 94-residue activation peptide, and a mature enzyme with predicted specificity for C-terminal aromatic and aliphatic amino acids. Computerized modeling was used to determine that the three-dimensional configurations of the mouse mast cell chymases are very similar to RMCP-II (27), a molecule of known tertiary structure (28). A similar analysis has been performed for the mast cell tryptases (29). The three-dimensional structures indicate that the mouse secretory granule proteases differ from chymotrypsin and trypsin by the presence of a deep substrate binding cleft and by the presence of additional residues on each side of the cleft, which are predicted to allow interaction with multiple amino acid residues adjacent to the cleavage site on the substrate. This is likely to account for the much narrower substrate specificities of the MMCPs compared with chymotrypsin and trypsin.

## TRANSCRIPTION OF PROTEASE GENES IN MAST CELL SUBSETS

Although the MMCP molecules and their encoding cDNAs are highly homologous, gene-specific cDNA or cRNA probes were generated to analyze the expression of each gene in different populations of mast cells by detection of mRNA. The pattern of protease gene expression was found to

**TABLE 2.** *Expression of neutral proteases in mouse mast cell subsets[a]*

| Protease | BMMC$_{IL-3}$ (in vitro) | MMC (helminth infection) | SMC (peritoneal) | CTMC (perivascular skin) |
|---|---|---|---|---|
| Chymases | | | | |
| MMCP-1 | − | + | − | − |
| MMCP-2[b] | − | + | − | + |
| MMCP-3[c] | ND | ND | + | ND |
| MMCP-4 | − | − | + | + |
| MMCP-5 | + | − | + | + |
| Tryptases | | | | |
| MMCP-6 | + | − | + | + |
| MMCP-7 | + | − | − | + |
| Exopeptidases | | | | |
| MC-CPA | + | − | + | + |

[a] Expression for all proteases except MMCP-3 determined by detection of mRNA.
[b] Expression in CTMC varies with mouse strain.
[c] Expression determined by resolution of protein and N-terminal amino acid sequence.
ND, not determined.

be a discriminating marker of mast cell heterogeneity in vivo. SMC are known to contain MMCP-3 protein (15) and were found to express transcripts encoding MMCP-4, -5, -6, and MC-CPA. In contrast, MMC enriched intestinal tissue from *T. spiralis*-infected mice selectively expressed MMCP-1 and -2 mRNA (16–21,23,30). Although SMC and tissue CTMC appear histochemically identical, the protease phenotype of CTMC had not previously been determined. Therefore, RNA isolated from skin and ear tissue of the congeneic +/+ littermates of *Sl/Sl*$^d$ and *W/W*$^v$ mast-cell–deficient mice was examined for MMCP transcripts by RNA blot and RNase protection analyses. RNA was also isolated from the mast cell-deficient animals as a control, to ensure the specificity of positive hybridizations in the +/+ samples. We found that perivascular CTMC present in skin and ear tissue of +/+ mice express MMCP-2 and MMCP-7 mRNA in addition to the SMC transcripts MMCP-4, -5, and -6 and MC-CPA. In the case of MMCP-2, the protein was localized to mast cell granules in skin, ear, and skeletal muscle with an anti–MMCP-2 peptide immunologic probe (see below) (31). Therefore, mouse mast cells comprise at least three subsets based on analysis of the expression of secretory granule proteases (Table 2), whereas only two were previously recognized based on histochemical or morphological criteria.

## REGULATION OF PROTEASE GENE TRANSCRIPTION BY SPECIFIC CYTOKINES

Because mast cell heterogeneity is considered to reflect microenvironmental regulation, we used an in vitro system to determine the factors responsible for induction of specific mast cell protease genes. A population of immature bone marrow–derived mast cells (BMMC) can be generated by culturing mouse bone marrow cells in medium enriched for interleukin (IL)-3 (32–35). BMMC cultured for 2 to 3 weeks in IL-3-enriched WEHI-3B cell-conditioned medium (WCM) were found to express mRNA encoding a chymase, MMCP-5, two tryptases, MMCP-6 and -7, and MC-CPA (16,17,19,20). Because BMMC repopulate all subclasses of mast cells when transplanted into mast-cell–deficient mice (36), it appears that BMMC can serve as precursors to all mast cell subsets. Therefore, protease genes expressed by BMMC generated with IL-3 have been termed early-expressed genes, whereas the other chymases, MMCP-1, -2, and -4, which are presumably induced by factors specific for different mast cell subsets, have been termed late-expressed genes. To investigate the factors that might induce activation of these late-expressed proteases, BMMC were generated using IL-3 and subsequently exposed to various cytokines. We found that the MMCP-4 gene is induced by exposure of BMMC to the c-kit protooncogene product KIT ligand (KL) (also known as stem cell factor) (37), whereas the MMCP-1 and -2 genes are activated by IL-10 (23,30). Inasmuch as IL-3 induces the early-expressed protease genes, it dominantly suppresses transcription of the late-expressed protease genes by KL or IL-10. In addition to inducing MMCP-4 gene expression, KL can elicit transcription of the early-expressed MMCP-5, MMCP-6, and MC-CPA genes in mast cells of low purity derived directly from bone marrow (37). The expression of MMCP-7 by BMMC cultured in WCM is transient, reaching a peak after 3 weeks of culture from bone marrow but decreasing significantly thereafter (16). However, transcription of the MMCP-7 gene can be maintained if IL-10 is added to the IL-3-enriched culture medium used to obtain a virtually pure immature mast cell population (McNeil, unpublished observations).

These findings provide an explanation for the selective expression of different protease genes by various mast cell subsets. The expression of MMCP-1 and -2 by MMC is consistent with the known role of $T_H2$ cell cytokines IL-3, IL-4, and IL-10 in helminth infections (2,38–40). The presence of MMCP-4 in SMC and CTMC is consistent with induction of this protease gene by the fibroblast-derived cytokine KL, as both SMC and CTMC are located within fibroblast-rich connective tissue. The expression of MMCP-2 and MMCP-7 in skin mast cells may be explained by the recent finding that keratinocytes produce IL-10 (41). Taken together, these results provide further evidence that the phenotype of mast cells is dependent on local exposure to tissue-specific cytokines, and it follows that there exists a close association between mast cell phenotype and local or autocrine cytokine production.

Complementary to these studies of protease gene transcription, we have recently produced probes that can specifically detect the translated gene products. Synthetic peptides derived from sequences unique to each protease were used as immunogens to produce antipeptide antibodies to

MMCP-2, MMCP-5, and MC-CPA (42,43). We have found that the CTMC in mouse ear, skin, and skeletal muscle are reactive with anti–MMCP-2 antibody as well as with anti–MMCP-5 and anti–MC-CPA antibodies (31), confirming the transcription analysis noted above. In the intestines of normal mice, MMCP-5$^+$ and MC-CPA$^+$ mast cells are situated in the submucosa on the serosal side of the muscularis mucosa. MMCP-2$^+$ mast cells are uncommon and are located in the lamina propria. During *T. spiralis* infection, MMC that are MMCP-2$^+$ expand in the lamina propria and extend into intraepithelial locations. The presence of MMC containing MMCP-2 is indicative that there is local production of a cytokine such as IL-10 during *T. spiralis* infection.

## MOUSE MAST CELL DIFFERENTIATION

Although at least five murine mast cell growth factors have been recognized [IL-3 (44), IL-4 (45), IL-9 (46), IL-10 (39), and KL (47)], the relative importance of each during differentiation of mast cells from bone marrow progenitors has been unclear. Murine mast-cell–progenitor cells are present in bone marrow as mononuclear cells mostly lacking FcεRI (48,49), which on stimulation with IL-3 proliferate to produce immature mast cell colonies. Once committed to the mast cell lineage, fibroblast-derived growth factors such as KL are able to stimulate further mast cell growth and differentiation (50–53). During initial IL-3 exposure, expression of FcεRI occurs before granule formation (49,54). Early expression of FcεRI may directly bring about mast cell proliferation, as IgE has been found to stimulate mast cell formation from bone marrow progenitors in the absence of IL-3, possibly via autocrine secretion of IL-3 (52). These findings indicating that IL-3 and KL act relatively early during mast cell differentiation are compatible with our observations that both cytokines induce transcription of the early-expressed protease genes in vitro, although only IL-3 favors the differentiation of mast cells over other cell types from the mononuclear progenitors. Since KL also induces the late-expressed MMCP-4 gene and IL-3 suppresses late-expressed gene transcription, our results predict that KL but not IL-3 is important for later stages of differentiation in vivo. KL is produced by fibroblasts as both secreted and membrane-bound forms. The extracellular domain of mast cell *KIT* interacts with fibroblast membrane bound KL to mediate attachment of mast cells to fibroblasts (55,56) and with soluble KL to elicit chemotaxis (57), which may be important in trafficking of mast cell precursors to tissue sites. When BMMC are co-cultured in vitro on 3T3 fibroblasts, the cells acquire multiple features characteristic of SMC, including a switch to heparin proteoglycan biosynthesis, and accumulation of approximately 50-fold more histamine and approximately 100-fold more MC-CPA activity (58,59). The lack of MMCP-4 transcription in this system (Eklund et al., unpublished observations) (Fig. 1) compared with the effects of recombinant KL may be due to the suppressive effect of IL-3 on KL-induced MMCP-4 gene transcription (37), which may occur via an IL-3-induced downregulation of the KL receptor *KIT* (60). Treatment of immature mast cells obtained from mesenteric lymph nodes of *Nippostrongylus brasiliensis*-infected mice with fibroblast-conditioned medium in the absence of IL-3 results in cells reactive with antibody to RMCP-I (53), which is presumptive evidence for the presence of MMCP-4 because RMCP-I is the rat homologue of MMCP-4 (18). Although mast cells generated using sequential IL-3 and KL express MMCP-4, they do not mature to the same extent as do BMMC co-cultured with 3T3 fibroblasts (37), suggesting that additional factors or presentation or bioactivity of KL are important in achieving full mast-cell maturation. Regardless of the lack of appreciable translation of secretory granule constituents in BMMC treated with sequential IL-3 and KL, the transcription phenotype of these cells is identical to that of SMC, suggesting that a similar pathway may operate in vivo. Differentiation of mast cell progenitors into the perivascular CTMC subtype may be similar to that for SMC but may also include the effect of IL-10, which would be predicted to induce MMCP-2 transcription and maintain MMCP-7 expression.

The lack of expansion of the MMC subtype in T-cell–deficient mice (1) indicates that T-cell–specific cytokines are involved. Although IL-3 is pro-

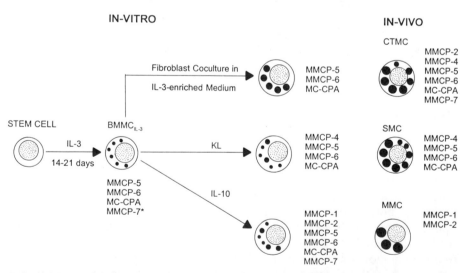

**FIG. 1.** Mouse mast cell phenotypes defined by protease expression of immature mast cells derived in vitro by culture from bone marrow stem cells (see refs. 23,30,37,58, and 59 for details of culture conditions) or of mature in vivo mast cell subtypes present in skin and ear (CTMC), the peritoneal cavity (SMC), or intestinal tissue from *T. spiralis*–infected mice (MMC).*, the expression of MMCP-7 in BMMC cultured in IL-3–enriched WCM is transient (see text).

duced predominantly by T cells, other cells, including mast cells themselves, presumably provide the IL-3 necessary to initiate differentiation of the CTMC subset in mice lacking T cells. Antibodies to IL-3 and IL-4 suppress the mastocytosis associated with helminth infection (2), suggesting that these two cytokines are clearly important. Because MMC express MMCP-1 and MMCP-2 (23,30), it is likely that IL-10 operates in vivo. However, the lack of MMC in mice with mutations causing a nonfunctional KL/*KIT* system indicates that KL is instrumental in the differentiation of MMC, possibly via a chemoattractant or cell-specific adherence function distinct from its role in the development of CTMC. A further critical deficiency in the schema depicted to date is the failure to recognize mechanisms for the suppression of the early-expressed MMCP-5, MMCP-6, and MC-CPA genes in elicited MMC, or the absence of induced MMCP-1 in CTMC if the latter are IL-10-dependent (Fig. 1).

## REGULATION OF OTHER MAST CELL GENES

The phenotyping of mouse mast cells by transcription and translation of secretory granule neutral proteases has provided an approach to defining tissue-specific heterogeneity in vivo and to identification of cytokine-regulated gene expression in vitro as the basis for heterogeneity. The functional implications of these findings are not available as regards the proteases, but there are initial data for arachidonic acid metabolism and surface expression and function of FcγRIII. Whereas mouse SMC synthesize prostaglandin $D_2$ as their major metabolite, mouse BMMC release predominantly $LTC_4$ and lesser amounts of $LTB_4$ and $PGD_2$ after activation via FcεRI, but they do not respond to stimulation of FcγRII/III. After co-culture with mouse 3T3 fibroblasts, the arachidonic acid product profile is unchanged but can be elicited by activation via either FcεRI or FcγRII/III. Fibroblast co-culture upregulates surface expression of FcγRIII (61,62) by attenuation of endoplasmic reticulum degradation of FcγRIII and enhanced cell surface association with the FcεRI γ-chain (63,64).

## ACKNOWLEDGMENT

The work described here was supported by grants AI 22531, AI 31599, AR 35907, AR 36308, HL 36110, and RR 05950 from the National Institutes of Health and by a grant from the Hyde and Watson Foundation. H. P. McNeil was a recipient of a Heald Fellowship from the Arthritis Foundation of Australia.

## REFERENCES

1. Mayrhofer G. *Cell Immunol* 1979;47:312–22.
2. Madden KB, Urban JF, Ziltener HJ, Schrader JW, Kinkelman FD, Katona IM. *J Immunol* 1991;147:1387–91.

3. Irani AA, Craig SS, DeBlois G, Elson CO, Schechter NM, Schwartz LB. *J Immunol* 1987;138:4381–6.
4. Strobel S, Miller HRP, Ferguson A. *J Clin Pathol* 1981;34:851–8.
5. Dobbins WO, Tomasini JT, Rollins EL. *Gastroenterology* 1969;56:268–79.
6. Caulfield JP, Lewis RA, Hein A, Austen KF. *J Cell Biol* 1980;85:299–312.
7. Friedman MM, Kaliner M. *J Allergy Clin Immunol* 1985;76:70–82.
8. Craig SS, Schechter NM, Schwartz LB. *Lab Invest* 1988;58:682–91.
9. Weidner N, Austen KF. *Lab Invest* 1990;63:63–72.
10. Irani AA, Schechter NM, Craig SS, DeBlois G, Schwartz LB. *Proc Natl Acad Sci USA* 1986;83:4464–8.
11. Irani AA, Goldstein SM, Wintroub BU, Bradford T, Schwartz LB. *J Immunol* 1991;147: 247–53.
12. Schechter NM, Irani AA, Sprows JL, Abernethy J, Wintroub B, Schwartz LB. *J Immunol* 1990;145:2652–61.
13. Weidner N, Austen KF. *J Invest Dermatol* 1991;96:26S–31S.
14. Miller JS, Moxley G, Schwartz LB. *J Clin Invest* 1990;86:864–70.
15. Reynolds DS, Stevens RL, Lane WS, Carr MH, Austen KF, Serafin WE. *Proc Natl Acad Sci USA* 1990;87:3230–4.
16. McNeil HP, Reynolds DS, Schiller V, et al. *Proc Natl Acad Sci USA* 1992;89:11174–8.
17. Reynolds DS, Stevens RL, Gurley DS, Lane WS, Austen KF, Serafin WE. *J Biol Chem* 1989;264:20094–9.
18. Serafin WE, Sullivan TP, Conder GA, et al. *J Biol Chem* 1991;266:1934–41.
19. McNeil HP, Austen KF, Somerville LL, Gurish MF, Stevens RL. *J Biol Chem* 1991;266: 20316–22.
20. Reynolds DS, Gurley DS, Austen KF, Serafin WE. *J Biol Chem* 1991;266:3847–53.
21. Serafin WE, Reynolds DS, Rogelj S, et al. *J Biol Chem* 1990;265:423–9.
22. Huang R, Blom T, Hellman L. *Eur J Immunol* 1991;21:1611–21.
23. Ghildyal N, McNeil HP, Stechschulte S, et al. *J Immunol* 1992;149:2123–9.
24. Chu W, Johnson DA, Musich PR. *Biochim Biophys Acta* 1992;1121:83–7.
25. Gurish MF, Nadeau JH, Johnson KR, et al. *J Biol Chem* 1993;268:11372–9.
26. Crosby JL, Bleackley RC, Nadeau JH. *Genomics* 1990;6:252–9.
27. Sali A, Matsumoto R, McNeil HP, Karplus M, Stevens RL. *J Biol Chem* 1993;268:9023–34.
28. Remington SJ, Woodbury RG, Reynolds RA, Matthews BW, Neurath H. *Biochemistry* 1988;27:8097–105.
29. Johnson DA, Barton GJ. *Protein Sci* 1992;1:370–7.
30. Ghildyal N, McNeil HP, Gurish MF, Austen KF, Stevens RL. *J Biol Chem* 1992;267: 8473–7.
31. Stevens RL, Friend DS, McNeil HP, et al. *Proc Natl Acad Sci USA* 1994;91:128–32.
32. Nabel G, Galli SJ, Dvorak AM, Dvorak HF, Cantor H. *Nature* 1981;291:332–4.
33. Schrader JW, Lewis SJ, Clark-Lewis I, Culvenor J-G. *Proc Natl Acad Sci USA* 1981;78: 323–7.
34. Razin E, Cordon-Cardo C, Good RA. *Proc Natl Acad Sci USA* 1981;78:2559–61.
35. Tertian G, Yung Y-P, Guy-Grand D, Moore MAS. *J Immunol* 1981;127:788–94.
36. Nakano T, Sonoda T, Hayashi C, et al. *J Exp Med* 1985;162:1025–43.
37. Gurish MF, Ghildyal N, McNeil HP, Austen KF, Gillis S, Stevens RL. *J Exp Med* 1992; 175:1003–12.
38. Sher A, Fiorentino D, Caspar P, Pearce E, Mosmann T. *J Immunol* 1991;147:2713–6.
39. Thompson-Snipes L, Dhar V, Bond MW, Mosmann T, Moore KW, Rennick DM. *J Exp Med* 1991;173:507–10.
40. Heinzel FP, Sadick MD, Mutha SS, Locksley RM. *Proc Natl Acad Sci USA* 1991;88: 7011–5.
41. Enk AH, Katz SI. *J Immunol* 1992;149:92–5.
42. McNeil HP, Frenkel DP, Austen KF, Friend DS, Stevens RL. *J Immunol* 1992;149: 2466–72.
43. Gurish MF, Stevens RL, Ghildyal N, Austen KF, McNeil HP, Nicodemus CF. *FASEB J* 1992;6:A1723 (Abstract).
44. Rennick DM, Lee FD, Yokata T, Arai KI, Cantor H, Nabel GJ. *J Immunol* 1985;134:910–4.
45. Smith CA, Rennick DM. *Proc Natl Acad Sci USA* 1986;83:1857–61.

46. Hultner L, Druez C, Moeller J, et al. *Eur J Immunol* 1990;20:1413–6.
47. Nocka K, Buck J, Levi E, Besmer P. *EMBO J* 1990;9:3287–4.
48. Seder RA, Paul WE, Dvorak AM, et al. *Proc Natl Acad Sci USA* 1991;88:2835–9.
49. Rottem M, Barbieri S, Kinet J-P, Metcalfe DD. *Blood* 1992;79:972–80.
50. Jarboe DL, Marshall JS, Randolph TR, Kukolja A, Huff TF. *J Immunol* 1989;142:2405–17.
51. Jarboe DL, Huff TF. *J Immunol* 1989;142:2418–23.
52. Ashman RI, Jarboe DL, Conrad DH, Huff TF. *J Immunol* 1991;146:211–6.
53. Leftwich JA, Westin EH, Huff TF. *J Immunol* 1992;148:2894–8.
54. Thompson HL, Metcalfe DD, Kinet J-P. *J Clin Invest* 1990;85:1227–33.
55. Flanagan JG, Leder P. *Cell* 1990;63:185–94.
56. Adachi S, Ebi Y, Nishikawa S, et al. *Blood* 1992;79:650–6.
57. Meininger CJ. *Blood* 1992;79:958–63.
58. Serafin WE, Dayton ET, Gravallese PM, Austen KF, Stevens RL. *J Immunol* 1987;139: 3771–6.
59. Levi-Schaffer F, Dayton ET, Austen KF, et al. *J Immunol* 1987;139:3431–41.
60. Welham MJ, Schrader JW. *Mol Cell Biol* 1991;11:2901–4.
61. Katz HR, Arm JP, Benson AC, Austen KF. *J Immunol* 1990;145:3412–7.
62. Katz HR, Raizman MB, Gartner CS, Scott HC, Benson AC, Austen KF. *J Immunol* 1992;148:868–71.
63. Kurosaki T, Gander I, Ravetch JV. *Proc Natl Acad Sci USA* 1991;88:3837–41.
64. Lobell RB, Arm JP, Raizman MB, Austen KF, Katz HR. *J Biol Chem* 1993;268:1207–12.

*Advances in Prostaglandin, Thromboxane,
and Leukotriene Research*, Vol. 22, edited by
S.-E. Dahlén et al. Raven Press, Ltd., New York © 1994

# Transport and Metabolism of Leukotrienes

Dietrich Keppler, Gabriele Jedlitschky, and Inka Leier

*Division of Tumor Biochemistry, Deutsches Krebsforschungszentrum,
D-69120 Heidelberg, Germany*

Transport, metabolism, and metabolic inactivation decisively influence the concentration of biologically active leukotrienes at their site of action (1,2). Transport processes mediate the release of these mediators from leukotriene-generating cells (3–5), the removal from the blood circulation by predominant uptake into hepatocytes (6–10), and the excretion from the liver into bile (11,12). In addition, transport during renal excretion and during the limited intestinal reabsorption of cysteinyl leukotrienes contributes to the control of leukotriene concentrations in body fluids (13). The pathways of elimination and inactivation also provide information on the compartments, the body fluids, and the metabolites that may be analyzed for an assessment of systemic leukotriene production in vivo (14–16).

## THE EXPORT PUMP MEDIATING LTC$_4$ RELEASE AFTER ITS BIOSYNTHESIS

The release of LTC$_4$ has been studied in cultured human eosinophils incubated with exogenous LTA$_4$ (3). This transport is saturable, temperature-dependent, and inhibited by intracellular LTC$_5$, suggesting a carrier-mediated process. The mechanism underlying the export of LTC$_4$ has been elucidated in plasma membrane vesicles prepared from murine mastocytoma cells and characterized as a primary-active, unidirectional ATP-dependent process with apparent $K_M$ values of 48 μ$M$ for ATP and 110 n$M$ for LTC$_4$ (5). Among the cysteinyl leukotrienes, LTC$_4$ is the best substrate for this ATP-dependent export pump (Fig. 1). The relative transport rates at a concentration of 10 n$M$ are 1.00, 0.31, 0.12, and 0.08 for LTC$_4$, LTD$_4$, LTE$_4$, and $N$-acetyl-LTE$_4$, respectively (5). LTC$_4$ transport is competitively inhibited by the glutathione S-conjugate S-(2,4-dinitrophenyl)glutathione and by low micromolar concentrations of several other amphiphilic anions, including LTD$_4$/LTE$_4$-receptor antagonists (5). Primary-active ATP-dependent transport is insignificant with LTB$_4$ as a substrate. Therefore, inhibition of the

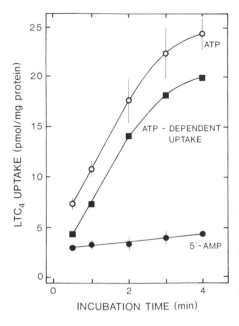

**FIG. 1.** ATP-dependent transport of [$^3$H]LTC$_4$ (50 n$M$) into inside-out plasma membrane vesicles prepared from murine mastocytoma cells. Methods for plasma membrane vesicle preparation were described earlier (5,12). An ATP-regenerating system was included to keep the ATP concentration at 4 m$M$ during transport; 5'-AMP instead of ATP was present in the control incubation.

LTC$_4$ export pump in leukotriene-synthesizing cells by structural analogues and LTD$_4$/LTE$_4$-receptor antagonists may serve as a novel pharmacologic approach to interfere selectively with LTC$_4$ production without influencing LTB$_4$ release. Isolation and molecular characterization of the LTC$_4$ export carrier from leukotriene-generating cells, such as mast cells, eosinophils, and monocytes, will answer the question of whether this pump is a member of the family of the ATP-dependent glutathione conjugate export pumps originally described in the erythrocyte plasma membrane (17) (see note added in proof).

## LEUKOTRIENE UPTAKE INTO HEPATOCYTES

Leukotrienes released into the blood circulation undergo rapid elimination from blood, predominantly owing to uptake by the liver (18,19). Albumin serves as transport protein in the blood circulation (20). Uptake by hepatocytes has been demonstrated both for cysteinyl leukotrienes (7,10) and for LTB$_4$ (9,10). Uptake of LTC$_4$, LTD$_4$, LTE$_4$, and $N$-acetyl-LTE$_4$ across the sinusoidal (basolateral) membrane into hepatocytes is independent of a Na$^+$ gradient and a K$^+$ diffusion potential (10). At a concentration of 10 n$M$, the relative uptake rates into rat hepatocytes for LTC$_4$, LTD$_4$, LTE$_4$, and LTB$_4$ were 1.0, 1.3, 1.6, and 1.6, respectively. The $K_M$ values for the leukotrienes ranged between 100 and 200 n$M$ (10). Kinetic studies in hepatocytes employing inhibitors indicate the existence of distinct uptake systems for the cysteinyl leukotrienes and LTB$_4$ in the sinusoidal membrane. The interaction of both cysteinyl leukotrienes and $LTB_4$ with hepatocytes does not lead to detectable receptor-mediated signal transduction if the mediators are added in the physiologic nanomolar concentration range. This indicates that the hepatocyte uptake systems are transporters and not receptors for the leukotrienes.

## THE EXPORT PUMP MEDIATING LEUKOTRIENE TRANSPORT ACROSS THE HEPATOCYTE CANALICULAR MEMBRANE

During vectorial transport across the hepatocyte, some of the leukotriene metabolites retain their structure and some undergo oxidative degradation from the ω-end (Fig. 2). Products of ω- and β-oxidation of $LTE_4$, N-acetyl-$LTE_4$, and $LTB_4$, as well as unmodified $LTC_4$, $LTD_4$, $LTE_4$, and N-acetyl-$LTE_4$, are substrates for the leukotriene export pump in the canalicular (apical) membrane of hepatocytes (11,12). The mechanism of this transport has been analyzed by use of plasma membrane vesicles enriched in canalicular membranes. The inside-out vesicles incubated in the presence of labeled cysteinyl leukotrienes and ATP showed primary-active, ATP-dependent uptake, corresponding to ATP-dependent export across the canalicular membrane into bile (12). Primary-active, ATP-dependent transport seems to be domain specific, with a location in the canalicular but not in the sinusoidal hepatocyte membrane (Fig. 2). This is indicated by transport studies in vesicle preparations from different membrane domains (12) and by photoaffinity labeling with the $^{35}$S-labeled ATP analogue ATP-γ-S of canalicular and sinusoidal membranes (21). Among the cysteinyl leukotrienes, $LTC_4$ is the best substrate for the canalicular export pump. Apparent $K_M$ values are 0.25, 1.5, and 5.2 $\mu M$ for $LTC_4$, $LTD_4$, and N-acetyl-$LTE_4$, respectively, whereas the $K_M$ value for the cysteine S-conjugate $LTE_4$ is more than 10 $\mu M$ (12). In addition, ω-carboxy-$LTB_4$, but not $LTB_4$ itself, is a substrate for ATP-dependent transport across the canalicular membrane. As indicated by the transport of $LTD_4$ and N-acetyl-$LTE_4$ via this ATP-dependent pump,

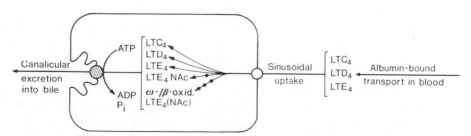

**FIG. 2.** Hepatobiliary cysteinyl leukotriene elimination. Transport across the hepatocyte is initiated by high-affinity uptake at the sinusoidal membrane that is not primary-active or directly ATP-dependent. Unidirectional export into bile, however, is mediated by an ATP-dependent export pump (12).

the glutathione moiety is not a structural requirement determining the substrate property, although it may be a property providing higher affinity for the active site of the pump. The pumps expressed in different tissues may be similar in substrate specificity but seem to be distinct, as evidenced by a hereditary deficiency of the leukotriene export pump in liver (11) and its simultaneous presence in erythrocyte membranes from mutant rats (22). The ATP-dependent leukotriene export carrier in the canalicular membrane was absent or inactive in a mutant strain of rats in which cysteinyl leukotriene excretion into bile is reduced to less than 2% of normal (11,12). These mutants are partially deficient in the hepatobiliary excretion of several other non-bile salt amphiphilic organic anions, such as bilirubin glucuronide and dibromosulfophthalein (23). Deficiency of the leukotriene export pump in the canalicular membrane is compensated by metabolic inactivation and degradation of the leukotrienes in the hepatocyte with a subsequent increase in renal excretion of leukotriene catabolites (1,11).

## ELIMINATION AND TRANSPORT IN VIVO

The pathways of elimination of leukotrienes in the intact organism were originally studied by autoradiographic (18) and invasive techniques, mostly by use of $^3$H-labeled leukotrienes (6,9,24). Using $N$-acetyl-LTE$_4$ as a representative tracer, half-lives in blood during the initial elimination period were 38 sec in the rat and 4 min in humans (2). The advantage of using $N$-acetyl-LTE$_4$, radioactively labeled in the $N$-acetylcysteine moiety, is the metabolic stability of the label as opposed to the extensive loss of tritium from leukotrienes labeled in the arachidonate-derived fatty acid moiety during β-oxidation from the ω-end (25). $N$-acetyl-LTE$_4$ is also an endogenous metabolite of LTC$_4$ in human urine (16,26) and in rodent bile (27). Moreover, $N$-acetyl-LTE$_4$ is eliminated and transported via the same routes and at comparable rates as the other cysteinyl leukotrienes LTC$_4$, LTD$_4$, and LTE$_4$. Within 1 hr, 80% of intravenously administered $N$-acetyl-LTE$_4$ is excreted in the rat with bile, either intact or after partial oxidative degradation from the ω-end of the fatty acid chain (25). At the same time, renal excretion in the rat amounts to about 2%.

Positron emission tomography using $^{11}$C-labeled, positron-emitting $N$-[$^{11}$C]acetyl-LTE$_4$ enables noninvasive analyses of elimination kinetics, organ distribution, and transport of this cysteinyl leukotriene (28). In rat, the initial distribution phase was characterized by a rapid disappearance of $^{11}$C radioactivity from the blood circulation. This was accompanied by an increase in the leukotriene concentration in liver reaching its maximum 4 min after intravenous injection. In the Cynomolgus monkey this maximum was reached after 12 min. Only negligible amounts of the leukotrienes were monitored in the urinary bladder of the rat within 50 min. Renal excretion was significant, however, in the monkey, which is in accordance with previous invasive tracer studies in this species (13). In the mutant rat strain with the hereditary defect of hepatobiliary transport of cysteinyl leukotrienes across the hepatocyte canalicular membrane (11,12), elimination of leukotriene radioactivity from the blood circulation was retarded, the mean transit time or storage period in the liver was extended from 17 to 54 min, and leukotriene excretion into the intestines was below detectable levels. This impaired hepatobiliary elimination was compensated by transport of $\omega$-/$\beta$-oxidized metabolites from the liver back into blood, with subsequent renal excretion. This was monitored by the sharp rise of [11]C radioactivity in the urinary bladder of the mutant rats. A similar shift from hepatobiliary to renal cysteinyl leukotriene elimination was observed in rats with extrahepatic cholestasis. Leukotrienes labeled with a short-lived, positron-emitting radioisotope thus provide quantitative insight into the pathways of their elimination and transport in vivo and into the relative contribution of liver and kidney to these processes under normal and pathophysiologic conditions.

## METABOLIC DEACTIVATION AND INACTIVATION OF LEUKOTRIENES

Enzyme-catalyzed chemical modification of the leukotrienes determines their biologic activity. Modification of the cysteinylglycine moiety of $LTD_4$ and $\omega$-oxidation followed by $\beta$-oxidation of $LTE_4$, $N$-acetyl-$LTE_4$, and $LTB_4$ result in deactivation and inactivation of these leukotrienes (29,30). Inactivation of potent mediators is equally important as their biosynthesis, because the relative rates of synthesis and inactivation determine the concentration of the biologically active leukotrienes. The liver converts $LTE_4$ and $N$-acetyl-$LTE_4$ to the respective $\omega$-hydroxy and $\omega$-carboxy metabolites (31,32). Further degradation by $\beta$-oxidation from the $\omega$-end yields $\omega$-carboxy-dinor, -tetranor, and -hexanor derivatives of $LTE_4$ and $N$-acetyl-$LTE_4$ (16,25,32,33). All these $\omega$-carboxy derivatives of $LTE_4$ and $N$-acetyl-$LTE_4$ are biologically inactive (30). The increased degradation of leukotrienes in the $\beta$-oxidation pathway after treatment of rats with clofibrate, an inducer of peroxisome proliferation, suggested that $\beta$-oxidation of leukotrienes may be localized in peroxisomes (1,25).

Direct evidence for an exclusive degradation of cysteinyl leukotrienes in peroxisomes has been obtained by use of isolated liver peroxisomes and direct photoaffinity labeling of the peroxisomal enzymes of $\beta$-oxidation with $\omega$-carboxy-$N$-[3H]acetyl-$LTE_4$ (25). In addition, isolated peroxisomes catalyze the $\beta$-oxidation from the $\omega$-end of $\omega$-carboxy-$LTB_4$, yielding the dinor and the tetranor catabolites (25). In vitro experiments indicate that the degradation of $LTB_4$ can also proceed in liver mitochondria, as indicated in Fig. 3. It is unlikely, however, that the mitochondrial $\beta$-oxidation of $\omega$-carboxy-

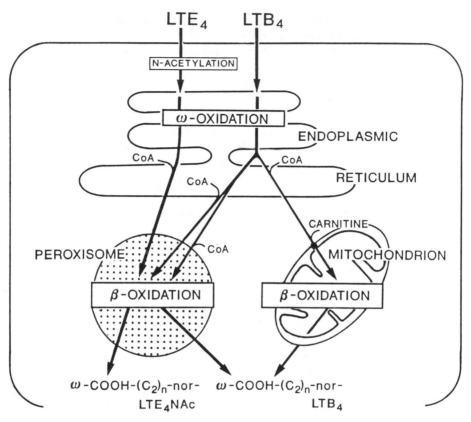

**FIG. 3.** Compartmentation of inactivation and degradation of $LTE_4$ and $LTB_4$ in the hepatocyte. Products of peroxisomal β-oxidation may be dinor, tetranor, or hexanor metabolites of $LTE_4$, *N*-acetyl-$LTE_4$, or $LTB_4$ [designated ω-COOH-$(C_2)_n$-nor-leukotriene). (From ref. 25 with permission.)

$LTB_4$ plays a major role in the intact organism, because $LTB_4$ degradation is severely impaired in patients with Zellweger syndrome, a disorder of peroxisome biogenesis (34). In this inherited disease, the defect of peroxisomal leukotriene degradation results in increased levels of the biologically active, proinflammatory mediators $LTE_4$ and $LTB_4$. In addition, the concentrations in urine of ω-carboxy-$LTE_4$ and ω-carboxy-$LTB_4$, which are the immediate substrates for peroxisomal β-oxidation, are greatly increased (34). These findings in humans with peroxisome deficiency underscore the essential role of peroxisomes in the catabolism of leukotrienes.

**Note added in proof:** Our recent work has demonstrated that ATP-dependent membrane transport of $LTC_4$ is mediated by the 190-kDa multidrug resistance-associated protein (MRP) (see ref. 35).

## REFERENCES

1. Keppler D, Huber M, Baumert T, Guhlmann A. *Adv Enzyme Regul* 1989;28:307–19.
2. Keppler D, Müller M, Klünemann C, et al. *Adv Enzyme Regul* 1992;32:107–16.
3. Lam BK, Owen WF Jr, Austen KF, Soberman RJ. *J Biol Chem* 1989;264:12885–9.
4. Lam BK, Gagnon L, Austen KF, Soberman RJ. *J Biol Chem* 1990;265:13438–41.
5. Schaub T, Ishikawa T, Keppler D. *FEBS Lett* 1991;279:83–6.
6. Hammarström S, Örning L, Bernström K. *Mol Cell Biochem* 1985;69:7–16.
7. Uehara N, Ormstad K, Örning L, Hammarström S. *Biochim Biophys Acta* 1983;732:69–74.
8. Keppler D, Hagmann W, Rapp S, Denzlinger C, Koch HK. *Hepatology* 1985;5:883–91.
9. Hagmann W, Korte M. *Biochem J* 1990;267:467–70.
10. Leier I, Müller M, Jedlitschky G, Keppler D. *Eur J Biochem* 1992;209:281–9.
11. Huber M, Guhlmann A, Jansen PLM, Keppler D. *Hepatology* 1987;7:224–8.
12. Ishikawa T, Müller M, Klünemann C, Schaub T, Keppler D. *J Biol Chem* 1990;265:19279–86.
13. Denzlinger C, Guhlmann A, Scheuber PJ, Wilker D, Hammer DK, Keppler D. *J Biol Chem* 1986;261:15601–6.
14. Keppler D, Huber M, Hagmann W, Ball HA, Guhlmann A, Kästner S. *Ann NY Acad Sci* 1988;524:68–74.
15. Maltby NH, Taylor GW, Ritter JM, Moore K, Fuller RW, Dollery CT. *J Allergy Clin Immunol* 1990;85:3–9.
16. Sala A, Voelkel N, Maclouf J, Murphy RC. *J Biol Chem* 1990;265:21771–8.
17. Kondo T, Dale GL, Beutler E. *Proc Natl Acad Sci USA* 1980;77:6359–62.
18. Appelgren LE, Hammarström S. *J Biol Chem* 1982;257:531–5.
19. Denzlinger C, Rapp S, Hagmann W, Keppler D. *Science* 1985;230:330–2.
20. Falk E, Müller M, Huber M, Keppler D, Kurz G. *Eur J Biochem* 1989;186:741–7.
21. Müller M, Ishikawa T, Berger U, et al. *J Biol Chem* 1991;266:18920–6.
22. Board P, Nishida T, Gatmaitan Z, Che M, Arias IM. *Hepatology* 1992;15:722–5.
23. Jansen PLM, Peters WH, Lamers WH. *Hepatology* 1985;5:573–9.
24. Hagmann W, Denzlinger C, Keppler D. *Circ Shock* 1984;14:223–5.
25. Jedlitschky G, Huber M, Völkl A, et al. *J Biol Chem* 1991;266:24763–72.
26. Huber M, Kästner S, Schölmerich J, Gerok W, Keppler D. *Eur J Clin Invest* 1991;19:53–60.
27. Hagmann W, Denzlinger C, Rapp S, Weckbecker G, Keppler D. *Prostaglandins* 1986;31:239–51.
28. Keppler D, Guhlmann A, Oberdorfer F, et al. *Ann NY Acad Sci* 1991;629:100–4.
29. Lewis RA, Drazen JM, Austen KF, et al. *Proc Natl Acad Sci USA* 1981;78:4579–83.
30. Samhoun MN, Conroy DM, Piper PJ. *Br J Pharmacol* 1989;98:1406–12.
31. Örning L. *Eur J Biochem* 1987;170:77–85.
32. Stene DO, Murphy RC. *J Biol Chem* 1988;263:2773–8.
33. Huber M, Müller J, Leier I, et al. *Eur J Biochem* 1990;194:309–15.
34. Mayatepek E, Lehmann W-D, Fauler J, et al. *J Clin Invest* 1993;91:881–8.
35. Jedlitschky G, Leier L, Buchholz U, Center M, Keppler D. *Cancer Res* 1994;54:4833–6.

*Advances in Prostaglandin, Thromboxane,*
*and Leukotriene Research,* Vol. 22, edited by
S.-E. Dahlén et al. Raven Press, Ltd., New York © 1994

# Microvascular Mechanisms in Inflammation

## Per Hedqvist, Lennart Lindbom, Ulla Palmertz, and Johan Raud

*Department of Physiology and Pharmacology, and Institute of Environmental Medicine, Karolinska Institutet, S-171 76 Stockholm, Sweden*

Acute inflammatory reactions are characterized by a series of vascular events, including changes in arteriolar caliber, increased vascular permeability, and accumulation of leukocytes. These events are triggered by inflammatory stimuli and are mediated by agents generated in tissue fluid or released from tissue cells either as preformed packages or as the result of de novo synthesis.

Among the many mediators of inflammatory processes that have been proposed over the years, the leukotrienes deserve special attention. These agents have a well-documented capacity, even in minute concentrations, to provoke two cardinal signs of inflammation: tissue edema and recruitment of phagocytizing cells. In addition, they have an almost ubiquitous distribution in the body, as they can be formed by blood-borne and tissue-residing cells of the white blood cell series. Moreover, there is considerable experimental evidence that leukotrienes are significant mediators in bronchial asthma, and circumstantial evidence for a mediator role can be presented for still other diseases of inflammatory origin.

This chapter summarizes recent work on microvascular actions and interactions of some eicosanoids and other autacoids with potential to mediate or modulate significant events in acute inflammation. Principally, the results are based on intravital microscopy of the terminal vascular bed of the hamster cheek pouch, which has been adopted for in vivo quantitation of mediator release and dynamic microvascular changes during immunologically induced mast-cell–dependent inflammation (1).

## MICROVASCULAR ACTIONS OF LEUKOTRIENES

Valuable contributions to the understanding of microvascular mechanisms behind leukotriene-induced inflammation have been made with intravital microscopy. Thus, the cysteinyl leukotrienes ($LTC_4$, $LTD_4$, $LTE_4$) elicit a dose-dependent extravasation of plasma in the hamster cheek pouch with a potency exceeding that of histamine by approximately 1,000-fold (2). The permeability increase is localized to postcapillary venules (2), and electron microscopy of tissues exposed to cysteinyl leukotrienes has shown that markers for plasma proteins leak out via gaps between apparently contracted endothelial cells (3,4). On the other hand, local administration of leukotriene $B_4$ (LTB$_4$) to the hamster cheek pouch or rabbit tenuissimus muscle causes leukocytes to adhere to the endothelium of venules of all sizes and subsequently to emigrate to the perivascular interstitium (5–8). This process is accompanied by plasma leakage which is entirely dependent on the presence and/or intact adhesive function of leukocytes (5,9).

## LEUKOTRIENES AS INFLAMMATORY MEDIATORS

The cheek pouch model has also been used to study the potential of leukotrienes as mediators of microvascular changes associated with acute allergic inflammation.

Hamsters are sometimes said to be resistant to allergic reactions. However, recent intravital microscopic studies in the hamster cheek pouch have clearly documented that immunized hamsters respond vigorously to local antigen challenge. Therefore, after immunization with either milligram doses of ovalbumin (OA) in Freund's adjuvant (FA) or microgram amounts of OA mixed with Al(OH)$_3$, topical challenge with OA in the hamster cheek pouch leads to a sequence of acute microvascular inflammatory events characterized by a brief phase of arteriolar constriction, followed by extensive postcapillary extravasation of plasma and arteriolar dilatation. With a slower onset, the antigen challenge is also accompanied by an increase in venular leukocyte adherence and subsequently emigration of leukocytes (10,11). Both types of allergic reactions involve mast cell activation and histamine release (10,11). However, mechanistically they are different, because OA challenge using the FA method leads to an immune complex-dependent response, whereas immunization with low doses of OA and Al(OH)$_3$ results in an immediate-type allergic reaction. Therefore, hamsters immunized with FA have increased serum levels of antigen-specific IgG, and FITC-labeled OA applied locally in the cheek pouch deposits specifically at the walls of postcapillary and small venules, a phenomenon typical of immune-complex reactions (12). By contrast, hamsters immunized with Al(OH)$_3$ showed no increase in serum IgG, and FITC-labeled OA deposited selectively on mast cells, indicating the presence of mast-cell–cytotropic antibodies, most likely of IgE type (1,11). The results presented below are based on the latter procedure unless otherwise stated.

That leukotrienes may play a role in allergic inflammation in the cheek pouch was first indicated in studies showing that an early generation of

5-lipoxygenase inhibitors (BW-755C, L-651,392) slightly reduced antigen-induced plasma leakage in animals immunized for either immune-complex reactions (13) or immediate-type allergic inflammation (1). More recently, using drugs that selectively interfere with the action of cysteinyl leukotrienes (ICI 198,615, SK&F 104 353) (14,15) or the biosynthesis of leukotrienes (MK-886, BAY X1005) (16,17) we have readdressed this question using immediate-type sensitized animals that were pretreated with an antihistamine inhibitor and a prostaglandin synthesis inhibitor to provide an experimental situation for histamine-independent microvascular anaphylaxis dissociated from the modulating influence of cyclooxygenase products (18,19). Based on the following lines of evidence, the results strongly indicate an important role for leukotrienes as mediators of microvascular inflammatory changes during type I reactions in the hamster cheek pouch. First, the mi-

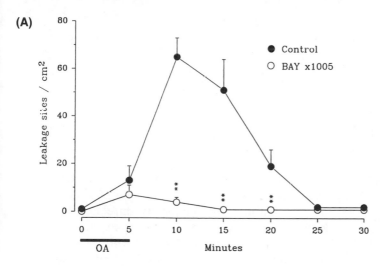

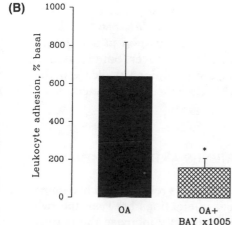

**FIG. 1.** Challenge of the hamster cheek pouch with specific antigen [ovalbumin (OA) 10 $\mu$g/ml topically for 5 min] provokes plasma leakage **(A)** and leukocyte adhesion **(B)** (filled symbols and column) which are substantially reduced after inhibition of leukotriene biosynthesis with BAY X1005 (1 mg/kg i.v. and 1 $\mu M$ topically to the pouch) (open symbols and cross-hatched column). Mean values ± SEM; $n$ = 7 or 8. *$p<0.05$; **$p<0.01$.

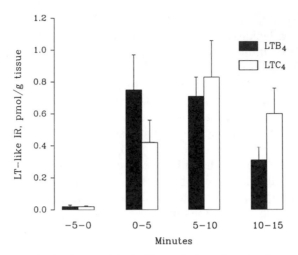

**FIG. 2.** Antigen-provoked release of leukotrienes in hamster cheek pouch in vivo. The buffer surrounding the pouch was collected at 5-min intervals before, during, and after challenge (OA 10 $\mu$g/ml topically at 0 to 5 min) and analyzed for immunoreactive $LTC_4$ and $LTB_4$ using an enzyme immunoassay kit (Cayman Chemical Co., Ann Arbor, MI, U.S.A.). Mean values $\pm$ SEM of duplicate determinations from 10 experiments.

crovascular inflammatory response to antigen challenge in cheek pouches pretreated to abolish the effects of histamine and prostaglandins is fully mimicked by the combined action of low nanomolar concentrations of $LTB_4$ and cysteinyl leukotrienes, i.e., arteriolar constriction followed by plasma extravasation and leukocyte accumulation. Second, these components of the antigen reaction were profoundly inhibited by chemically unrelated drugs that either selectively block the action of cysteinyl leukotrienes at the receptor level (ICI 198,615, SK&F 104 353), or interfere with production of both $LTB_4$ and the cysteinyl leukotrienes (MK-886, BAY X1005). Therefore, ICI 198,615 and SK&F 104 353 virtually abolished the arteriolar constriction and plasma leakage induced by antigen, and MK-886 and BAY X1005 reduced the antigen-induced leukocyte accumulation in addition to suppressing the leakage of plasma (18,19) (Fig. 1). Moreover, both $LTB_4$ and $LTC_4$ were released, albeit in small amounts, during antigen challenge in the cheek pouch, and this release was suppressed below the level of detection by MK-886 and BAY X1005 (Fig. 2).

## SYNERGISM BETWEEN LEUKOTRIENES AND HISTAMINE

In acute allergic inflammation, activated mast cells release both histamine and $LTC_4$, thus making possible subsequent interactions between the two mediators. At the microvascular level they uniformly increase the permeability for plasma by causing endothelial cell contraction and formation of gaps between adjacent cells in postcapillary venules (8,20,21). Like other vasodilators, e.g., prostaglandins $E_2$ and $I_2$ (PGE$_2$, PGI$_2$), nitroprusside, and forskolin, histamine is expected to potentiate LTC$_4$-induced extravasation of plasma as a direct consequence of increased blood flow and hydrostatic pressure in the venules (1,22). However, recent observations indicate that histamine and LTC$_4$ can act synergistically to greatly increase vascular permeability by a mechanism that is independent of changes in arteriolar tone and blood flow (23). Thus, concentrations of histamine (0.3 1 $\mu M$) and LTC$_4$ (10 to 100 p$M$) that per se caused only minimal increases in venule permeability when applied individually (10 min of topical application) strikingly enhanced vascular permeability when co-administered (Fig. 3). Moreover, the H$_1$-receptor antagonist chlorpheniramine (3 $\mu M$ topically) abolished the plasma extravasation of combined challenge with histamine and LTC$_4$. In contrast to histamine, the vasodilator PGE$_2$ (3 n$M$), which caused an increase in blood flow very similar to that caused by histamine, failed to enhance the vascular permeability response to LTC$_4$.

These results imply that threshold concentrations of histamine and LTC$_4$ together evoke considerable endothelial cell contraction and gap formation by a mechanism that requires intact H$_1$ receptors. Furthermore, the concentrations of histamine and LTC$_4$ used to document the striking synergism are of the same order of magnitude as those recovered from the interstitial fluid of the cheek pouch after antigen challenge. Consequently, the results add further weight to the consideration that leukotrienes and histamine are major mediators of acute allergic inflammation.

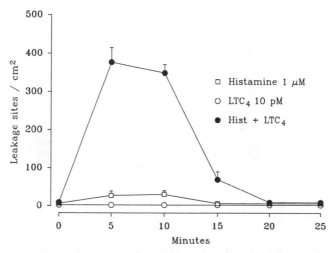

**FIG. 3.** Plasma leakage provoked by 10-min topical challenge with LTC$_4$ (10 p$M$, O—O) or histamine (1 $\mu M$ □—□) alone and in combination (●—●). Mean values ± SEM; $n = 7$.

## VASODILATORS AS MODULATORS OF INFLAMMATION

Since the discovery that aspirin and other nonsteroidal anti-inflammatory drugs (NSAIDs) inhibit prostaglandin biosynthesis (24), interest has been focused on the actions and roles of arachidonic acid derivatives in microvascular control and in inflammation. In particular the vasodilating $PGE_2$ and $PGI_2$ have been in focus, and it is generally believed that these eicosanoids are proinflammatory mainly because they induce arteriolar dilatation and increased blood flow (22).

During the initial pharmacologic characterization of immediate-type allergic inflammation in the cheek pouch, we found that indomethacin treatment caused a marked and reproducible potentiation of the antigen response, despite reducing the vasodilatation (25) (Fig. 4). Likewise, indomethacin and another potent NSAID, diclofenac, potentiated the inflammatory effects of the mast cell secretagogue compound 48/80 (26). By measuring the in vivo release of histamine to the buffer surrounding the cheek pouch, we found that both indomethacin and diclofenac enhanced the histamine release evoked by mast cell activation (Fig. 4).

When the hamster cheek pouch was challenged with antigen and both $PGE_2$ (30 n$M$) and indomethacin (or diclofenac) were present in the superfusion buffer, the NSAID-induced potentiation of plasma leakage and leukocyte accumulation was prevented, despite a marked increase in arteriolar diameter and blood flow (25,26) (Fig. 4). Moreover, a similar inhibitory effect on the antigen reaction was exerted by $PGI_2$ (27). By contrast, both $PGE_2$ and $PGI_2$ potentiated the effects of different individual inflammatory mediators, including the plasma leakage induced by topical histamine or

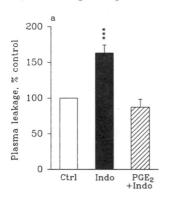 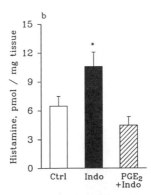

**FIG. 4.** Plasma leakage **(a)** and histamine release **(b)** after challenge with specific antigen (ovalbumin 10 µg/ml topically for 5 min) in cheek pouches of hamsters sensitized to give rise to mast cell cytotropic antibodies and immediate-type allergic reaction. Figures show control responses to antigen alone (open bars), effect of indomethacin treatment (5 mg/kg i.v. and 6 µ$M$ topically) (filled bars), and reversal of indomethacin effect by $PGE_2$ (30 n$M$ topically) (hatched bars). Mean values ± SEM; $n$ = 5 to 7. *$p<0.05$, ***$p<0.001$ versus antigen alone.

$LTC_4$, as well as the leukocyte emigration and associated plasma extravasation in response to local challenge with $LTB_4$ (25,27). Therefore, although being in agreement with the concept of synergism between vasodilating compounds and permeability-increasing mediators, these findings indicate that $PGE_2$ and $PGI_2$ inhibited the mast-cell–dependent reactions at the level of mediator release and not by reducing mediator target action. Accordingly, further experiments showed that $PGE_2$ (30 n$M$ topically) completely reversed the enhanced histamine release both in indomethacin-treated hamsters challenged with antigen (25) and in diclofenac-treated animals challenged with compound 48/80 (26).

It seems clear from what has been presented here that vasodilating prostaglandins can operate via two distinct and independent mechanisms to strengthen or suppress inflammation in vivo. The balance between pro- and anti-inflammatory prostaglandin effect, i.e., enhancement of mediator target action and inhibition of mediator release, is likely to depend on local conditions and circumstances such as basal blood flow and the site of prostaglandin production (or route of administration). Such variability may help to explain why NSAIDs and prostaglandins have been reported to enhance, suppress, or be without effect on different types of inflammatory reactions.

In this context it should be noted that there are exceptions to the rule that vasodilators enhance the target action of inflammatory mediators. One example is lipoxin $A_4$ ($LXA_4$), representative of a group of arachidonic acid derivatives whose biosynthesis involves interaction between different lipoxygenases that are abundant in mammalian tissues (28). In the cheek pouch, $LXA_4$ elicits vasodilatation and increased blood flow without changing vascular permeability or leukocyte behavior (29,30). However, $LXA_4$ was found to competitively inhibit $LTB_4$-induced extravasation of plasma and diapedesis of leukocytes. Similar observations were made with $LXB_4$ and the lipoxin precursor 15-HETE. Because plasma leakage provoked by $LTB_4$ occurs secondary to accumulation and diapedesis of leukocytes and because the two effects were inhibited in parallel, it is likely that lipoxins interfere with mechanisms for leukocyte-dependent alteration of microvascular permeability.

Another example is given by calcitonin gene-related peptide (CGRP), an exceedingly potent vasodilator which is assumed to mediate neurogenic inflammation together with substance P (SP) (31). CGRP has been reported to enhance tissue edema evoked by SP and several other inflammatory mediators (32,33). However, others have found no synergism (34–36), and a recent report instead indicates antagonism (37). Therefore, in spite of causing marked vasodilatation, CGRP inhibited edema-promoting actions in vivo of the inflammatory mediators histamine, $LTB_4$, and 5HT in human skin, hamster cheek pouch, and rat paw (Fig. 5). Similar findings were made with sensory nerve activation and release of endogenous CGRP, indicating that sensory nerves may play an anti-inflammatory role.

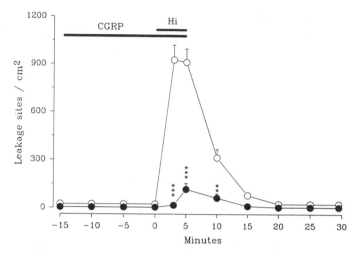

**FIG. 5.** Plasma leakage provoked by histamine (10 μ*M* topically, 0 to 5 min) (open symbols), and histamine in the presence of CGRP (10 n*M*, −15 to 5 min) (filled symbols) in hamster cheek pouch. Mean values ± SEM; *n* = 8. \*\**p*<0.01; \*\*\**p*<0.001, Student's *t* test.

## CONCLUSIONS

It is well established that eicosanoids are deeply involved in the control of microvascular functions. With regard to mast-cell–dependent allergic inflammation, as seen in the hamster, leukotrienes account for virtually all extravasation of plasma that is not due to liberated histamine. The dramatic synergism between histamine and $LTC_4$ can be regarded as a substrate-saving amplifier of inflammation, but it also offers a most effective tool for its control. Furthermore, the leukotriene family is responsible for the early vasoconstriction, and in the guise of $LTB_4$ it accounts for at least part of leukocyte recruitment. In addition, the vasodilating prostaglandins contribute to the dynamics of inflammation. However, as distinct from the leukotrienes, they function primarily as modulators of inflammation with the capacity to cause both up- and downregulation. Similarly, agents such as lipoxins and CGRP, which because of their vasodilating properties can enhance the target action of liberated mediators, may also act to restrain specific events in the inflammatory process.

## ACKNOWLEDGMENT

The authors are supported by the Swedish Medical Research Council (14X-4342, O4P-8865), the Swedish Society for Medical Research, the Institute of Environmental Medicine, the Knut and Alice Wallenberg Foundation, the L. Hierta Foundation, and the Karolinska Institutet.

# REFERENCES

1. Raud J. *Acta Physiol Scand* 1989;135(suppl 578):1–58.
2. Dahlén S-E, Björk J, Hedqvist P, et al. *Proc Natl Acad Sci USA* 1981;78:3887–91.
3. Hedqvist P, Thureson-Klein Å, Öhlén A, Raud J, Lindbom L, Dahlén S-E. In: Nobin A, Owman C, Arneklo-Nobin B, eds. *Neuronal messengers in vascular function.* Amsterdam: Elsevier; 1987:435–6.
4. Joris I, Majno G, Corey EJ, Lewis RA. *Am J Pathol* 1987;126:19–24.
5. Björk J, Hedqvist P, Arfors K-E. *Inflammation* 1982;6:189–200.
6. Lindbom L, Hedqvist P, Dahlén S-E, Lindgren J-A, Arfors K-E. *Acta Physiol Scand* 1982a; 116:105–8.
7. Thureson-Klein Å, Hedqvist P, Lindbom L. *Tissue Cell* 1986;18:1–12.
8. Thureson-Klein Å, Hedqvist P, Öhlén A, Raud J, Lindbom L. *Pathol Immunopathol Res* 1987;6:190–206.
9. Arfors K-E, Lundberg C, Lindbom L, Lundberg K, Beatty PG, Harlan JM. *Blood* 1987; 69:338–40.
10. Björk J, Smedegård G. *Int Arch Allergy Appl Immunol* 1984;74:178–85.
11. Raud J, Dahlén S-E, Smedegård G, Hedqvist P. *Acta Physiol Scand* 1989a;135:95–105.
12. Crawford JP, Movat HZ, Minta JO, Opas M. *Exp Mol Pathol* 1985;42:175–93.
13. Björk J, Smedegård G. *Inflammation* 1987;11:47–58.
14. Hay DWP, Muccitelli RM, Tucker AA, et al. *J Pharmacol Exp Ther* 1987;243:474–81.
15. Snyder DW, Giles RE, Keith RA, Yee YK, Krell RD. *J Pharmacol Exp Ther* 1987;243: 548–56.
16. Ford-Hutchinson AW. In: Samuelsson B, Dahlén S-E, Fritsch J, Hedqvist P, eds. *Advances in prostaglandin, thromboxane, and leukotrine research*, Vol. 20. New York; 1990:161–9.
17. Hatzelman A, Fruchtmann R, Mohs KH, et al. In: Dahlén S-E, Hedqvist P, Samuelsson B, Taylor WA, Fritsch J, eds. *Advances in prostaglandin, thromboxane, and leukotriene research*, Vol. 22. New York: Raven Press; 1993:23–31 (this volume).
18. Hedqvist P, Raud J, Dahlén S-E. In: Samuelsson B, Dahlén S-E, Fritsch J, Hedqvist P, eds. *Advances in prostaglandin, thromboxane, and leukotriene research*, Vol. 20. New York: Raven Press; 1990:153–60.
19. Hedqvist P, Raud J, Palmertz P, Kumlin M, Dahlén S-E. In: Samuelsson B, Ramwell PW, Paoletti R, Folco G, Granström E, eds. *Advances in prostaglandin, thromboxane, and leukotriene research*, Vol. 21. New York: Raven Press 1990:537–43.
20. Majno G, Palade GE. *J Biophys Biochem Cytol* 1961;11:571–605.
21. Clough G. *Prog Biophys Mol Biol* 1991;55:47–69.
22. Williams TJ. *Br Med Bull* 1983;39:239–42.
23. Raud J, Lindbom L, Hedqvist P. *Acta Physiol Scand* 1992;146:545–6.
24. Vane JR. *Nature* 1971;231:232–5.
25. Raud J, Dahlén S-E, Sydbom A, Lindbom L, Hedqvist P. *Proc Natl Acad Sci USA* 1988; 85:2315–9.
26. Raud J, Sydbom A, Dahlén S-E, Hedqvist P. *Agents Actions* 1989b;28:108–4.
27. Raud J. *Br J Pharmacol* 1990;99:449–54.
28. Serhan CN, Samuelsson B. *Adv Exp Med Biol* 1988;229:1–14.
29. Hedqvist P, Raud J, Palmertz U, Haeggström J, Nicolaou KC, Dahlén S-E. *Acta Physiol Scand* 1989;137:571–2.
30. Raud J, Palmertz U, Dahlén S-E, Hedqvist P. *Adv Exp Med Biol* 1991;354:185–92.
31. Holzer P. *Neuroscience* 1988;24:739–68.
32. Brain SD, Williams TJ, Tippins JR, Morris HR, MacIntyre I. *Nature* 1985;313:54–6.
33. Buckley TL, Brain SD, Rampart M, Williams TJ. *Br J Pharmacol* 1991;103:1515–9.
34. Barnes PJ, Brown MJ, Dollery CT, Fuller RW, Heavey DJ, Ind PW. *Br J Pharmacol* 1986;88:741–5.
35. Gamse R, Posch M, Saria A, Jancsó G. *Acta Physiol Hung* 1987;69:343–54.
36. Alving K, Matran R, Lundberg JM. *Naunyn Schmiedebergs Arch Pharmacol* 1991;343:37–45.
37. Raud J, Lundeberg T, Brodda-Jansen G, Theodorsson E, Hedqvist P. *Biochem Biophys Res Commun* 1991b;180:1429–35.

*Advances in Prostaglandin, Thromboxane, and Leukotriene Research*, Vol. 22, edited by S.-E. Dahlén et al. Raven Press, Ltd., New York © 1994

# Prostaglandin E₂ Regulation of the Immune Response

Rachel L. Roper and *Richard P. Phipps

*National Institute of Allergy and Infectious Disease, National Institutes of Health, Bethesda, Maryland 20892; and *Medical Center, University of Rochester, School of Medicine, Rochester, New York 14642*

Study of prostaglandins of the E series (PGE) has shown that these arachidonic acid metabolites profoundly affect the cells of the immune system: accessory cells such as macrophages that present antigens to the immune system, B lymphocytes that synthesize protective antibodies (humoral response), and T lymphocytes that kill tumor cells or virally infected cells (cell-mediated response) and provide help to B cells for immunoglobulin production. The interplay among these three key cell types provides the host with protection against a plethora of environmental and internal insults. In health, the regulation of these interactions allows efficacious responses to foreign invaders and avoids or curtails inappropriate (e.g., autoimmune) reactions. A wealth of literature supports the hypothesis that the type and physiologic state of the cell that presents an antigen to the system determines the substance and subtleties of the ensuing immune response. Our laboratory has explored the regulatory role of antigen-presenting cells with emphasis on the arachidonic acid metabolites (e.g., prostaglandins) secreted by accessory cells. This review first presents a brief history of the suppressive effects of PGE, followed by a discussion of the more recent advances in understanding PGE regulation of the immune response. In particular, we focus on the ability of PGE to *enhance* B-cell immunoglobulin class switching to IgE, IgG₁, and IgG₂ₐ and on the importance of the second-messenger cAMP and PGE-inducible regulatory proteins (PIRP).

## BACKGROUND: PGE CAN BE IMMUNOSUPPRESSIVE

### PGE Inhibits B-Lymphocyte Functions

In the study of accessory cell regulation of immunity, it was noted that certain accessory cells presented an immunogenic moiety in a manner that enhanced immunity, whereas other cell types presented the same protein in a manner that resulted in specific hyporesponsiveness or tolerance. A break-through in understanding this difference came with the discovery that PGE-secreting antigen-presenting cells decreased the antibody response in vivo and in vitro, whereas non–PGE-secreting cells induced augmented immunity (1–5). Purified PGE has been found to be immunosuppressive in many tissue culture and animal models.

In a model in which deaggregated human immunoglobulin was used to specifically tolerize mice (induce a deficient IgM response), inhibition of PG production by indomethacin or aspirin blocked the induction of unresponsiveness (6). In the presence of PG synthesis inhibitors, hyporesponsiveness could be restored by the administration of $PGE_2$, demonstrating the importance of PGE in mechanisms of tolerance in vivo. In another system, antigen-pulsed accessory cells injected into mice delivered an enhancing or suppressive effect depending on whether they produced $PGE_2$ (3). PGE-secreting accessory cells depressed the antibody response in an MHC-restricted, antigen-specific manner, and non–PGE-secreting cells enhanced immunoglobulin synthesis measured in the direct IgM plaque assay. $PGE_2$ delivered via the anus resulted in an increase in blood PGE-derivative levels and induced hyporesponsiveness (7,8). This may be of particular importance in the transmission of HIV, because $PGE_2$ concentrations in human semen are extremely high ($10^{-4}$ $M$). Furthermore, $PGE_2$ allows greater HTLV-III replication in tissue culture (9).

Many of the effects of PGE on the immune response have been dissected in vitro. PGE interferes with the humoral immune response by directly inhibiting IgM production (the first line of defense) by B lymphocytes under a variety of conditions (3–6,10–14). $PGE_2$ and $PGE_1$ significantly diminish IgM synthesized in response to polyclonal B cell activators (mitogens) such as bacterial lipopolysaccharide (LPS) and *Staphylococcus aureus* Cowan I strain, as well as to specific protein antigens (1,2,4,5,11,12,14). Macrophages pulsed with haptenated immunoglobulin induce hapten-specific B-cell unresponsiveness in a PGE-dependent manner. PGE can synergize with immune complexes or other model tolerogens (4,5,11,13) to reduce B-cell IgM synthesis. PGE also possesses mild antiproliferative effects on B cells in murine and human systems (12,14), and inhibits B-cell activation events, including class II MHC upregulation, enlargement, and induction of the low-affinity IgE receptor, FcεRII/CD23 (15–17). Because most experiments employ heterogeneous B lymphocytes purified from, e.g., spleen and tonsil, PGE effects on homogeneous populations of B lymphoma cells, which are believed to mimic developmental B-cell stages, have also been studied. PGE can itself inhibit lymphoma proliferation, or it can synergize with anti-immunoglobulin to block proliferation and can even induce programmed cell death, or apoptosis, in certain lymphomas (18,19). The phenotype of these lymphomas suggests that "immature" B cells are more sensitive to the inhibitory actions of PGE. The immunomodulatory characteristics of PGE are contrasted with $PGF_{2\alpha}$, which has few reported effects on immune cells (12–14,18,19).

### PGE Inhibits T-Lymphocyte Responses

PGE inhibits the production of interleukin 2 (IL-2), the major autocrine growth factor of T cells, and reduces the activation-induced IL-2 receptor and transferrin receptor upregulation on T cells (20–22). In this way, PGE blunts the proliferation of T lymphocytes, a crucial step in the expansion of T-cell clones that respond to a specific stimulus. Recent evidence suggests that increases in PGE in humans (such as occur after thermal or mechanical trauma) are responsible for depressed T-cell responses in patients (23). PGE also inhibits the secretion of interferon-$\gamma$ (IFN-$\gamma$), a cytokine that has anti-viral activity and is important in activating T cells and macrophages, thus promoting the cellular immune response (24,25). In addition, PGE mitigates the ability of cytotoxic T lymphocytes and natural killer cells to kill their target cells (virally infected or tumor cells) (26,27). Furthermore, certain tumors elaborate PGE, and PGE may be involved in promoting metastasis (28).

### PGE Inhibits Accessory Cell Functions

Macrophages secrete PGE as the major product of arachidonic acid metabolism, but they are not refractory to its effects. For example, PGE inhibits class II MHC expression of macrophages (29). This has profound implications for the antigen-presenting capacity of these cells, because effective antigen presentation requires dense class II MHC expression (30). PGE also blunts IL-1 synthesis, another signal required for robust antigen presentation (31).

The experiments described here led researchers to believe that PGE inhibits all lymphocyte and antigen-presenting cell responses and to hypothesize that PGE was a crucial element in "horror autotoxicus," or the body's failure (in most situations) to attack itself, i.e., self-tolerance. Recent evidence, however, clearly demonstrates that PGE has both enhancing and suppressing activities.

## PGE CAN UPREGULATE ELEMENTS OF THE IMMUNE RESPONSE

### PGE Enhances Cytokine Synthesis

PGE regulates T cell and macrophage cytokine production, which controls cell-mediated responses and enhances and shapes the immunoglobulin production of B cells. $T_H1$ and $T_H2$ subsets of helper T cells have been described based on the production of lymphokines that either enhance a cell-mediated response (IL-2 and IFN-$\gamma$) or promote B-cell differentiation and immunoglobulin synthesis (IL-4 and IL-5) (32). Although PGE inhibits IL-2 and IFN-$\gamma$ production by $T_H1$ lymphocytes (20,21,25), $T_H2$ lymphokines are not inhibited and may even be enhanced by PGE. Synthesis of IL-4, the hallmark $T_H2$ lymphokine, is unaffected by PGE (5,24,33–35), and cAMP-inducing agents (such as PGE) increase IL-5 production (24,36). Because PGE inhibits IL-2 and IFN-$\gamma$ production and spares IL-4 and IL-5 synthesis, the presence of PGE would promote the humoral response and B-cell isotype differentiation (3,32). In addition, T cells stimulated with IL-2 and PGE dramatically upregulate their production of granulocyte/macrophage colony stimulating factor (20). This cytokine promotes phagocytosis and the development of macrophages from the bone marrow. PGE can also induce the synthesis by macrophages of tumor necrosis factor $\alpha$ (TNF$\alpha$), a cytokine that activates macrophages and can cause tumor regression in mice (37,38).

## PGE Promotes Immunoglobulin Class Switching

Our laboratory was the first to report that PGE can promote the production of certain immunoglobulin isotypes by B lymphocytes (12). $PGE_1$ and $PGE_2$, as well as other cAMP-inducing agents, enhanced the IgE and $IgG_1$ synthesis of B cells activated with IL-4 and LPS up to 26-fold, whereas $PGF_{2\alpha}$ had no effect on immunoglobulin production (5,10,12,15). This surprising finding was confirmed with a report of PGE promoting IgE synthesis in an antigen-specific system in the mouse and in the human (39,40), although there is also a mention of PGE inhibiting IgE synthesis in a complex tissue culture system (41). Inclusion of indomethacin in tissue culture to inhibit endogenous PGE production can reduce IgE synthesis by 60% (39). These data suggested that PGE may play a role in promoting allergy in vivo. In addition to enhancing the effects of IL-4, PGE synergized with IFN-$\gamma$ to increase $IgG_{2a}$ synthesis (13). PGE enhances immunoglobulin production in spite of a mild inhibitory effect of B-cell proliferation (12). Figure 1 summarizes the known immunoglobulin-enhancing effects of PGE. Therefore, PGE is not an obligate inhibitor but rather is a regulator, with impressive immune-enhancing capacity. Interestingly, PGE was found to diminish IgM synthesis and activation-induced responses (class II MHC upregulation, enlargement, and FcεRII/CD23 expression) in B cells stimulated under the same circumstances in which isotype switching was enhanced (15). Several lines of evidence also suggested that there was a PGE-resistant subset of B lymphocytes (10,15,18). Sorting experiments determined that PGE was inhibiting activation in the *same subset* of B cells that were enhanced by PGE for IgE and $IgG_1$ synthesis (15). These results suggest that PGE encourages certain

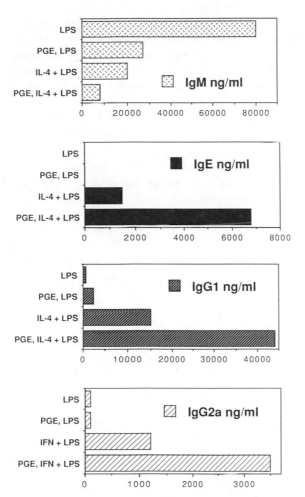

**FIG. 1.** PGE inhibits IgM synthesis but increases switching to IgE, IgG$_1$ and IgG$_{2a}$ in LPS-stimulated cells. PGE at $10^{-6}$ to $10^{-8}$ $M$ significantly inhibits IgM synthesis in response to LPS in the presence or absence of IL-4 (1,000 U/ml). PGE significantly enhances IgE production (20,000 U/ml IL-4 is shown), IgG$_1$ synthesis (100 U/ml IL-4 shown), and IgG$_{2a}$ synthesis (50 U/ml IFN-γ). Immunoglobulins were measured by specific ELISA (12,13).

lines of B-cell development (isotype differentiation) at the expense of other responses (activation, proliferation, and IgM synthesis).

Recent data indicate that PGE (and other cAMP-inducing agents) act by enhancing the molecular DNA rearrangement event of class switching to IgE and IgG$_1$ synthesis (10,42,43). First, ELISA spot data indicate that PGE significantly increases the frequency of B cells that undergo class switching to IgE and IgG$_1$. Although PGE increases the number of cells secreting IgE and IgG$_1$, it does not appear to increase the rate of synthesis. Second, PGE acts on surface IgM-positive cells, which are uncommitted B cells (44), to encourage differentiation to IgE and IgG$_1$ production. Third, by semiquantitative PCR, PGE synergizes with IL-4 and LPS to induce germline epsilon transcripts. Germline transcripts through the switch region precede class switching and are believed to be important for inducing the class-switching mechanism (45). Fourth, in the presence of PGE, mature epsilon mRNA transcripts are detectable earlier than with IL-4 and LPS alone, indicating that PGE not only induces germline transcripts, but also allows enhanced rearrangement of the heavy chain genes and ultimately the expression of IgE. Cholera toxin (which induces cAMP) has been shown to enhance switch differentiation to IgG$_1$, although the role of cAMP in this system is unclear (42). These results indicate that T-cell products are not the only important elements in inducing class switching in B lymphocytes.

## MECHANISM OF PGE ACTION: CYCLIC AMP AND INDUCTION OF PGE-INDUCIBLE REGULATORY PROTEINS

Many laboratories had shown that PGE actions could be mimicked by cAMP-elevating agents (12,20–22,24,37,38,46). Therefore, we determined whether pharmacologic agents that increase intracellular cAMP mimic the actions of PGE. Cholera toxin and dibutyryl cAMP inhibit B lymphocyte activation events (15), proliferation, and IgM synthesis, and enhance IgE and IgG$_1$ synthesis in a manner very similar to PGE (12). In addition, we showed that PGE$_2$ and PGE$_1$ induce a significant cAMP response in purified resting B cells, whereas PGF$_{2\alpha}$ and cholera toxin B-subunit (which are not immunomodulatory) do not (12,13). These data provided strong evidence that PGE signaling occurred through a cAMP-dependent pathway. Formal proof of this hypothesis was gained by the use of RpcAMP, a nonhydrolyzable cAMP analogue, which is a competitive inhibitor of cAMP-dependent protein kinase A (PKA). RpcAMP was able to totally block the action of PGE on B cell enlargement (Fig. 2) and class II MHC and FcεRII/CD23 upregulation, as well as promotion of IgG$_{2a}$ synthesis (13,46,47). Interestingly, antibodies binding to class II MHC also cause an increase in cAMP and can enhance class switching similar to PGE (46,48). Although RpcAMP inhibits the action of PKA and implicates PKA in PGE action, it remains possible that other cAMP-responsive proteins are responsible for PGE signaling. For example, protein kinase C, which is important in B and T lymphocyte activation, translocates to the nuclei of B cells that are treated with various cAMP-inducing agents, including PGE (48). It has been hypothesized that protein kinase C regulates transcription in this compartment.

Initially, we noted that a preincubation with cAMP or PGE (16 hrs) was required for maximal activity (inhibition of activation events and enhancement of IgE synthesis). On further investigation, we determined that PGE

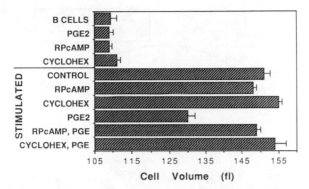

**FIG. 2.** PGE inhibition of activation-induced B-cell enlargement occurs through cAMP signaling pathways and requires protein synthesis. B cells were pretreated $\pm$ PGE$_2$ $10^{-6}$ $M$ in the absence or presence of cycloheximide (0.5 $\mu$g/ml) or RpcAMP (500 $\mu M$). PGE, RpcAMP, and cycloheximide do not affect the volume of resting B cells. However, PGE significantly inhibits enlargement and RpcAMP and cycloheximide block the effects of PGE, restoring B-cell enlargement. In experiments using cycloheximide, cells were washed with media three times before stimulation with IL-4 at 50 U/ml and LPS at 5 $\mu$g/ml. Cell volume was measured 24 hr after activation.

had maximal activity even if it was washed out of the culture after 1 hr, provided that the B cells had a period of incubation time after exposure to PGE before stimulation. This indicated that the signal from PGE to the B cell occurred rapidly (cAMP is increased within 10 minutes) but that the cell required time to change in response to PGE. To clarify the events occurring after PGE treatment that were responsible for the PGE-treated phenotype (lessened activation, increased isotype differentiation), we used cycloheximide to reversibly inhibit protein synthesis during the preincubation period (47). Inhibition of protein synthesis after PGE treatment, before stimulation, blocked the effect of PGE completely in both activation models (Fig. 2) and class switching. Therefore, protein synthesis is required for the action of PGE on B lymphocytes. Because protein synthesis is required both for inhibition of activation and for enhancement of IgE synthesis, we termed the responsible entities PGE-inducible regulatory protein(s), or PIRP. Two-dimensional gel analysis of $^{35}$S-labeled PGE-treated B lymphocytes showed consistent up-regulation of three putative PIRP (47). Figure 3 shows a diagram of PGE action in B cells. PGE is believed to bind a specific cell surface receptor (49). A PGE receptor has been characterized for macrophages, but lymphocyte PGE receptors are elusive and in a field where imagination dwarfs the available scientific data. The lymphocyte PGE receptor has not been cloned or characterized beyond Scatchard analysis (49,50).

## PROSTAGLANDIN SYNTHESIS

Many immunologic stimuli induce the synthesis of PGE by epithelial cells, follicular dendritic cells, fibroblasts, monocytes, and macrophages (3,51–

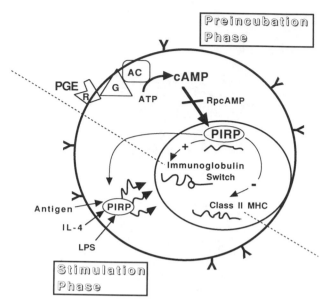

**FIG. 3.** Mechanism of PGE action in inhibiting B-lymphocyte activation and enhancing immunoglobulin class switching. During preincubation, PGE is believed to bind an uncharacterized cell surface receptor (R), activating a GTP binding protein (G), which in turn stimulates adenylate cyclase (AC) to catalyze the formation of cAMP (PGE second messenger). RpcAMP, a cAMP analogue that is a competitive inhibitor of protein kinase A (PKA), can block the action of PGE. PGE and other agents that increase cAMP induce the synthesis of PIRP (PGE-inducible regulatory proteins). Cycloheximide blocks the action of PGE, indicating that synthesis of PIRP is required for PGE regulation of B-cell function. During the stimulation phase, PIRP affects the response of B cells to antigen, interleukin 4 (IL-4), and/or the mitogen LPS (bacterial lipopolysaccharide), either altering stimulation signaling pathways or gene expression. PGE inhibits B-cell class II MHC upregulation and other activation events but enhances immunoglobulin class switching in the same subset of B cells.

54). Crosslinking of surface IgG, IgA, and IgE receptors, IL-1, TNFα, LPS, components of the complement cascade, and IL-6 all can induce PGE synthesis (51,53–57). Interestingly, macrophages secrete PGE, which can enhance granulocyte macrophage colony stimulating factor production, in turn increasing the production of macrophages from the bone marrow, a potential source of PGE synthesis (20). This is one example of several complex feedback loops of PGE synthesis. PGE can induce TNFα synthesis in macrophages, and TNFα upregulates PGE synthesis (37,38). IL-1 induces PGE synthesis, which feedback-inhibits IL-1 production, and PGE increases IL-1 receptor expression (57). PGE also increases $IgG_{2a}$ Fc receptor expression (58) on macrophages, and crosslinking of $IgG_{2a}$ Fc receptors promotes PGE synthesis. Almost certainly, regulatory loops and mechanisms of PGE production and regulation will be discovered.

## CLINICAL RELEVANCE: PGE AND TYPE I HYPERSENSITIVITY

PGE acts to inhibit B cell activation and enhance immunoglobulin isotype differentiation to IgE synthesis (the antibody class responsible for allergy). In human disease, it is interesting that increased PGE synthesis is linked to overproduction of IgE in vivo in several cases. Monocytes from patients with hyper-IgE syndrome constitutively secrete high levels of PGE (59). In another case, it was found that patients with Hodgkin's disease have approximately nine times the serum IgE levels of the normal population (60). Monocytes from patients with Hodgkin's disease produce fourfold the PGE of normal monocytes in 48 hr culture (61). This PGE production was found to be the source of the hyporesponsiveness of Hodgkin's lymphocytes to phytohemagglutinin. Moreover, in synovial fluid of patients with rheumatoid arthritis, PGE levels are elevated (62) and IgE is apparently produced by lymphocytes in the synovium (63). Synovial fluid and serum IgE levels are significantly elevated in the majority of patients with rheumatoid arthritis (63,64). Furthermore, high levels (400% of controls) of PGE are secreted by monocytes from trauma patients (23). Significantly, these patients mirror our in vitro system, developing elevated serum IgE and markedly depressed IgM levels (65). A similar scenario exists in a septic rat model and in septic patients: PGE secretion by monocytes and macrophages is increased, PGE levels in serum are elevated, and patients with sepsis have significantly increased IgE and lowered IgM levels in plasma (65,66). Parasites elicit an IgE response and parasitic worms secrete PGE (67). Finally, in a person sensitized to one allergen, cAMP-inducing agents released during each allergic episode (*e.g.*, PGE and histamine) (68) may feed back in to the system and promote B cell isotype switching to IgE, thus contributing to the allergic subject's tendency to rapidly become hypersensitive to a host of antigens. In conclusion, PGE is a powerful regulator of the immune response in vivo.

## ACKNOWLEDGMENT

This research was supported by grants CA42739, DE11390, CA55305, and CA11198 from the National Cancer Institute. R. Roper was supported by NIAID training grant T32AI07285. The authors thank M. Borello and M. Felch for helpful discussions concerning this manuscript.

## REFERENCES

1. Saito-Taki T, Nakano M. *J Immunol* 1983;130:2022–6.
2. Goldings EA. *J Immunol* 1986;136:817–22.
3. Phipps RP, Illig K, Schad V, Bhimani K. *J Leukocyte Biol* 1988;43:271–8.
4. Schad VC, Phipps RP. *J Immunol* 1989;143:2127–32.

5. Phipps RP, Roper RL, Stein SH. *Immunol Rev* 1990;117:135–58.
6. Scheuer WV, Hobbs MV, Weigle WO. *Cell Immunol* 1987;104:409–18.
7. Alexander NJ, Tarter TH, Fulgham DL, Ducsay CA, Novy MJ. *Am J Reprod Immunol Microbiol* 1987;15:47–51.
8. Kuno S, Ueno R, Hayaishi O. *Proc Natl Acad Sci USA* 1986;83:2682–3.
9. Kuno S, Ueno R, Hayaishi O, Nakashima H, Harada S, Yamamoto N. *Proc Natl Acad Sci USA* 1986;83:3487–90.
10. Phipps RP, Stein SH, Roper RL. *Immunol Today* 1991;12:349–52.
11. Stein SH, Phipps RP. *Eur J Immunol* 1990;20:403–7.
12. Roper RL, Conrad DH, Brown DM, Warner GL, Phipps RP. *J Immunol* 1990;115:2644–51.
13. Stein SH, Phipps RP. *J Immunol* 1991;147:2500–6.
14. Simkin NJ, Jelinek DF, Lipsky PE. *J Immunol* 1987;138:1074–81.
15. Roper RL, Phipps RP. *J Immunol* 1992;149:2984–91.
16. Polla BS, Ohara J, Paul WE, et al. *J Mol Cell Immunol* 1988;3:363–73.
17. Galizzi JP, Cabrillat H, Rousset F, Ménétrier C, DeVries JE, Banchereau J. *J Immunol* 1988;141:1982–8.
18. Phipps RP, Lee D, Schad V, Warner GL. *Eur J Immunol* 1989;19:995–1001.
19. Brown DM, Warner GL, Ales-Martinez JE, Scott DW, Phipps RP. *Clin Immunol Immunopathol* 1992;63:221–9.
20. Quill H, Gaur A, Phipps RP. *J Immunol* 1989;142:813–8.
21. Chouaib S, Welte K, Mertelsmann R, Dupont B. *J Immunol* 1985;135:1172–9.
22. Rincon M, Tugores A, Lopez-Rivas A, et al. *Eur J Immunol* 1988;18:1791–6.
23. Faist E, Mewes A, Baker CC, et al. *J Trauma* 1987;27:837–48.
24. Betz M, Fox BS. *J Immunol* 1991;146:108–13.
25. Hasler F, Bluestein H, Zvaifler N, Epstein LB, *J Immunol* 1983;131:768–72.
26. Wolf M, Droege W. *Cell Immunol* 1982;72:286–93.
27. Lang NP, Ortaldo JR, Bonnard GD, Herberman RB. *J Natl Cancer Inst* 1982;69:339–43.
28. Fulton AM, Zhang SZ, Chong YC. *Cancer Res* 1991;51:2047–50.
29. Snyder DS, Beller DI, Unanue ER. *Nature* 1982;299:163–5.
30. Matis LA, Glimcher LH, Paul WE, Schwartz RH. *Proc Natl Acad Sci USA* 1983;80:6019–23.
31. Bonnefoy J-Y, Denoroy M-C, Guillot O, Martens CL, Banchereau J. *J Immunol* 1989;143:864–9.
32. Mosmann TR, Coffman RL. *Annu Rev Immunol* 1989;7:145–73.
33. Munoz E, Zubiaga AM, Merrow M, Sauter NP, Huber BT. *J Exp Med* 1990;172:95–103.
34. Novak TJ, Rotherberg EV. *Proc Natl Acad Sci USA* 1990;87:9353–7.
35. Gajewski TF, Schell SR, Fitch FW. *J Immunol* 1990;144:4110–20.
36. Munoz E, Beutner U, Zubiaga A, Huber BT. *J Immunol* 1990;144:964–9.
37. Lehmmann V, Benninghoff B, Droge W. *J Immunol* 1988;141:587–91.
38. Renz H, Gong J-H, Schmidt A, Nain M, Gemsa D. *J Immunol* 1988;141:2388–93.
39. Ohmori H, Hikida M, Takai T. *Eur J Immunol* 1990;20:2499–2503.
40. Shah TP, Lichtenstein LM, Undem B, MacDonald SM. *J Allergy Clin Immunol* 1992;89:173 (Abstract 115).
41. Pene J, Rousset F, Briere F, et al. *Proc Natl Acad Sci USA* 1988;85:6880–4.
42. Lycke N, Severinson E, Strober W. *J Immunol* 1990;145:3316–24.
43. Roper RL, Phipps RP. (Submitted.)
44. Snapper CM, Finkelman FD. *J Immunol* 1990;145:3654–60.
45. Rothman P, Li SC, Alt FW. *Immunology* 1989;1:65–77.
46. Stein SH, Phipps RP. *J Immunol* 1992;148:3943–9.
47. Roper RL, Ludlow J, Phipps RP. *Cell Immunol* 1994;154:296–308.
48. Cambier JC, Newell MK, Justement LB, McGuire JC, Leach KL, Chen ZZ. *Nature* 1987;327:629–32.
49. Brown DM, Phipps RP. *Proceedings of the 8th Intl Conference on Prostaglandins and Related Compounds* 1992;69 (Abstract 263).
50. Coleman RA. In: Benedetto C, McDonald-Gibson RG, Nigam S, Slater TF, eds. *Prostaglandins and related substances: a practical approach.* Washington, DC: IRL Press; 1987:267–303.
51. Mitchell MD, Dudley DJ, Edwin SS, Schiller SL. *Eur J Pharmacol* 1991;192:189–91.

52. Heinen E, Cormann N, Braun M, Kinet-Denoël C, Vanderschelden J, Simar LJ. *Ann Inst Pasteur* 1986;137D:369–82.
53. Bernheim HA. *Yale J Biol Med* 1986;59:151–8.
54. Kurland JI, Bockman R. *J Exp Med* 1978;147:952–7.
55. Ferreri NR, Howland WC, Spiegelberg HL. *J Immunol* 1986;136:4188–93.
56. Hsueh W, Arroyave CM, Jordan RL. *Prostaglandins* 1984;28:889–904.
57. Akahosi TJ, Oppenheim J, Matsushima K. *J Clin Invest* 1988;82:1219–24.
58. Zimmer T, Jones PP. *J Immunol* 1990;145:1167–75.
59. Leung DYM, Key L, Steinberg JJ, et al. *J Immunol* 1988;140:84–8.
60. Amlot PL, Slaney J, *Int Arch Allergy Appl Immunol* 1981;64:138–45.
61. Goodwin JS, Messner RP, Bankhurst AD, Peake GT, Saiki JII, Williams RC. *N Engl J Med* 1977;297:963–8.
62. Trang LE, Granstrom E, Lovgren O. *Scand J Rheumatol* 1977;6:151–4.
63. Gruber B, Ballan D, Gorevic PD. *Clin Exp Immunol* 1988;71:289–94.
64. Gioud-Paquet M, Auvinet M, Raffin T, et al. *Ann Rheum Dis* 1987;46:65–71.
65. DiPiro JT, Hamilton RG, Howdieshell TR, Adkinson NF Jr, Mansberger AR Jr. *Ann Surg* 1992;215:460–6.
66. Ertel W, Morrison MH, Wang P, Ba ZF, Ayala A, Chaudry IH. *Ann Surg* 1991;214:141–8.
67. Liu LX, Serhan CN, Weller PF. *J Exp Med* 1990;172:993–6.
68. Fogh K, Herlin R, Kragballe K. *J Allergy Clin Immunol* 1989;83:450–5.

*Advances in Prostaglandin, Thromboxane,
and Leukotriene Research*, Vol. 22, edited by
S.-E. Dahlén et al. Raven Press, Ltd., New York © 1994

# 5-Lipoxygenase Inhibitors in the Treatment of Inflammatory Bowel Disease

Jørgen Rask-Madsen, *Klaus Bukhave,
†Laurits Stærk Laursen, and †Karsten Lauritsen

*Department of Medical Gastroenterology 261, Hvidovre Hospital, University of
Copenhagen, DK-2650, Hvidovre, Denmark; *Department of Biochemistry and
Nutrition, The Technical University of Copenhagen, DK 2800 Lyngby, Denmark;
and †Department of Medical Gastroenterology S, Odense University Hospital,
DK-5000 Odense, Denmark*

During the past decade, considerable progress has been made in elucidating the immunologic changes that occur in inflammatory bowel disease (IBD). Furthermore, advances in understanding of the immunopharmacologic mechanisms of drug action have allowed the development of new therapeutic approaches to IBD. This review briefly discusses the present knowledge of immunoregulatory changes in IBD, the biology of leukotrienes (LTs) and their relation to IBD, and the rationale for inhibiting LTs in IBD, before focusing on the evidence for potential beneficial effects of 5-lipoxygenase (5-LO) inhibitors in the treatment of IBD.

## IMMUNOREGULATION IN IBD

In the pathophysiology of IBD, the mucosal immune system is involved in a sequence of events beginning with antigen processing (1). Over the last few years, several groups have presented data suggesting that class II antigen-bearing gastrointestinal epithelial cells are capable of antigen presentation to lymphocytes (2–5). If this occurs in vivo, the HLA-DR expression seen in IBD may augment the inflammatory response by increasing the amount of antigen presented to the mucosal immune system (1). There is also convincing evidence that intestinal differentiation of T cells is disturbed in IBD owing to an immunoregulatory defect in which T cells produce an abnormal cytokine profile with $T_H^1/T_H^2$ cell imbalance and selective proliferation of IgG-producing B cells. The precise nature of the antigens that initiate IBD is unknown, but a major focus is presently being placed on the possible etiologic role of bacterial cell wall products, including peptidoglycans, formylmethionyl-leucyl-phenylalanine (fMLP), and lipopolysaccharides (LPS), which nonspecifically activate macrophages, polymorphonuclear leukocytes (PMNs), and lymphocytes in the colonic mucosa. Therefore, common bacterial cell wall products and molecules capable of initiating and activating an inflammatory immune response in a genetically predisposed individual may initiate a sequence of immunologic processes that are not appropriately downregulated (1).

To summarize the sequence of events that lead to the inflammatory processes that occur in IBD, the cytokine- and cell-mediated regulation of immunoglobulin production appears more important because of its ability to trigger the complement pathway and macrophage activation. A variety of processes may account for the large influx of macrophages and PMNs, including cytokines, such as generation of interleukin (IL)-1, IL-6, IL-8, IL-10, and tumor necrosis factor-$\alpha$ (TNF$\alpha$), complement activation, and eicosanoid synthesis. Once the influx of macrophages and PMNs occurs, a markedly increased production of free oxygen radicals, proteases, LTs (in particular LTB$_4$), platelet-activating factor (PAF-acether), and other soluble mediators of inflammation results in the secondary amplification of the inflammatory response, which provides the clinical manifestations of the final inflammatory processes in the intestine (6). Although eicosanoids are far down the pathogenetic pathway of IBD and are relatively nonspecific, they are important because they may be considered key mediators of inflammation and belong to the portion that actually causes the damage to the intestine, in addition to being more readily approachable by drug therapy (6). This impression is emphasized by the fact that most of our current drug therapy, such as corticosteroids, anti-inflammatory salicylates, and immunosuppressive agents, inhibit the nonspecific inflammatory processes observed in IBD.

## LEUKOTRIENE BIOLOGY

Eicosanoids are a family of molecules derived from arachidonic acid. The products of this pathway have been implicated in a large number of physiologic functions and disease processes (7). Among them are the cyclooxygenase products [prostaglandins (PGs), thromboxanes (TXs), and prostacyclin], the 5-LO products, including LTs, the products of 12- or 15-lipoxygenases, and lipoxins, which are products of 5- or 15-lipoxygenases. Both cyclooxygenase and lipoxygenases are enzymes that catalyze the stereospecific insertion of molecular oxygen into various positions in arachidonic acid. They are named according to the position of the carbon atom into which the oxygen is inserted. The insertion of oxygen provides the energy potential for this large family of molecules, and each of the reactions of arachidonic acid with oxygen results in a molecule with a unique spectrum of biologic activities (8). Enzymes metabolizing arachidonic acid are selectively distributed in different cell types, thus further increasing the diversity of the eicosanoids that can be produced.

## RATIONALE FOR INHIBITING LEUKOTRIENES IN IBD

Chronic IBD is associated with excess eicosanoid formation in the target tissue of inflammation (6). The first inflammatory mediator examined was $PGE_2$, which is produced in markedly increased amounts in IBD (9). However, the use of cyclooxygenase inhibitors appears to worsen IBD, to provoke a relapse (10), or even to induce ulcerative disease of the colon indistinguishable from ulcerative colitis (11). The explanation for this was not entirely clear until studies were carried out examining the inhibition of the 5-LO pathway by 5-aminosalicylic acid (5-ASA) and, more importantly, the markedly increased production of $LTB_4$ in IBD (12,13). It therefore appears very important which parts of the arachidonic acid metabolism pathway are blocked by pharmacologic agents.

It is now well established that LTs, and in particular $LTB_4$, are generated and released in vitro from colonic mucosa obtained from patients with ulcerative colitis or Crohn's disease (14,15). The large bowel also produces LTs in vivo, as assessed by rectal equilibrium dialysis in patients with active ulcerative colitis (16). Because these products are not produced by peripheral blood leukocytes in vitro after the addition of an activating stimulus, the responsible cells must be activated in situ. The rationale for using anti-LT drugs in IBD is based, therefore, on markedly increased generation of $LTB_4$, potent proinflammatory actions of $LTB_4$, and clinical efficacy of established drugs [corticosteroids, sulfasalazine, and its metabolite 5-aminosalicylic acid (5-ASA)], all of which, among other pharmacologic properties unrelated to LT biosynthesis, inhibit LT formation.

## ANTILEUKOTRIENE AGENTS IN IBD

The compounds that inhibit LT formation and function can be conveniently separated into agents that reduce substrate arachidonic acid availability, agents that inhibit the 5-LO, and agents that blockade LT receptors (17,18).

### Agents That Reduce Substrate Arachidonic Acid Availability

The basic strategies to block LT biosynthesis are shown in Fig. 1. The first enzymatic step in the biosynthesis of LTs in the inflamed mucosa is the liberation of free arachidonic acid from membrane phospholipids by the

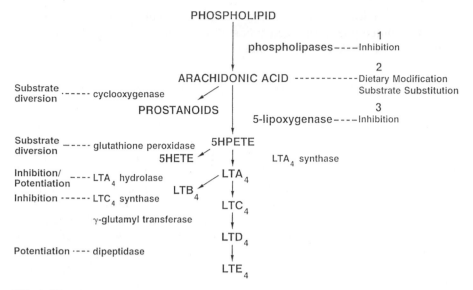

**FIG. 1.** The three enzymatic steps (right 1–3) that provide the basic strategies to block leukotriene (LT) biosynthesis.

hydrolytic enzyme phospholipase $A_2$ (18). Drugs that act at this point can generally be divided into three types: those interacting with phospholipase $A_2$; those interacting with the substrate for phospholipase $A_2$; and those modulating intracellular calcium levels. Most important are the corticosteroids, which belong to the first type, but they have no direct interaction with the enzyme. Instead, a receptor–drug complex is formed that induces synthesis and release of proteins with antiphospholipase properties (18). Thus, the corticosteroids prevent formation of free arachidonic acid by promotion of the phospholipase $A_2$ inhibitor lipocortin (19–23), and in patients with active IBD prednisolone causes a prompt reduction in the generation of $LTB_4$ and $PGE_2$ (13). However, corticosteroids also have effects on lymphocyte differentiation, cytokine synthesis, and interferon production (1,24, 25). It is therefore still unclear which of the pharmacologic properties account for the therapeutic efficacy of corticosteroids.

The second type includes a wide range of drugs, most of which have other actions and therefore inhibit phospholipase $A_2$ indirectly, such as the antimalarial agents mepacrine and chloroquine and the local anaesthetic lidocaine.

The third group comprises calcium antagonists, but the concentrations required far exceed those necessary for inhibition of "slow" calcium channels. Nevertheless, the calcium-channel antagonist verapamil has recently been shown to inhibit mucosal 5-LO activity in therapeutic concentrations by 30% in rectal biopsies from patients with active ulcerative colitis without affecting mucosal $PGE_2$ release (26). This effect is explained by the calcium dependence of 5-LO. The observation awaits therapeutic evaluation.

Incorporation of alternative fatty acid substrates may also affect biosynthesis of LTs. If the dietary intake of arachidonic acid is decreased and/or the intake of eicosatrienoic and eicosapentaenoic acid is increased, LTs of the 3 and 5 series are produced instead. $LTB_3$ is only slightly less potent than $LTB_4$ as a chemotactic and chemokinetic agent of human PMNs, but the structurally analogous product $LTB_5$ (5,12-dihydroxyeicosapentaenoic acid) is less efficiently produced and is a markedly weaker stimulator of PMN function. As a consequence, the therapeutic potential of dietary precursor modulation by a fish oil-supplemented diet [ω-3 fatty acids, such as eicosapentaenoic acid ($C20:5,ω-3$) and docosahexaenoic acid ($C22:6,ω-3$)] in the treatment of IBD has been shown to result in a 35% to 50% decrease in PMN production of $LTB_4$ (27–29). Significant improvement in symptoms and histologic appearance of the rectal mucosa has been observed in several small series of patients with Crohn's disease (28) and ulcerative colitis (30–32) given fish oil (Max EPA) 3 to 4 g daily for 2 to 6 months in uncontrolled studies, as well as in small double-blind crossover studies in ulcerative colitis (33,34). However, a larger, randomized, double-blind trial comprising 96 patients with ulcerative colitis failed to reveal any benefit in remission maintenance or treatment of relapse on 4.5 g of eicosapentaenoic acid daily, although $LTB_4$ synthesis by blood peripheral PMNs in response to ionophore stimulation was reduced by 49%, 53%, and 59% after 2, 6, and 12 months, respectively (35). It should be emphasized, however, that the anti-inflammatory actions of fish oils, in addition to their inhibition of $LTB_4$, include suppression of IL-1 and PAF-acether synthesis and scavenging of free oxygen radicals. Several explanations for the lack of efficacy in remission maintenance exist. Probably more than 50% inhibition of $LTB_4$ biosynthesis is required to obtain clinical efficacy, but it is also possible that placebo olive oil has therapeutic activity or acts as a scavenger of free oxygen radicals (35). The results of an as yet unpublished study demonstrating that, e.g., concentrations of docosahexaenoic acid are abnormally high in patients with IBD may be more important, because these patients have an increased metabolism of polyunsaturated fatty acids and normal plasma levels of arachidonic acid and linoleic acid (personal communication). These observations, therefore, question the rationale for using fish oil in the treatment in IBD.

### Agents That Inhibit 5-Lipoxygenase

At present, the greatest amount of effort is being assigned to the identification of compounds that specifically and effectively inhibit the 5-LO enzyme. In addition to calcium-channel antagonists mentioned above, sul-

**TABLE 1.** *Examples of experimental 5-lipoxygenase (5-LO) inhibitors*

| Agent | Chemical structure | Selected references |
|---|---|---|
| Zileuton | *N*-(1-(benzo-(b)-thien-2-yl)ethyl)-*N*-hydroxyurea | 76,77 |
| BW 4AC | *N*-(3-phenoxycinnamyl)acetohydroxamic acid | 35,94 |
| BW A137C | *N*-(4-benzyloxybenzyl)acetohydroxamic acid | 94 |
| BW A797C | *N*-(3-(5,6,7,8-tetrahydro-2-naphthyl)prop-2-enyl)acetohydroxyamic acid | 94 |
| EP10045 | Methyl-2-butyl-mercapto-4-catechol | 95 |
| L-651,392 | 4-Bromo-2,7-dimethoxy-3H-phenothiazin-3-one | 96,97 |
| MK-0591 | 3-(1-((4-chlorophenyl)methyl)-3((1,1-dimethyl-ethyl)thio)-5(quinolin-2-ylmethyloxy)-1H-indol-2-yl)-2,2-dimethyl-propanoate | |
| ONO-RS-085 | *N*-(2E,11Z,14Z-eicosatrienoyl)-anthranilic acid | 98 |
| S-26431 | 3-(3,5-di-*t*-butyl-4-hydroxyanilino)-benzoic acid | 99 |
| SC41930 | 7-(3-(4-acetyl-3-methoxy-2-propylphenoxy)-propoxyl)-3,4-dihydro-8-propyl-2H-1-benzopyran-2-carboxylic acid | 75,100 |

fasalazine and its active moiety 5-ASA (mesalazine) are also weak 5-LO inhibitors (15,24,36–42), but they may also reduce inflammation by modulating PMN leukocyte function (43–47) and by acting as inhibitors of PGs (9,48–50), TXs (51), PAF-acether (52), IL-1 (25,53), TNFα (54), intestinal mast cell and basophil-stimulated histamine release (55), and fMLP-receptor binding (56), in addition to being scavengers of free oxygen radicals (57–69). As was the case with corticosteroids, it is still unclear which of the above properties account for the therapeutic efficacy of sulfasalazine and 5-ASA.

The compounds identified as inhibitors of 5-LO can be divided into three main types. First, there are antioxidants (70). Classical examples comprise the phenyl pyrazoline BW755C, nordihydroguaiaretic acid, and vitamin E (7). They do inhibit the 5-LO enzyme, but it should be recognized that they are not well-defined, selective enzyme inhibitors but rather are dual inhibitors of the cyclooxygenase and the 5-LO enzyme. Second, there are substrate analogues, such as 5,6-dehydro-arachidonic acid. Third, there is a large miscellaneous group of inhibitors with differing mechanisms of action (Table 1), among which hydroxamic acids (71,72) are potent and more selective inhibitors of 5-LO, but 20 to 30 times less potent as cyclooxygenase inhibitors.

### *Experimental 5-Lipoxygenase Inhibitors*

A number of 5-LO inhibitors have been studied in animal models. Although no model of IBD exactly mimics human disease, many features of the models can be used to investigate the role of particular inflammatory cells and mediators in the underlying inflammatory processes. However, studies with 5-LO inhibitors in models of IBD have yielded variable effects, but this notion also applies to the effects of corticosteroids and sulfasalazine (73). Hence, the relevance of models for selection of novel therapeutic agents should be viewed with caution, although such studies may allow selection of potent, selective, and bioavailable 5-LO inhibitors for clinical evaluation.

In vitro data on human colitis tissue have also begun to accumulate. The acetohydroxamic acid BWA4C inhibited basal and ionophore stimulated in vitro formation of $LTB_4$ synthesis by colorectal biopsy specimens obtained from patients with ulcerative colitis, without significantly inhibiting $PGE_2$ or $TXB_2$ synthesis (74). The $IC_{50}$ for inhibition of $LTB_4$ formation by BWA4C was 0.03 μmol/L compared with an $IC_{50}$ of 0.08 μmol/L for nordihydroguaiaretic acid. In a fairly similar design, SC41930 and SC45662 inhibited mucosal $LTB_4$ release by 17% and 41%, respectively, compared with an inhibition by 5-ASA of 18% (75).

Until now, clinical data on 5-LO inhibition in patients with IBD are available only for zileuton (Abbott-64077). Another compound, MK-886, was withdrawn from clinical development pending evaluation of observed animal toxicity but has already been replaced by MK-0591, which is presently undergoing phase I clinical evaluation in patients with mild-to-moderate ulcerative colitis (personal communication). MK-0591 is a potent $LTB_4$ biosynthesis inhibitor that binds to the 5-LO-activating protein (FLAP) and thereby inhibits the translocation of 5-LO. The compound appears able to inhibit calcium ionophore-stimulated $LTB_4$ biosynthesis ex vivo in whole blood by more than 99% after a single oral dose of 125 mg MK-0591 in healthy volunteers, and 24 hr after dosing the mean percentage inhibition of a single 500-mg dose was still more than 90% (personal communication).

### Zileuton

Zileuton (Table 1) strongly inhibits 5-LO activity in rat basophilic leukemia-1 cells and in rat and human PMNs. In rat leukocytes the drug is 28-fold more potent in inhibiting 5-LO than cyclooxygenase (76).

In a single-dose study, $LTB_4$ and $PGE_2$ concentrations in rectal dialysis fluid from 10 patients with active ulcerative colitis were measured before and after oral administration of 800 mg of zileuton (76). Figure 2 shows that the median $LTB_4$ level fell significantly, from 4.9 (range 0.6 to 20.4) ng/ml before treatment to 1.6 (0.3 to 5.7) ng/ml after 4 hr and 0.7 (0.1 to 8.0) ng/ml after 8 hr; it returned to pretreament levels after 24 hr. The concentrations of $PGE_2$ did not change significantly. These findings in patients with ulcerative colitis indicate that zileuton is a specific (i.e., without effect on the cyclooxygenase) and efficient inhibitor of $LTB_4$ formation in the target tissue of inflammation (76).

Two studies on the use of zileuton in the treatment of ulcerative colitis have been published. First, in an open trial patients given zileuton 800 mg once a day for 4 weeks showed a trend toward symptomatic improvement (77). Second, the results of a randomized, double-blind, placebo-controlled, multicenter trial [the first of two scheduled interim analyses (78)] of zileuton 800 mg orally twice daily for up to 4 weeks in patients with mild-to-moderate

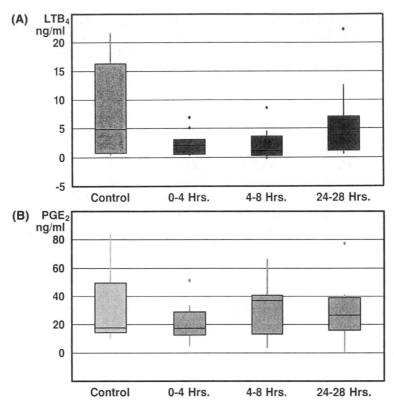

**FIG. 2.** Box plots of $LTB_4$ **(A)** and $PGE_2$ **(B)** concentrations in rectal dialysates from 10 patients with mild to moderately active ulcerative colitis before (control) and after administration of a single dose (800 mg) of zileuton. The central horizontal line in each box represents the group median, the box encloses the middle 50% of the data values, and the tails extend to the most extreme values within a border or "fence" at 1.5 times the interquartile range. The dots denote outliers. Adapted from ref. 76.

disease activity showed that zileuton treatment resulted in significant improvement in symptoms, in addition to significant inhibition of $LTB_4$ in the target tissue of inflammation (79). Briefly, a primary stratification was performed for patients with ($n = 45$) or without ($n = 31$) concomitant sulfasalazine or 5-ASA. The patients were evaluated before entry, after 2 and 4 weeks, and at follow-up after week 5. Efficacy evaluation was based on symptoms, sigmoidoscopy, and histology. The safety assessments included physical examination and laboratory screening. Seventy-six patients entered the study. Forty patients were randomized to zileuton and 36 to placebo. A clinical response with combined improvement in both symptom and sigmoidoscopy scores occurred more often in the zileuton group and significantly so in the subset of patients without concurrent sulfasalazine. Furthermore, zileuton significantly improved total symptom score and scores of rectal bleeding, stool character, abdominal/rectal pain, and urgency. A statistically significant improvement in histology score was also noted when patients receiving zileuton without concomitant sulfasalazine were compared with those receiving placebo. No adverse events or toxicity indicating an unfavorable benefit-to-risk ratio were observed. The $LTB_4$ concentrations in rectal dialysates were significantly inhibited by zileuton, with a median percentage inhibition of 70%.

These data offer encouraging therapeutic insights into the control of the inflammatory response in IBD, but a higher degree of 5-LO inhibition and a prolonged treatment should be assessed in future studies. Nevertheless, the results provide direct evidence for the hypothesis that selective inhibition of the synthesis of a single mediator may result in clinical response, although more than a hundred different inflammatory mediators are involved in the pathogenesis of ulcerative colitis (6).

### Agents That Blockade Leukotriene Receptors

Antagonism of the actions of LT can also be obtained by using selective receptor antagonists (80,81). The number and specificity of LT receptors remain a matter of debate (82–84). Since the discovery of the first LT antagonist, FPL 55712 (85), several new agents have been described. Most experience has been obtained with cysteinyl LT-receptor antagonists, the $LTD_4$ receptors being considered an important target for pharmacologic intervention. Less effort has been given to the search for $LTB_4$ antagonists because of the complexity of the in vitro assays (86), among other things owing to changes in receptor expression modulated by protein kinase C (87). Such changes may account for changes in PMN responsiveness to $LTB_4$.

Some agents with purported LT receptor antagonism [e.g., CGP 34064A (88) and CGP 35949 (89)] not only block the action of LTs at the receptor level but also block the biosynthesis of the LTs by inhibiting phospholipase $A_2$. Furthermore, some of the antagonists also possess 5-LO inhibitory activity [e.g., FPL 55712 (90), SC41930 (75), and Wy-49911 (90)].

### CONCLUSIONS AND PROSPECTS

A large number of anti-LT drugs are presently under development. Selective interventions that target other mediators of inflammation [e.g., PAF-acether receptor antagonists (91–93), IL-1–receptor antagonists, in addition to antibodies to IL-1 or IL-1Rs, and bradykinin-receptor antagonists (93)] will soon follow. In this connection it should be emphasized that blocking 5 LO is a highly effective way of inhibiting cytokine synthesis. In addition, several kinin antagonists were synthesized years ago, and it was shown that $B_2$-receptor antagonists (D-Arg-Arg-Pro-Hyp-Gly-Thi-Ser-D-Phe-Thi-Arg-

TFA and D-Pro-Phe-Arg-heptylamide) cause significant antagonism of bradykinin-induced inflammatory reactions (93). However, medical intervention focusing on inhibition of the 5-LO, LT receptors, the terminal enzymes responsible for the formation of $LTB_4$, cysteinyl LTs, and PAF-acether receptors presently appears the most promising therapeutic approach in IBD. The main disadvantage of existing new LT inhibitors relates to the high potency of the LTs. Unless a high degree of inhibition can be achieved, endogenous LTs may still be present in sufficient amounts to produce their effects. Because a physiologic role for LTs is generally accepted, the possibility that effective long-term inhibition may be associated with side effects should also be ruled out before placing regulation of the LT pathway within the realm of clinical medicine.

## REFERENCES

1. MacDermott RP, Stenson WF. *Adv Immunol* 1988;42:285–328.
2. Bland PW, Warren LG. *Immunology* 1986;58:1–7.
3. Bland PW, Warren LG. *Immunology* 1986;58:9–14.
4. Mayer L, Schlien R. *J Exp Med* 1987;166:1471–83.
5. Kaiserlian D, Vidal K, Revillard J-P. *Eur J Immunol* 1989;19:1513–6.
6. Lauritsen K, Laursen LS, Bukhave K, Rask-Madsen J. *Int J Color Dis* 1989;4:75–90.
7. Rask-Madsen J. *Clin Gastroenterol* 1986;15:545–66.
8. Lewis RA, Austen KF, Soberman RJ. *N Engl J Med* 1990;323:645–55.
9. Sharon P, Ligumsky M, Rachmilewitz D. *Gastroenterology* 1978;75:638–40.
10. Rampton DS, Sladen E. *Postgrad Med J* 1981;57:297–9.
11. Gibson GR, Whitacre EB, Ricotti CA. *Arch Intern Med* 1992;152:625–32.
12. Sharon P, Stenson WF. *Gastroenterology* 1984;86:453–60.
13. Lauritsen K, Laursen LS, Bukhave K, Rask-Madsen J. *Gut* 1987;28:1095–9.
14. Sharon P, Stenson WF. *Gastroenterology* 1984;86:453–60.
15. Peskar BM, Dreyling KW, Peskar BA. *Agents Actions* 1986;18:381–3.
16. Lauritsen K, Laursen LS, Bukhave K, Rask-Madsen J. *Gastroenterology* 1986;91:837–44.
17. Lauritsen K. *Dan Med Bull* 1989;36:378–93.
18. Rask-Madsen J, Bukhave K, Laursen LS, Lauritsen K. *Agents Actions* 1992;C37–46.
19. Hirata F. *J Biol Chem* 1981;256:7730–3.
20. Cloix JF, Colard O, Rothhut B, Russo-Marie F. *Br J Pharmacol* 1983;79:313–21.
21. DiRosa M, Flower RJ, Hirata F, Parente L, Russo-Marie F. *Prostaglandins* 1984;28: 441–2.
22. Wallner BP, Mallatiano RJ, Hesion C, et al. *Nature* 1986;320:77–81.
23. Sakanoue Y, Kusunoki M, Hatada T, et al. *Horm Metab Res* 1990;22:453–4.
24. Mahida YR, Lamming CE, Gallagher A, Hawthorne AB, Hawkey CJ. *Gut* 1991;32:50–4.
25. Ligumsky M, Simon PL, Karmeli R, Rachmilewitz D. *Gut* 1990;31:686–9.
26. Gertner DJ, Rampton DS, Stevens TRJ, Lennard-Jones JE. *Aliment Pharm Ther* 1992;6: 163–8.
27. Hawthorne AB, Edwards T, Filopowicz B, Daneshmend TK, Hawkey CJ. *Gut* 1989;30: A738.
28. Scheurlen M, Daiss W, Steinhilber D, Clemens M, Jaschonek K. *Scand J Gastroenterol* 1989;24(suppl 158):100–1.
29. Hawthorne AB, Edwards T, Filipowicz B, Daneshmend TK, Hawkey CJ. *Gastroenterology* 1989;96:A201.
30. McCall TB, O'Leary D, Bloomfield J, O'Morain CA. *Aliment Pharmacol Ther* 1989;3: 415–24.
31. Salomon P, Kornbluth AA, Janowitz HD. *J Clin Gastroenterol* 1990;12:157–61.
32. Salomon P, Kornbluth AA, Janowitz HD. *Gastroenterology* 1990:98:A201.

33. Tobin A, Suzuki Y, O'Morain CA. *Gastroenterology* 1990;98:A207.
34. Stenson WF, Cort D, Rodgers J, Burakoff R, et al. *Ann Intern Med* 1992;116:609–14.
35. Hawthorne AB, Daneshmend TK, Hawkey CJ, et al. *Gut* 1992;33:922–8.
36. Stenson WF, Lobos E. *J Clin Invest* 1982;69:494–7.
37. Sircar JC, Schwender CF, Carethers ME. *Biochem Pharmacol* 1983;32:170–2.
38. Allgayer H, Eisenburg J, Paumgartner G. *Eur J Clin Pharmacol* 1984;26:449–51.
39. Nielsen OH, Bukhave K, Elmgreen J, Ahnfelt-Rønne I. *Dig Dis Sci* 1987;32:577–82.
40. Nielsen ST, Beninati L, Buonato CB. *Scand J Gastroenterol* 1988;23:272–6.
41. Allgayer H, Stenson WF. *Immunopharmacology* 1988;15:39–46.
42. Peskar BM, Dreyling KW, May B, Schaarschmidt K, Goebell H. *Dig Dis Sci* 1987;32: 51S–6S.
43. Rubinstein A, Das KM, Melamed J, Murphy RA. *Clin Exp Immunol* 1978;33:217–24.
44. Molin L, Stendahl O. *Acta Med Scand* 1979;206:451–7.
45. Rhodes JM, Bartholomew TC, Jewell DP. *Gut* 1981;22:642–7.
46. MacDermott RP, Kane MG, Steele LL, Stenson WF. *Immunopharmacology* 1986;11: 101–9.
47. Aparicio-Pages MN, Verspaget HW, Hafkenscheid JC, et al. *Gut* 1990;31:1030–2.
48. Ligumsky M, Karmeli F, Sharon P, Zor U, Cohen F, Rachmilewitz D. *Gastroenterology* 1981;81:444–9.
49. Smith PR, Dawson DJ, Swan CH. *Gut* 1979;20:802–5.
50. Hawkey CJ, Karmeli F, Rachmilewitz D. *Gut* 1983;24:881–5.
51. Stenson WF, Lobos E. *Biochem Pharmacol* 1983;32:2205–9.
52. Eliakim R, Karmeli F, Razin E, Rachmilewitz D. *Gastroenterology* 1988;95:1167–72.
53. Remvig L, Andersen B. *Scand J Rheumatol* 1990;19:11–6.
54. Shanahan F, Niederlehner A, Carramanzana N, Anton P. *Immunopharmacology* 1990; 20:217–24.
55. Fox CC, Moore WC, Lichtenstein LM. *Dig Dis Sci* 1991;36:179–84.
56. Stenson WF, Mehta J, Spilberg I. *Biochem Pharmacol* 1984;33:407–12.
57. Miyachi Y, Yoshioka A, Imamura S, Niwa Y. *Gut* 1987;28:190–5.
58. Dull BJ, Salata K, Langehove A, Goldman P. *Biochem Pharmacol* 1987;36:2467–72.
59. Craven PA, Pfanstiel J, Saito R, DeRubertis. FR. *Gastroenterology* 1987;92:1998–2008.
60. Neal TM, Winterbourn CC, Vissers MC. *Biochem Pharmacol* 1987;36:2765–8.
61. Ahnfelt-Rønne I, Nielsen OH. *Agents Actions* 1987;21:191–4.
62. Aruoma OI, Wasil M, Halliwell B, Hoey BM, Butler J. *Biochem Pharmacol* 1987;36:3739–42.
63. Williams JH, Hallett MB. *Biochem Pharmacol* 1989;38:149–54.
64. Carlin G, Djursäter R, Smedegård G. *Pharmacol Toxicol* 1989;65:121–7.
65. Williams JG, Hallett MB. *Gut* 1989;30:1581–7.
66. Dallegri F, Ottonello L, Ballestrero A, Bogliolo F, Ferrando F, Patrone RF. *Gut* 1990; 31:184–6.
67. Kanerud L, Hafström I, Ringertz B. *Ann Rheum Dis* 1990;49:296–300.
68. Gionchetti P, Guarnieri C, Campieri M, et al. *Dig Dis Sci* 1991;36:174–8.
69. Tamai H, Kachur JF, Grisham MB, Gaginella TS. *Biochem Pharmacol* 1991;41:1001–6.
70. Hammond ML, Kopka IE, Zambias RA, et al. *J Med Chem* 1989;32:1006–20.
71. Summers JB, Gunn BP, Mazdiyasni H, et al. *J Med Chem* 1988;31:3–5.
72. Summers JB, Gunn BP, Martin JG, et al. *J Med Chem* 1988;31:1960–4.
73. Boughton-Smith NK. *Eur J Gastroenterol Hepatol* 1989;1:140–4.
74. Hawthorne AB, Boughton-Smith NK, Whittle BJR, et al. *Gut* 1992;33:513–7.
75. Gertner DJ, Rampton DS, Lennard-Jones JE. *Gastroenterology* 1990;96:A450.
76. Laursen LS, Naesdal J, Bukhave K, Lauritsen K, Rask-Madsen J. *Lancet* 1990;335:683–5.
77. Collawn C, Rubin P, Perez N, et al. *Am J Gastroenterol* 1989;84:1178.
78. Lauritsen K, Laursen LS, Rask-Madsen J, et al. *Gastroenterology* 1990;98:A185.
79. Bukhave K, Laursen LS, Lauritsen K, et al. *Gastroenterology* 1991;100:A200.
80. Snyder DW, Fleisch JH. *Annu Rev Pharmacol Toxicol* 1989;29:123–43.
81. Brown FJ, Bernstein PR, Cronk LA, et al. *J Med Chem* 1989;32:807–26.
82. Lewis RA, Austen KF, Soberman RJ. *N Engl J Med* 1990;323:645–55.
83. Austen KF, Soberman RJ. *Ann NY Acad Sci* 1988;524:xxi–xxv.

84. Crooke ST, Mong S, Clark M, et al. In: Litwack G, ed. *Biochemical actions of hormones.* New York: Academic Press; 1987:81–139.
85. Augstein J, Farmer JB, Lee TB, Sheard P, Tattersall ML. *Nature [New Biol]* 1973;245: 215–7.
86. Goetzl EJ, Sherman JW, Ratnoff, WD, et al. *Ann NY Acad Sci* 1988;524:345–55.
87. Goldman DW. *Ann NY Acad Sci* 1988;524:187–95.
88. von Sprecher A, Ernest I, Main A, et al. In: Samuelsson B, Paoletti R, Ramwell PW, eds. *Advances in prostaglandin, thromboxane, and leukotriene research,* Vol. 17A. New York: Raven Press; 1987:519–25.
89. Bray MA, Beck A, Wenk P, et al. *Advances in prostaglandin, thromboxane, and leukotriene research,* Vol. 17A. 1987:526–31.
90. Musser JH, Kubrak DM, Chang J, Lewis AJ. In: Samuelsson B, Paoletti R, Ramwell PW, eds. *Advances in prostaglandin, thromboxane, and leukotriene research,* Vol. 17A. New York: Raven Press; 1987:536–9.
91. Coffier E, Borrel MC, Lefort J, et al. *Eur J Pharmacol* 1986;131:179–88.
92. Szpejda M. *Lab Invest* 1986;54:275–81.
93. Braquet P, Touqui L, Shen TY, Vargaftig BB. *Pharmacol Rev* 1987;39:97–145.
94. Bhattacherjee P, Boughton-Smith NK, Follenfant RL. *Ann NY Acad Sci* 1988;524:307–20.
95. Lavaud P, Touvay C, Etienne A, et al. *Ann NY Acad Sci* 1988;524:454–5.
96. Guindon Y, Girard Y, Maycock A, et al. In: Samuelsson B, Paoletti R, Ramwell PW, eds. *Advances in prostaglandin, thromboxane, and leukotriene research,* Vol. 17A. New York: Raven Press; 1987:554–7.
97. Wallace JL, MacNaughton WK, Morris GP, Beck BL. *Gastroenterology* 1989;96:29–36.
98. Toda M, Nakai H, Sakuyama S, et al. In: Samuelsson B, Paoletti R, Ramwell PW, eds. *Advances in prostaglandin, thromboxane, and leukotriene research,* Vol. 17B. New York: Raven Press; 1987:768–70.
99. Hammerbeck DM, Bell RL, Stelzer VL, et al. *Ann NY Acad Sci* 1988;524:398–401.
100. Fretland DJ, Levin S, Tsai BS, et al. *Agents Actions* 1989;27:395–7.

*Advances in Prostaglandin, Thromboxane, and Leukotriene Research*, Vol. 22, edited by S.-E. Dahlén et al. Raven Press, Ltd., New York © 1994

# Summary:
# Eicosanoid Effector Sites

Robert A. Lewis and *Peter C. Weber

*Syntex Research, Palo Alto, California 94304; and *University of Munich, 80336 Munich 2, Germany*

The previous five chapters, with their diverse topics, cannot be easily integrated under a unitary theme. However, one area of unanswered questions is: Do 5-lipoxygenase products or other oxygenated arachidonic acid metabolites have intracellular regulatory functions in addition to their effector functions as intercellular mediators?

In the process of assessing the distal products of the 5-lipoxygenase pathway, i.e., the cysteinyl leukotrienes and $LTB_4$, the potential biological actions of the less stable precursors, 5-HPETE and $LTA_4$, or of other oxygenated arachidonic acid metabolites, such as EETs (1), are often forgotten. It has been shown, for example, by Chang et al. (2) that tumor necrosis factor-$\alpha$-dependent induction of manganous superoxide dismutase in a murine adipogenic cell line $TA_1$ is dependent on 5-HPETE production. The mechanism by which this effector function occurs appears to require the induction of *c-fos* transcription by the lipid hydroperoxide; the induction does not appear to be regiospecific and thus apparently reflects the effector function of the hydroperoxy domain rather than a more complicated signal specifically related to the fact that it is a 5- rather than a 12- or 15-lipoxygenase product. Likewise, Peppelenbosch and colleagues (3) have shown that epidermal growth factor brings about a 5-lipoxygenase-dependent transcription of the early response gene *junB* in P19 8-39 cells (murine P19 embryonal carcinoma cells stably transfected with human EGF receptor).

Similarly, the role of noncyclooxygenase products of arachidonic acid as modulators of the growth response to mitogenic agents may rely on their intracellular functions as stimulatory factors for gene activation. This can be concluded from a study by Sellmayer et al. (4) in which increased mRNA levels of the immediate early response genes *c-fos* and Egr-1 in proliferating mesangial cells have been reported in association with increased levels of i.c. EET-like compounds. Results by Bernstrom et al. (5) imply that such products, derived, e.g., from the cytochrome P-450 monooxygenase pathway, are incorporated into specific intracellular phospholipid pools in a distinctive pattern that is different from that of most other eicosanoids. They suggest that these arachidonic acid metabolites may modulate physicochemical properties of cell membranes (e.g., ion channels) or receptors and subsequent signal transduction events.

It is further possible that some of the various observations on agonist-activated ion channels, including $Ca^{2+}$, $K^+$, and $Na^+$ ligand-operated channels, being regulated by distal 5-lipoxygenase product second messengers, could involve the leukotriene interactions on either the cytoplasmic or the extracellular face of the plasma membranes in a leukotriene-generative cell. The observations that Dietrich Keppler and colleagues presented (*this volume*) on leukotriene transport, particularly in the hepatocyte model, demonstrate both uptake and export mechanisms that are located basolateral or apical, respectively. Such transporters, as well as the export system for $LTC_4$ in eosinophils and that in murine mastocystoma cells, which ligate leukotrienes on the cytoplasmic side, raise the possibility that cells that generate cysteinyl leukotrienes might not require feedback through a cell surface receptor as part of an autocrine mechanism to cause LT-induced ion-channel opening.

On the same topic, the various immunomodulatory effects postulated for $LTB_4$ in lymphocyte subpopulations [especially the work of M. Rola-Pleszczynski and colleagues (5)] need not necessarily involve $LTB_4$ production by other cells in the microenvironment acting on lymphocyte $LTB_4$ receptors. Alternatively, these effects could result from transcellular metabolism, providing $LTA_4$ to T cells with the $LTA_4/LTB_4$ epoxide hydrolase, and immunomodulation affected in the $LTB_4$-generative lymphocyte itself without requiring leukotriene export. Again, whether this occurs by export and receptor-mediated activation on the extracellular side of the plasma membrane as part of an autocrine feedback loop or whether the effect begins and ends on the cytoplasmic side of the cell membrane for any of these $LTB_4$ effects, including augmentation of natural cytotoxic T-cell activity against *Herpes*-infected target cells and induction and activation of $CD^{8+}$ suppressor T cells, is still moot. These issues relating to cell biology of immunomodulation might be considered in the context of the contribution by Phipps (*this volume*), in which $PGE_2$ effects are logically presumed to act from the cell surface via classical receptor-mediated transduction.

In the context of microcirculatory processes in inflammation addressed by Hedquist (*this volume*), the role of oxidatively modified membrane phospholipids (6) to activate adhesion processes of immune-competent cells, such as neutrophils, to the endothelium via the receptor for platelet-activating factor (7) needs to be considered. Such mechanisms could contribute to the pathophysiology of asthma and/or ulcerative colitis.

# REFERENCES

1. Oliw EH, Guengerich FP, Oates JA. *J Biol Chem* 1982;257:3771–81.
2. Chang DJ, Ringold GM, Heller RA. *Biochem Biophys Res Commun* 1992;188:538–46.
3. Peppelenbosch MP, Tertoolen LGJ, den Hertog J, de Laat SW. *Cell* 1992;69:295–303.
4. Sellmayer A, Uedelhoven WM, Weber PC, Bonventre JV. *J Biol Chem* 1991;266:3800–7.
5. Rola-Pleszczynski M, et al. *Adv Exp Med* 1991;314:205–21.
6. Bernstrom K, Kayganich K, Murphy RC, Fitzpatrick FA. *J Biol Chem* 1992;267:3686–90.
7. Smiley PL, Stremler KE, Prescott SM, Zimmerman GA, McIntyre TM. *J Biol Chem* 1991;266:11104–10.

# 3. Mediators and Mechanisms in Asthma and Airway Inflammation

Advances in Prostaglandin, Thromboxane,
and Leukotriene Research, Vol. 22, edited by
S.-E. Dahlén et al. Raven Press, Ltd., New York © 1994

# The Interaction Among Granulocyte Lipid Mediators and the Generation of Oxygen Radicals in Antigen-Induced Airway Hyperresponsiveness

William M. Abraham

*Department of Research, Mount Sinai Medical Center,
Miami Beach, Florida 33140*

Mechanisms that contribute to allergen-induced late responses and the prolonged airway hyperresponsiveness that follow are of potential clinical importance because they may be linked to factors that heighten the severity of asthma (1). The airways of asthmatic subjects and experimental animals can remain inflamed for prolonged periods of time after antigen challenge, and this inflammatory state is associated with airway hyperresponsiveness (2). The inflammation is characterized by neutrophils, eosinophils, activated macrophages, and lymphocytes (3). The eosinophil is a potent source of leukotrienes (LTs) and platelet-activating factor (PAF), putative mediators of late responses and airway hyperresponsiveness. Eosinophils also release major basic protein (MBP), eosinophil cationic protein, and eosinophil peroxidase. MBP damages respiratory epithelium (4,5), and instillation of MBP into the airways causes airway hyperresponsiveness (6,7). The neutrophil, via the generation of cyclooxygenase products of arachidonic acid metabolism, especially thromboxane ($TxA_2$), has been linked to antigen- and ozone-induced airway hyperresponsiveness (8–10). Depletion and/or inactivation of these granulocytes, either by chemical means (11) or by use of specific monoclonal antibodies (12), prevents the airway hyperresponsiveness associated with antigen challenge, underscoring the importance of these inflammatory cells. A number of recent studies have examined the relationship between airway inflammation, as assessed by either bronchial biopsy or bronchoalveolar lavage (BAL), and airway responsiveness. The findings indicate that numbers of eosinophils, epithelial cells, metachromatic cells (mast cells/basophils), and macrophages can all be correlated with airway hyperresponsiveness (13–19). Such observations suggest that hyperresponsiveness is a multicellular process. Therefore, it is not surprising that soluble factor(s)- or granule-mediated interactions among neutrophils, eosinophils, and macrophages result in enhanced responses to exogenous stimuli (20–25). Stimulated neutrophils, eosinophils, and other cells release a variety of mediators, including arachidonic acid metabolites. In addition, these cells also generate free oxygen radicals: superoxide $O_2^-$, hydrogen peroxide ($H_2O_2$), and their metabolites, including the extremely reactive and toxic hydroxyl radical (OH•) which is formed through the Haber–Weiss reaction (26). The pathophysiologic effects of these toxic oxygen species have been an intense area of study in experimental models of the adult respiratory distress syndrome (27). However, because these radicals can initiate eicosanoid synthesis and because of the important role of arachidonic acid metabolites in the pathophysiology of asthma, it is possible that these radicals contribute to abnormalities of the conducting airways, such as airway hyperresponsiveness.

There is evidence to support a role for oxygen radicals in airway hyperresponsiveness. In anesthetized cats, inhaled xanthine–xanthine oxidase (a reaction that produces free oxygen radicals) caused a short-lived bronchoconstriction and increased airway responsiveness (28). These effects were blocked by the $O_2^-$ scavenger superoxide dismutase (SOD) and by the $H_2O_2$ scavenger catalase (CAT), but further studies into the mechanisms of this response were not performed. In patients with chronic airflow obstruction, a correlation was found between the production of $O_2^-$ by peripheral PMNs stimulated with phorbol ester and the degree of airway hyperresponsiveness (29). Alveolar macrophages, obtained by BAL from subjects challenged with cotton bract extract, released increased amounts of $O_2^-$ and $TxA_2$ compared with BAL cells from saline-challenged controls (30). Although the in vitro parameters of BAL cell activation did not correlate with the degree of extract-induced bronchoconstriction, there was a relationship between the pulmonary response and the concentration of $TxA_2$ in BAL. That $H_2O_2$ caused selective stimulation of $TxA_2$ in rat alveolar macrophages (31) agrees with these in vivo observations. Because $TxA_2$ is a putative mediator of airway hyperresponsiveness (32), this pathway may have important implications for the control of airway tone. Free oxygen radicals also cause smooth-muscle contraction and enhance smooth-muscle responsiveness in vitro (33,34). In guinea pig trachealis muscle, $LTD_4$ potentiated the contractile response to histamine (35). As expected, this effect was blocked by the LT antagonist FPL-55712, but surprisingly the potentiation was also blocked by SOD, indicating that $LTD_4$ stimulated the release of $O_2^-$. The LT–oxygen radical interaction may be an important factor in the pathophysiology of asthma because of the recent data implicating $LTD_4$ as a mediator of the late response in human subjects (36) and studies implicating $LTE_4$ in the development of airway hyperresponsiveness (37,38).

These data suggest that, in asthma, oxygen free radicals generated by airway inflammatory cells could act as an intercellular signal controlling the release of lipid mediators which, in turn, mediate the airway hyperresponsiveness associated with allergen challenge. To prove this hypothesis, however, we need to show evidence that: granulocyte and lipid mediators contribute to airway hyperresponsiveness that follows antigen challenge; the airway hyperresponsiveness is an active process; toxic oxygen radicals can cause airway hyperresponsiveness and that this is linked to the generation of lipid mediators; and toxic oxygen radical scavengers can block antigen-induced airway hyperresponsiveness.

## METHODS

The sheep model of allergic bronchoconstriction was used for these studies. All sheep were sensitive to inhaled *Ascaris suum* antigen. In most studies described, sheep with a history of dual responses (i.e., both early and late airway responses) were used. Measurements of airway mechanics (specific lung resistance, $SR_L$) and airway responsiveness ($PC_{400}$) were obtained as described previously (30–42).

## RESULTS AND DISCUSSION

### Evidence That Lipid Mediators Derived from Activated Granulocytes Contribute to Antigen-Induced Airway Hyperresponsiveness

Analysis of BAL for cells and mediators was performed before and 24 hr after antigen challenge in 13 allergic sheep that developed late responses (40). Twenty-four hours after antigen challenge, $PC_{400}$ fell from a baseline value of $22.0 \pm 2.2$ BU to $13.9 \pm 1.5$ BU ($p < 0.05$), indicating that the sheep were hyperresponsive. Associated with this airway hyperresponsiveness was an increase in lung granulocytes and lipid mediators (Table 1). Correlation coefficients ($r$) were calculated for different pairs of variables to de-

**TABLE 1.** *Changes in lipid mediators, granulocytes, and airway responsiveness before and 24 hr after antigen challenge in allergic sheep with late responses*

| Agent | Before | After |
|---|---|---|
| $TxB_2$ (pg/ml) | $0 \pm 0$ | $24.1 \pm 2.9^*$ |
| $LTB_4$ (pg/ml) | $0 \pm 0$ | $14.3 \pm 2.6^*$ |
| $LTC_4$ (pg/ml) | $0 \pm 0$ | $24.8 \pm 3.1^*$ |
| Granulocytes/ml BAL[a] | $0.37 \pm 0.12$ | $2.22 \pm 0.24^*$ |
| $PC_{400}$[b] | $22.0 \pm 2.2$ | $13.9 \pm 1.5^*$ |

Values are mean $\pm$ SE for 13 sheep.
[a] Values for granulocytes are expressed in log units.
[b] $PC_{400}$ is expressed in breath units (BU). $PC_{400}$ is defined as the cumulative breaths of carbachol that cause a 400% increase in specific lung resistance ($SR_L$). One breath unit is equivalent to one breath of 1% (w/v) carbachol solution (41,42).
* $p < 0.05$.

**TABLE 2.** *Correlation coefficients for lipid mediators, granulocytes, and airway responsiveness before and 24 hr after antigen challenge in allergic sheep with late responses*

| Variables | Correlation (r) | p values |
|---|---|---|
| $TxB_2$ vs. $LTC_4$ | 0.611 | <0.01 |
| $TxB_s$ vs. $LTB_4$ | 0.770 | <0.01 |
| $LTC_4$ vs. $LTB_4$ | 0.765 | <0.01 |
| $TxB_2$ vs. granulocytes | 0.762 | <0.01 |
| $LTC_4$ vs. granulocytes | 0.713 | <0.01 |
| $LTB_4$ vs. granulocytes | 0.697 | <0.01 |
| $TxB_2$ vs. $PC_{400}$ | 0.589 | <0.01 |
| $LTD_4$ vs. $PC_{400}$ | 0.314 | NS |
| $LTB_4$ vs. $PC_{400}$ | 0.296 | NS |
| Granulocytes vs. $PC_{400}$ | 0.497 | <0.02 |

*p* Values were based on 24 degrees of freedom. Measurements made in 13 sheep before and 24 hr after antigen challenge.
NS, not significant.

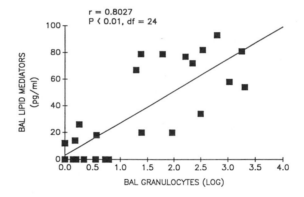

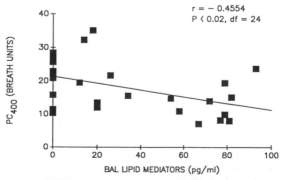

**FIG. 1.** Relationship between BAL granulocytes (expressed as log) and the total of the BAL lipid mediators ($TxB_2$, $LTC_4$, and $LTB_4$) from Table 1 **(top)** and between $PC_{400}$ and total BAL lipid mediators **(bottom).**

termine if any significant relationships existed (Table 2). Significant correlations were obtained between the lipid mediators analyzed, the lipid
mediators and the number of granulocytes found in the airways, and $PC_{400}$
and the number of granulocytes and the concentration of $TxB_2$ found in
BAL. Interestingly, there was no significant relationship between the $PC_{400}$
and the concentrations of $LTC_4$ or $LTB_4$ found, but using the total concentration of all mediators in BAL increased the relationships (Fig. 1). These
observations suggest that in an inflamed lung there is a relationship among
different lipid mediators, that these mediators are associated with activated
granulocytes, and that these variables affect airway responsiveness. Although these data do not prove cause and effect, the findings are consistent
with the hypothesis that lipid mediators generated from activated granulocytes recruited to the lungs contribute to antigen-induced airway hyperresponsiveness. Furthermore, the data are consistent with in vivo studies
showing that the cyclooxygenase inhibitor indomethacin blocks the postchallenge airway hyperresponsiveness but not the late response (10),
whereas LT antagonists and 5-LO inhibitors (43,44) block both the late
response and the airway hyperresponsiveness. Therefore, the generation of
LTs during the late response could cause the release of cyclooxygenase
metabolites (e.g., $TxA_2$), which then could mediate the hyperresponsiveness. Such a mechanism would be consistent with the ability of thromboxane
antagonists to reduce but not to block the late response (45,46).

To better understand the influence of the individual lipid mediators in the
development of airway hyperresponsiveness, sheep were challenged with
aerosolized 100 µg $LTD_4$ ($n = 6$), 1,250 µg PAF ($n = 4$), and 200 µg $LTB_4$

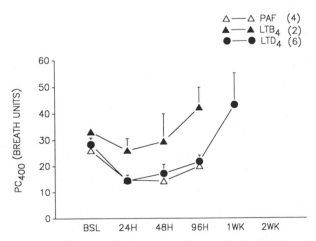

**FIG. 2.** Effects of inhaled lipids on airway responsiveness in allergic sheep. $LTD_4$ (100 mg)
and PAF (1,250 mg), but not $LTB_4$ (200 mg), caused prolonged airway hyperresponsiveness. Values are mean ± SE; (4), (2), (6) = number of animals.

($n = 2$), and the time course of the airway hyperresponsiveness was followed (Fig. 2). The sheep became hyperresponsive 24 hr after antigen challenge and remained so for 96 hr. Both PAF and $LTD_4$ induced a prolonged decrease in $PC_{400}$, whereas $LTB_4$ did not. These results provide further evidence that lipid mediators can initiate processes leading to prolonged airway hyperresponsiveness.

### Evidence That the Prolonged Airway Hyperresponsiveness That Follows Antigen Challenge Is an Active Process

The data from the first series of experiments suggested to us that the development of prolonged airway hyperresponsiveness was a cyclic process initiated by antigen challenge but mediated by activated inflammatory cells continuously recruited to the lung. If this were true, then the hyperresponsiveness could be treated after the late response had developed. We tested this hypothesis in two separate experiments. In the first study, dual responders were treated 7.5 hr, 24 hr, and 48 hr after antigen challenge, once with placebo and once with 30 mg nedocromil sodium on two separate occasions. (This dose of nedocromil does not affect basal airway responsiveness.) Nedocromil was used because it has been shown to reduce a variety of cell functions, including mediator release (47) and oxygen radical production (48). The early and late responses were similar for both the drug and the placebo trial. However, nedocromil given after the late response blocked the airway hyperresponsiveness. Twenty-four and 48 hr after antigen challenge (mean $\pm$ SE), $PC_{400}$ was 9.4 $\pm$ 1.5 and 9.4 $\pm$ 1.2 BU compared with 21.4 $\pm$ 1.6 and 20.9 $\pm$ 2.2 BU in the nedocromil trial.

We then determined if the post–antigen-induced airway hyperresponsiveness could be reversed. To do this, we treated sheep with a new anti-allergy agent, TYB-2285, after the airway hyperresponsiveness was already developed. For these studies, the sheep ($n = 7$) were challenged with antigen on two occasions, each separated by at least 21 days. The sheep were then treated with placebo or 100 mg/kg TYB-2285, p.o., *after* the 24-hr, 48-hr, and 72-hr determinations of $PC_{400}$. The dose of TYB-2285 chosen for these studies was based on the compound's ability to block late responses in this model. Respective early and late increases in $SR_L$ were (mean $\pm$ SE) 427 $\pm$ 62% and 179 $\pm$ 15% during the placebo trial and 398 $\pm$ 67% and 222 $\pm$ 27% during the drug trial. These changes were not different from each other. Likewise, both challenges resulted in a similar degree of airway hyperresponsiveness 24 hr after challenge (see below). However, this hyperresponsiveness was abolished from 48 to 96 hr by initiating treatment with TYB-2285, as seen in Table 3.

These results indicate that the airway hyperresponsiveness that follows the development of late responses can be reversed by acute treatment with

**TABLE 3.** *Prolonged airway hyperresponsiveness*

|  | BSL | 24 hr | 48 hr | 72 hr | 96 hr |
|---|---|---|---|---|---|
| Placebo | $23.2 \pm 2.1$ | $9.1 \pm 1.3^*$ | $9.9 \pm 1.8^*$ | $11.6 \pm 1.2^*$ | $13.3 \pm 1.2^*$ |
| Treated | $19.5 \pm 1.5$ | $7.8 \pm 1.1^*$ | $20.5 \pm 2.9^+$ | $26.1 \pm 2.8^+$ | $29.5 \pm 5.5^+$ |

Values are mean $\pm$ SE $PC_{400}$ (BU); $p < 0.05$: *versus baseline (BSL); $^+$versus placebo.

anti-allergy agents, supporting the hypothesis that this hyperresponsiveness is an active process.

## Evidence That Radicals Can Cause Airway Hyperresponsiveness

If oxygen radicals are involved in the propagation of airway hyperresponsiveness, then we should be able to show that oxygen radicals produce airway hyperresponsiveness and that there is a link between these radicals and the generation of lipid mediators. To do this, we generated oxygen radicals in the airways of allergic sheep ($n = 7$) by giving aerosols of xanthine (x; 0.1%)–xanthine oxidase (xo; 4.1 U) and determining the effect of x–xo on airway responsiveness (49). Measurements were made on a control day and on different experimental days, 1 hr after x–xo challenge when $SR_L$ had returned to baseline. Inhaled x–xo caused an immediate increase in $SR_L$ of $162 \pm 36\%$ (mean $\pm$ SE; $p < 0.05$) over baseline. The calculated $PC_{400}$ decreased to $16.6 + 1.7$ BU ($p < 0.05$) from a baseline value of $32.5 \pm 5.0$ BU. In separate experiments, the x–xo challenge was repeated after pretreatment with inhaled catalase (CAT, 38 mg; $H_2O_2$ scavenger), methylprednisolone succinate (MS, 1 mg/kg i.v.), indomethacin (IND, 2 mg/kg i.v.; cyclooxygenase inhibitor), WEB-2086 (3 mg/kg i.v.; PAF antagonist), MK-571 (5 mg aerosol; leukotriene $D_4$ antagonist), and nedocromil sodium (NS, 1 mg/kg aerosol; anti-asthma agent). Except for MK-571, pretreatment with all agents significantly blocked the x–xo-induced increase in $SR_L$. All agents significantly inhibited the x–xo-induced decrease in $PC_{400}$ (i.e., blocked airway hyperresponsiveness), although MK-571 was the least effective. Mean BUs were 27, 32, 34, 25, 31, 31, after CAT, WEB-2086, IND, MK-571, NS, and MS, respectively (all $p < 0.05$ versus x–xo alone) (Fig. 3). In a cell-free system in vitro, x–xo produced $755 \pm 43$ ng OH/ml ($n = 9$). CAT (50 $\mu$g/ml) inhibited this reaction by $74 \pm 11\%$ ($n = 7$; $p < 0.05$); all other drugs were ineffective, indicating that they did not have nonspecific radical scavenging action. In subsequent experiments, CAT pretreatment had no effect on PAF-induced bronchoconstriction or airway hyperresponsiveness, suggesting that the radical-induced generation of lipid mediators occurs first. These results suggest that, in sheep, the secondary generation of PAF and other arachidonic acid metabolites contributes to x–xo-induced bronchoconstriction and airway hyperresponsiveness.

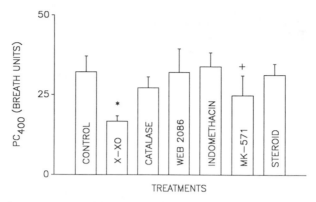

**FIG. 3.** Effect of pretreatment with pharmacological agents on x–xo-induced airway hyperresponsiveness values are mean ± SE; $n = 7$ for all except $n = 6$ for steroid. *$p < 0.05$ versus all others; †$p < 0.05$ versus control. Steroid, methylprednisolone succinate. (From ref. 49.)

## Evidence That Oxygen Radical Scavengers Can Block Antigen-Induced Airway Hyperresponsiveness

If oxygen radicals can initiate airway hyperresponsiveness and if this mechanism is involved in antigen-induced airway hyperresponsiveness, then we need to show that radical scavengers block this effect. To do this, we first determined baseline airway responsiveness in seven sensitized sheep and then, on a different day, the sheep underwent inhalation challenge with antigen. $SR_L$ was measured before and immediately after challenge and then hourly for 2 hr, at which time $SR_L$ had returned to prechallenge values. The postchallenge $PC_{400}$ was then measured. This procedure was repeated on separate occasions, each at least 14 days apart, except that the sheep were treated with an aerosol of the hydrogen peroxide ($H_2O_2$) inhibitor catalase (CAT, 38 mg in 3 ml milli Q water) at three different times (Table 4): given before antigen and then every 30 min after antigen challenge for 2 hr (A); given 1 hr and 2 hr after antigen challenge (B); and given only at 2 hr after antigen challenge (C). Results (mean ± SE) of the antigen-induced bronchoconstriction (AIB, % increase) and postchallenge $PC_{400}$ (BU) are given in Table 4.

CAT had no effect on AIB but blocked the airway hyperresponsiveness

**TABLE 4.** *Oxygen radical scavengers and airway hyperresponsiveness*

| Trial | Control | A | B | C |
|---|---|---|---|---|
| AIB | 303 ± 48 | 311 ± 22 | 324 ± 35 | 290 ± 25 |
| $PC_{400}$ | 11.0 ± 1.7* | 22.3 ± 2.5 | 23.1 ± 1.8 | 9.8 ± 1.2* |

Baseline (BSL) $PC_{400}$ was 21.8 ± 1.9 BU; *$p < 0.05$ versus BSL.

when given during the time (0 to 1 hr) of putative inflammatory cell recruitment. These results provide indirect evidence that the oxygen radicals contribute to antigen-induced airway hyperresponsiveness. That CAT given only 2 hr after challenge failed to block the airway hyperresponsiveness suggests that $H_2O_2$ is not the end-stage radical/metabolite but that it may initiate secondary mechanisms that contribute to this response (50). These data would be consistent with the hypothesis that radicals could act to stimulate the release of lipid mediators and that these lipids were responsible for the airway hyperresponsiveness.

## CONCLUSION

The results of this study provide indirect evidence for interactions among granulocytes, lipid mediators, and oxygen radicals in the propagation of antigen-induced airway hyperresponsiveness. The prolonged hyperresponsiveness observed after antigen challenge is probably the result of the continuous recruitment of new inflammatory cells to the airway and the subsequent activation of these and/or other resident cells, such as the macrophage. Our data suggest that radicals act as an intermediary in this process, probably contributing to the generation of these mediators. This conclusion is based on the inability of radical scavengers (e.g., CAT) to prevent PAF-induced airway hyperresponsiveness and the observation that CAT is effective only within a certain period of time after antigen challenge. These data suggest that once the active mediators are generated, receptor-mediated events are responsible for the end-organ response, in this case airway hyperresponsiveness.

## REFERENCES

1. O'Byrne PM, Dolovich J, Hargreave FE. *Am Rev Respir Dis* 1987;136:740–51.
2. March WR, Irvin CG, Murphy KR, Behrens BL, Larsen GL. *Am Rev Respir Dis* 1985; 131:875–9.
3. Metzger WJ, Richerson HB, Worden K, et al. *Chest* 1986;89:477–83.
4. Frigas E, Loegering DA, Gleich GJ. *Lab Invest* 1980;42:35–42.
5. Motojima S, Frigas E, Loegering DA, Gleich GJ. *Am Rev Respir Dis* 1989;139:801–5.
6. Brofman JD, White SR, Blake JS, Munoz NM, Gleich GJ, Leff AR. *J Appl Physiol* 1989; 66:1867–73.
7. Isakson PC, Raz A, Denny SE, Wyche A, Needleman P. *Prostaglandins* 1977;14:853–71.
8. O'Byrne PM, Walters EH, Gold BD, et al. *Am Rev Respir Dis* 1984;130:220–4.
9. Kirby JG, Hargreave FE, Cockcroft DW, O'Byrne PM. *J Appl Physiol* 1989;66:578–83.
10. Lanes S, Stevenson JS, Codias E, et al. *J Appl Physiol* 1986;61:864–72.
11. Larsen GL, Wilson MC, Clark RAF, Behrens BL. *Fed Proc* 1987;46:105–12.
12. Wegner CD, Gundel RH, Reilly P, Haynes N, Letts LG, Rothlein R. *Science* 1990;247: 456–9.
13. Beasley R, Roche WR, Roberts JA, Holgate ST. *Am Rev Respir Dis* 1989;139:806–17.
14. Ferguson AC, Wong FWM. *Chest* 1989;96:988–91.
15. Wardlaw AJ, Dunette S, Gleich GJ, Collins JV, Kay AB. *Am Rev Respir Dis* 1988;137:62–9.
16. Kelly C, Ward C, Stenton CS, Bird G, Hendrick DJ, Walters EH. *Thorax* 1988;43:684–92.

17. Kirby J, Hargreave FE, Gleich GJ, O'Byrne PM. *Am Rev Respir Dis* 1987;136:379–83.
18. Lozewicz S, Wells C, Gomez E, et al. *Thorax* 1990;45:12–5.
19. Jeffery PK, Wardlaw AJ, Nelson FC, Collins JV, Kay AB. *Am Rev Respir Dis* 1989;140: 1745–53.
20. Kloprogge E, De Leeuw AJ, de Monchy JGR, Kauffman HF. *Int Arch Allergy Appl Immunol* 1989;90:20–3.
21. Wilkinson JRW, Crea AEG, Clark TJH, Lee TH. *J Clin Invest* 1989;84:1930–41.
22. Howell CJ, Pujol J-L, Crea AEG, et al. *Am Rev Respir Dis* 1989;140:1340–7.
23. Moy JN, Gleich GJ, Thomas LL. *J Immunol* 1990;145:2626–32.
24. Yuo A, Kitagawa S, Ohsaka A, Saito M, Takaku F. *Biochem Biophys Res Commun* 1990; 171:491–7.
25. Lopez AF, Williamson DJ, Gamble JR, et al. *J Clin Invest* 1986;78:1220–8.
26. Klebanoff SJ. In: Gallin JI, Goldstein IM, Snyderman R, eds. *Phagocytic cells: products of oxygen metabolism.* New York: Raven Press; 1988:391–444.
27. Olson NC. *Mol Aspects Med* 1988;10:551–629.
28. Katsumata U, Miura M, Ichinose M, et al. *Am Rev Respir Dis* 1990;141:1158–61.
29. Postma DS, Renkema TEJ, Noordhoek JA, Faber H, Sluiter HJ, Kauffman H. *Am Rev Respir Dis* 1988;137:57–61.
30. Cooper JAD, Merrill WW, Rankin JA, Sibille Y, Buck MG. *J Appl Physiol* 1988;64:1615–23.
31. Sporn PHS, Peters-Golden M, Simon RH. *Am Rev Respir Dis* 1988;137:49–56.
32. Fujimura M, Sasaki F, Nakatsumi Y, et al. *Thorax* 1986;41:955–9.
33. Nishida Y, Suzuki S, Miyamoto T. *Inflammation* 1985;9:333–7.
34. Szarek JL, Schmidt NL. *Am J Physiol* 1990;258:L232–7.
35. Weiss EB, Bellino JR. *Chest* 1986;89:709–16.
36. Sladek K, Dworski R, Fitzgerald GA, et al. *Am Rev Respir Dis* 1990;141:1441–5.
37. Arm JP, O'Hickey SP, Spur BW, Lee TH. *Am Rev Respir Dis* 1989;140:148–53.
38. O'Hickey SP, Hawksworth RJ, Fong CY, Arm JP, Spur BW, Lee TH. *Am Rev Respir Dis* 1991;144:1053–7.
39. Abraham WM, Delehunt JC, Yerger L, Marchette B. *Am Rev Respir Dis* 1983;128:839–44.
40. Abraham WM, Burch RM, Farmer SG, Sielczak MW, Ahmed A, Cortes A. *Am Rev Respir Dis* 1991;143:787–96.
41. Soler M, Sielczak MW, Abraham WM. *J Appl Physiol* 1989;67:406–13.
42. Soler M, Sielczak M, Abraham WM. *J Appl Physiol* 1991;70:617–23.
43. Ahmed A, Cortes A, Sielczak MW, Abraham WM. *Am Rev Respir Dis* 1992;145:A288 (abst).
44. Abraham WM, Ahmed A, Coetes A, et al. *Eur J Pharmacol* 1992;217:119–26.
45. Ahmed A, Cortes A, Abraham WM. *FASEB J* 1989;3:A438 (Abstract).
46. Abraham WM, Ahmed A, Cortes A, Sielczak MW. *Am Rev Respir Dis* 1992;145:A291 (abst).
47. Wells E, Jackson CG, Harper ST, Mann J, Eady RP. *J Immunol* 1986;137:3941–5.
48. Rubin RP, Thompson RH, Naps MS. *Agents Actions* 1990;31:237–42.
49. Lansing MW, Mansour E, Ahmed A, et al. *Am Rev Respir Dis* 1991;144:1291–6.
50. Lansing MW, Ahmed A, Coetes A, et al. *Am Rev Respir Dis* 1993;147:321–6.

Advances in Prostaglandin, Thromboxane,
and Leukotriene Research, Vol. 22, edited by
S.-E. Dahlén et al. Raven Press, Ltd., New York © 1994

# The Role of Eicosanoids and Selectins in Experimental Asthma in Monkeys

Robert H. Gundel and *L. Gordon Letts

*Miles Preclinical Research, Miles Inc., West Haven, Connecticut 06516-4175; and
*Department of Pharmacology, Boehringer Ingelheim Pharmaceuticals, Inc,
Ridgefield, Connecticut 06877*

Asthma is a disease that affects approximately 5% of the population, and despite the availability of more potent and selective therapy, the incidence of asthma morbidity and mortality is on the rise (1). The acute symptoms of allergic asthma include shortness of breath and wheezing, which are largely the result of the action on airway smooth muscle of mast cell-derived mediators (e.g., histamine) that are released after exposure to specific allergen. These acute symptoms can be adequately controlled with $\beta_2$-agonist bronchodilators (2). However, the chronic symptoms of asthma, such as persistent airway obstruction and bronchial hyperresponsiveness, are less well understood and are often refractory to most presently available therapies (3). Current research suggests that chronic symptoms may be a manifestation of the development of airway inflammation involving a variety of cells and mediators. The development of airway inflammation involves a complex series of events occurring at both the cellular and the tissue level, one of which is the adherence of circulating leukocytes to pulmonary vascular endothelium, followed by transendothelial migration into the lungs in response to a chemotactic gradient (4).

We have developed a primate model of allergic asthma to study the role of lipid mediators and adhesion molecules involved in the induction and maintenance of pulmonary inflammation and associated changes in pulmonary function. In this communication, we present a brief introduction to adhesion molecules involved in the development of pulmonary inflammation, followed by a description of our primate model and our experimental results.

## ADHESION MOLECULES

Adherence of leukocytes to vascular endothelium represents a critical step in the movement of leukocytes from the circulation to sites of inflammation (5). The importance of adhesion molecules in cell recruitment is illustrated in leukocyte adhesion deficiency (LAD) patients who have an inability to express normal numbers of leukocyte adhesion molecules on their cell surfaces (6,7). These patients are unable to recruit neutrophils to sites of infection and therefore suffer from frequent life-threatening infections. Early studies utilizing monoclonal antibodies to adhesion molecules as antagonists demonstrated their ability to inhibit lymphocyte-mediated events such as cytotoxic T-cell activity, natural killer cell activity (8,9), T-cell proliferation, and the mixed lymphocyte response (10–13) as well as lymphocyte trafficking processes (5,14). In addition, these antibodies can inhibit granulocyte functions such as adherence to endothelium and homotypic aggregation (15,16). For an in-depth description of adhesion molecules the reader is referred to reviews by Albelda (17), Kishimoto et al. (18), and Larson and Springer (19).

### Endothelial/Epithelial Cell Adhesion Molecules

Exposure of cultured endothelial cells to various cytokines or inflammatory mediators induces or upregulates the expression of several adhesion ligands including E-selectin, P-selectin, intercellular adhesion molecule-1 (ICAM-1), and vascular cell adhesion molecule-1 (VCAM-1) (Table 1) (5, 21–23). It is the inducible expression of these molecules on endothelium that directs the adherence of leukocytes to endothelium for extravasation at specific sites of tissue inflammation.

P-selectin is a member of the selectin family of adhesion molecules characterized by their amino terminal carbohydrate binding (lectin) domain (24,25). P-selectin is not constitutively expressed on endothelium. However, its induced expression is extremely rapid (maximal expression within 5 min) and transient (26). P-selectin is stored in Weibel–Palade bodies of endothelial cells and, on activation, is rapidly mobilized to the cell surface (25,27). Another member of the selectin family of adhesion molecules found on activated endothelium is E-selectin. In contrast to P-selectin, expression of E-selectin requires protein synthesis and therefore occurs 4 to 6 hr after

**TABLE 1.** *Granulocyte–endothelial/epithelial cell adhesion molecules*

| Tissue/cell | Adhesion molecule | Family | Distribution | Ligand |
|---|---|---|---|---|
| Endothelium | P-selectin | Selectin | Endothelial cells, platelets | Sialylated Lewis$^x$ |
| | E-selectin | Selectin | Endothelial cells | Sialylated Lewis$^x$ |
| | ICAM-1 | Immunoglobulin | Endothelial cells, epithelial cells | LFA-1, Mac-1 |
| | VCAM-1 | Immunoglobulin | Endothelial cells | VLA-4 |
| Leukocyte | LFA-1 | Integrin | Leukocytes | ICAM-1 |
| | Mac-1 | Integrin | Myeloid cells | ICAM-1 |
| | p150,95 | Integrin | Myeloid cells | Unknown |

stimulation (22). Because of their relatively rapid upregulation, the selectins are believed to mediate acute inflammatory responses (28). The leukocyte receptors for E-selectin and P-selectin are not well defined. E-selectin binds to a carbohydrate group, sialyl Lewis$^X$, which is found on cell surface glycoproteins and glycolipids of neutrophils and monocytes (29), whereas P-selectin binds to the CD15 antigen lacto-$N$-fucopentaose III on neutrophils and monocytes (26).

In addition to selectins, members of the immunoglobulin supergene family, including (ICAM-1, ICAM-2, and VCAM-1, are also inducible on endothelial cells (13,30). Like E-selectin, the induced expression of these adhesion molecules requires protein synthesis and therefore is delayed. However, in contrast to E-selectin, maximal expression occurs after 12 to 24 hr and is maintained for up to 72 hr (31). Because of the prolonged expression on stimulated endothelial cells, these adhesion molecules may play an important role in the development and maintenance of chronic inflammation. In addition to the endothelium, ICAM-1 is also expressed on airway and alveolar epithelial cells. The leukocyte counterreceptors for ICAM-1 and VCAM-1 are members of the integrin supergene family LFA-1 (CD11a/CD18), Mac-1 (CD11b/CD18), and VLA-4 (CD49/CD29), respectively (17).

### Granulocyte Adhesion Molecules

Adhesion receptors on granulocytes are members of two supergene families, the selectins and the integrins (17). Selectins include L-selectin (LeCAM-1) and other undefined sialyl Lewis$^X$ CD15-containing glycoproteins (32). L-selectin contains an amino terminal $Ca^{2+}$ requiring a carbohydrate binding (lectin) domain, an epidermal growth-factor–like domain, and short consensus repeat units like those found in complement regulatory proteins (33–35). Integrins include the $B_2$, CD18 family and the $B_1$, CD29 family of receptors. The integrins are composed of transmembrane glycoprotein heterodimers ($\alpha$- and $\beta$-chains), which are noncovalently associated and require the presence of divalent cations and an intact cytoskeleton to mediate adhesion (19). Members of the CD18 family have a common $\beta$-chain (CD18) and three variants of the $\alpha$-chain: CD11a, CD11b, and CD11c (27). $B_1$ integrins also possess a common $\beta$-chain (CD29), and at least six variants of the $\alpha$-chair have been identified (CD49a–f) (17,36). These receptors bind to the extracellular matrix components fibronectin, laminin, and collagen, as well as to VCAM-1 on vascular endothelium.

### THE ROLE OF AIRWAY INFLAMMATION

Characteristics of asthmatic airways include tissue eosinophilia, deposition of eosinophil major basic protein (MBP) in and around the airways,

areas of epithelial cell damage or denudation, and bronchial hyperresponsiveness (37–40). Bronchial hyperresponsiveness, defined as an exaggerated
bronchoconstrictor response to a variety of physiologic, pharmacologic, or
mechanical stimuli, is an important component of the pathophysiology of
asthma (41–43). The importance of airway hyperresponsiveness is reflected
by studies demonstrating that its severity correlates with the intensity of
asthmatic symptoms, diurnal variations in peak flow rates, and the amount
of therapy required to control asthmatic symptoms (44–47). Although the
exact mechanisms(s) leading to the development of hyperresponsive airways
is unknown, recent evidence suggests that chronic airway inflammation
probably plays a major role.

Mast cells are present at mucosal surfaces and represent a first-line defense against infection. Crosslinkage of mast cell surface-bound IgE with
allergen leads to activation of the cell, resulting in the release of preformed
granule-associated mediators (e.g., histamine) and in de novo synthesis of
lipid mediators such as prostaglandins, leukotrienes, PAF, and others. The
release of these mediators from mast cells is responsible for the acute symptoms observed after allergen exposure in asthmatic subjects. The immediate
bronchoconstriction induced by allergen inhalation is maximal at 10 to 15
min after provocation and usually resolves within 2 hr. The immediate response is associated with mucous hypersecretion and with vasodilatation
and edema in the lung tissue. The immediate response is followed by an
influx of inflammatory cells (neutrophils and eosinophils) into the lungs as a
result of the synthesis and release of potent chemotactic substances. This
influx of inflammatory cells into the lungs can be associated with the occurrence of a second airway-obstructive response, the late-phase response. The
late-phase response is typically of longer duration and is more severe than
the immediate-phase bronchoconstriction. The late-phase response is associated with an increase in airway responsiveness to inhaled bronchoactive
agents (airway hyperresponsiveness). The simultaneous occurrence of inflammatory cell infiltration, the late-phase response, and increased airway
responsiveness suggests a link with events that occur during the immediate
response. Therefore, the activation of mast cells and other cells in the lungs,
resulting in the release of potent bronchoactive and chemotactic mediators,
may play a central role in the development of chronic airway inflammation
in allergic asthma.

Recent work suggests that mast cells are a source of proinflammatory
cytokines such as IL-3, IL-4, IL-5, IL-6, and TNF (48). These cytokines,
which were previously thought to be mostly associated with T helper lymphocytes, cause an upregulation of allergic inflammation. For example, IL-4
induces the switch of B-cell immunoglobulin synthesis to IgE and up-regu-
lates endothelial cell expression of VCAM-1. IL-3 and IL-4 promote basophil and mast cell differentiation and maturation, and IL-5 selectively
induces eosinophil proliferation, migration, and activation. The release of

cytokines from mast cells provokes a rapid and localized initiation of allergic inflammation. Therefore, the mast cell may play a pivotal role in the initiation of chronic airway inflammation, in addition to its role in the immediate response to inhaled allergen.

## THE PRIMATE MODEL OF ALLERGIC ASTHMA

We have developed a primate model of allergic asthma to study the role of inflammation in chronic airway dysfunction. Our studies involve the use of adult male cynomolgus monkeys (*Macaca fascicularis*) that have a naturally occurring IgE-mediated respiratory hypersensitivity to protein extracts of the nematode *Ascaris suum*. The methods of assessing airway cellular composition by bronchoalveolar lavage (BAL) or bronchial biopsy, airway responsiveness to inhaled methacholine, administration of inhaled antigen, and measurement of pulmonary function have been described in detail elsewhere (49,50).

### Acute and Chronic Lung Inflammation Models

The acute lung inflammation model involves the use of dual-responder primates (i.e., animals that respond to a single antigen inhalation with an immediate and late-phase airway obstructive response) (51). Dual-responder primates have an existing baseline airway eosinophilia and high levels of eosinophil peroxidase activity (EPO) in bronchoalveolar lavage (BAL) fluid, and have hyperresponsive airways. A single antigen inhalation induces an acute pulmonary inflammatory response characterized by a large influx of neutrophils into the airways and increased BAL fluid concentrations of myeloperoxidase (MPO), which occurs superimposed on the existing eosinophilic airway inflammation. Immunohistochemical staining for adhesion glycoproteins has demonstrated that ICAM-1 is constitutively expressed on pulmonary vascular endothelium and airway epithelium. In contrast, little or no staining for E-selectin is evident before antigen inhalation. However, a marked up-regulation of E-selectin occurs on vascular endothelium 6 hr after antigen inhalation.

The same animals are utilized for the chronic lung inflammation model, in which the baseline intrinsic airway eosinophila and airway hyperresponsiveness are examined. The protocols for both the acute model and the chronic model are outlined in Fig. 1.

### Acute Airway Inflammation and Late-Phase Airway Obstruction

Antigen inhalation causes the release of preformed and newly synthesized mediators that contribute to the acute bronchoconstriction and neutrophil

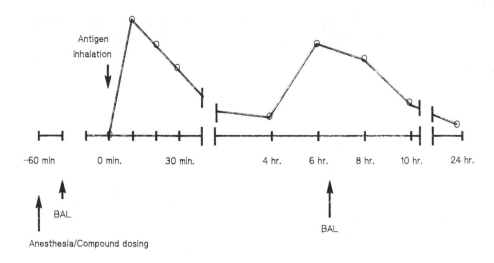

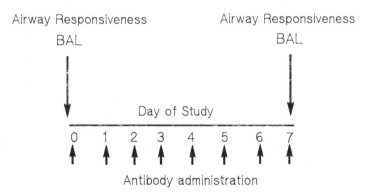

**FIG. 1.** Acute **(top)** and chronic **(bottom)** lung inflammation model.

infiltration into the lungs (52). Our suggestion of a possible effector cell role for newly recruited neutrophils in the late-phase response is supported by data from pharmacologic evaluation of the late-phase response. Treatment with 5-lipoxygenase inhibitors or glucocorticoids before antigen inhalation leads to a dose-related inhibition of the late-phase response (53). The efficacy of these compounds in blocking the late-phase response parallels their ability to inhibit the production and release of leukotrienes in the lungs during the acute response. Inhibition of leukotriene biosynthesis in the lungs blocks the acute influx of neutrophils into the airways associated with the late-phase response (53,54). These data suggest that the production and release of leukotrienes during the acute-phase response (immediately after

**TABLE 2.** *Effects of monoclonal antibody treatment on antigen-induced acute airway inflammation*

| Treatment | No. of infiltrating cells[a] | | | BAL fluid levels of | | % inhibition of |
|---|---|---|---|---|---|---|
| | Total cells | Eos | Neutros | MPO | EPO | LPR |
| Control | 7.6 ± 3.6 | −2.4 ± 1.7 | 3.3 ± 2.1 | 423 ± 87 | 590 ± 52 | − |
| Anti–E-selectin | −2.2 ± 0.9* | −1.2 ± 0.3 | 0.6 ± 0.9* | 101 ± 20* | 315 ± 110 | 72 ± 8* |
| Anti–ICAM-1 | 3.9 ± 3.7 | −3.1 ± 1.1 | 3.6 ± 2.3 | 388 ± 92 | 409 ± 97 | 19 ± 15 |

[a] Number of cells ($\times 10^5$/ml) recovered in BAL fluid 6 hr after antigen challenge.
* $p < 0.05$.

antigen inhalation) can both contribute to and trigger the events that lead to acute neutrophil infiltration and activation in the lungs. Once in the lungs, activated neutrophils may contribute to the late-phase airway obstruction via products of de novo synthesis (i.e., lipid mediators, oxidative products following respiratory burst) that can affect airway and vascular smooth muscle, resulting in a prolonged "obstructive" response (55). Several groups have demonstrated that eosinophil granule products (i.e., MBP) are capable of activating neutrophils (56, 57). We have shown that the levels of eosinophil-derived proteins are significantly increased during the late-phase response. Therefore, exposure of the newly recruited neutrophils to eosinophil

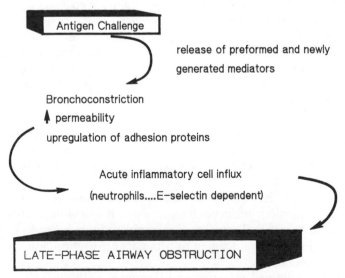

**FIG. 2.** Proposed mechanism of antigen-induced acute and late-phase response. Antigen challenge causes the release of preformed and newly generated broncho- and vasoactive mediators from resident cells in the lung resulting in the immediate bronchoconstriction response. Cellular infiltration (2–6 hr postchallenge) into the lungs is promoted by the upregulation of E-selectin on pulmonary vascular endothelin mediate the late-phase response by the release/generation of toxic oxygen radicals and other mediators.

granule proteins may act to stimulate the neutrophils to produce mediators that influence airway function. Further evidence for an effector cell role for the neutrophil comes from a recent study with a monoclonal antibody against the endothelial adhesion glycoprotein E-selectin (58). In this study, animals were pretreated with anti–E-selectin (CL2) or anti–ICAM-1 (R6.5) intravenously (2 mg/kg) 1 hr before antigen inhalation. Anti–ICAM-1 treatment had no effect on neutrophil influx into the lungs and the associated late-phase response (Table 2). In contrast, anti–E-selectin treatment significantly blocked both the acute neutrophil influx into the airways and the late-phase obstructive response. These data support the concept that newly recruited neutrophils infiltrate into the lung via an E-selectin–dependent mechanism and come in contact with mediators (i.e., MBP) and other cells that trigger a further activation of the neutrophils and synthesis of vasoactive and bronchoactive substances, resulting in airway smooth-muscle constriction and edema in lung tissue (Fig. 2).

### Chronic Airway Inflammation and Airway Hyperresponsiveness

As described above, dual-responder primates have an existing baseline chronic airway eosinophilia. In addition to airway eosinophilia, dual responders have increased numbers of activated T lymphocytes (identified by flow cytometry in BAL fluid) and their airways are hyperresponsive to inhaled methacholine. The levels of eosinophil-derived proteins present in BAL fluid before antigen inhalation are higher in dual-responder primates compared with single responders, suggesting that the eosinophils are activated and degranulating in the airways. It may be that the accumulation of activated eosinophils in the airways is the result of T lymphocyte activation and cytokine release. This leads to the development of airway hyperresponsiveness and contributes to the late-phase airway obstruction after antigen inhalation. Evidence to support this contention comes from studies in which we have demonstrated that multiple antigen inhalations by monkeys with normal airway cell composition and airway responsiveness induce a profound and selective eosinophilia that is associated with damage to the airway epithelium and a striking increase in airway responsiveness (31,49,50). Other studies have shown that direct intratracheal instillation of purified human MBP causes a transient bronchoconstriction and a 10-fold increase in airway responsiveness (59). Therefore, eosinophil granule proteins have direct effects on airway function, leading to bronchoconstriction and increases in airway responsiveness.

Recently we examined the effects of treatment with systemic or inhaled corticosteroids on the airway eosinophilia and airway hyperresponsiveness in late-phase responder primates (60). In a vehicle-controlled crossover study design, six primates were treated with dexamethasone (0.2 mg/kg, i.m.) or vehicle once a day for 7 consecutive days. Dexamethasone signifi-

**TABLE 3.** *Effects of monoclonal antibody treatment on chronic airway inflammation*[a]

| Treatment | No. of cells in BALF | | | BAL fluid levels of | | Methacholine $PC_{100}$ (mg/ml) |
|---|---|---|---|---|---|---|
| | Total cells ($\times 10^5$/ml) | Eos ($\times 10^5$/ml) | Neutros ($\times 10^5$/ml) | MPO (optical density) | EPO (optical density) | |
| Control | 7.1 ± 1.1 | 3.3 ± 0.8 | 0.1 ± 2.4 | 192 ± 41 | 389 ± 53 | 0.32 ± 1.5 |
| Anti–E-selectin | 7.8 ± 1.9 | 4.1 ± 1.3 | 0.4 ± 1.9 | 165 ± 49 | 240 ± 78 | 0.25 ± 1.6 |
| Anti–ICAM-1 | 7.9 ± 1.7 | 4.6 ± 1.0 | 0.4 ± 0.9 | 178 ± 37 | 310 ± 105 | 0.79 ± 2.3 |
| Dex | 3.3 ± 0.6 | 0.6 ± 0.2 | 0.1 ± 0.2 | 43 ± 10* | 52 ± 14* | 6.31 ± 2.0* |

[a] Parameters measured after 7 consecutive days of treatment.
* $p < 0.05$.

cantly reduced the total number of leukocytes and the numbers of eosinophils recovered by BAL. Moreover, the amount of EPO in BAL fluid was significantly decreased and there was a reduction in airway hyperresponsiveness (Table 3). Therefore, treatment with corticosteroids reduces the baseline airway eosinophilia, lowers the number of activated eosinophils, and reduces the airway responsiveness to inhaled methacholine. In contrast, treatment with a 5-lipoxygenase inhibitor had no effect on the existing eosinophilia or airway hyperresponsiveness.

Further studies were conducted to examine the role of adhesion molecules in chronic airway inflammation and hyperresponsiveness. The daily administration for 7 days of either anti–E-selectin or anti–ICAM-1 monoclonal antibodies did not significantly reduce the airway eosinophilia or airway hyperresponsiveness in monkeys with chronically inflamed airways.

## DISCUSSION

Features typical of the pathology of asthma include an intense infiltration of eosinophils and deposition of eosinophil-derived proteins in and around the airway mucosa (61). Areas of epithelial damage or desquamation are also common in asthma, as well as airway edema and mucous hypersecretion that lead to considerable plugging of the peripheral airways (62,63). Studies from our laboratory with a primate model of allergic asthma have demonstrated that, before antigen inhalation, dual-responder monkeys have higher numbers of activated eosinophils and T lymphocytes in the airways relative to single-responder monkeys. Antigen inhalation induces a transient neutrophil influx in both single and dual responders. However, the magnitude of the neutrophil influx is much greater in dual responders. In addition to a temporal relationship between neutrophil infiltration and the late-phase response, there is a modest but significant correlation between the magnitude of the neutrophil influx and the magnitude of the late-phase response, suggesting an effector cell role for the neutrophil. The level of BAL eosinophil-derived EPO is also increased 6 hr after antigen challenge during the late-phase response. Our results imply possible roles for both the eosinophil and the neutrophil in the development of the late-phase response. Therefore, in the primate model, the development of an acute neutrophil inflammation is superimposed on the chronic eosinophilic inflammation and is temporally related to the late-phase airway obstruction. We suggest that in this primate model of allergic asthma the increased number of eosinophils in the airways may have, in addition to contributing to the late-phase response, the potential to prime the airways for the occurrence of late-phase obstruction. Our studies with corticosteroids support this hypothesis. Chronic treatment with either dexamethasone or beclomethasone reduced the number of eosinophils in the airways as well as the level of eosinophil-derived proteins recovered in BAL fluid. In addition, this treatment regimen resulted in significant inhibition of both the acute and the late-phase airway responses.

Pharmacologic data indicate that the antigen-induced acute airway inflammation (neutrophil infiltration) and subsequent late-phase response are, in part, dependent on the generation of 5-lipoxygenase products of arachidonic acid metabolism. In addition, the acute influx of neutrophils into the airways occurs via an E-selectin–dependent mechanism, as pretreatment with monoclonal antibodies against E-selectin inhibited both the neutrophil influx and the late-phase response. Earlier work by several investigators has suggested a role for the neutrophil in asthma and in late-phase airway responses. For example, increased levels of high molecular weight neutrophil chemotactic activity (HMW-NCA) have been detected in the blood of asthmatic patients after antigen-induced acute and late-phase reactions (64,65). More recently, these observations have been confirmed in a study with severe asthmatics (66). These data support the hypothesis of acute airway inflammation and an effector cell role for the neutrophil in the late-phase response.

In contrast to acute neutrophilic airway inflammation and the late-phase response, our studies of chronic airway inflammation imply a dominant role of eosinophils in the onset and maintenance of airway hyperresponsiveness. For many years, the association between blood and sputum eosinophilia with bronchial asthma has been recognized. Eosinophil MBP has been identified on lung tissue taken from patients who have died from asthma (61). More recent studies have demonstrated an association between blood eosinophilia and dual asthmatic responses, as well as a direct correlation between blood eosinophilia and the degree of nonspecific airway hyperresponsiveness (67). In addition, MBP and other eosinophil granule proteins alter airway smooth muscle function in vitro and in vivo (59). It is well known that eosinophils can also generate membrane-derived lipid mediators (i.e., LTC4 and PAF) that are postulated to play a role in the pathogenesis of asthma and airway hyperresponsiveness (68,69).

Treatment with dexamethasone significantly reduced the airway inflammation and airway hyperresponsiveness in all animals. Interestingly, a 5-lipoxygenase inhibitor that was effective in blocking the acute airway inflammation and the late-phase response was ineffective against chronic inflammation and hyperresponsiveness. These data suggest that 5-lipoxygenase products contribute to acute inflammation and the late-phase response but do not influence the maintenance of chronic airway inflammation and hyperresponsiveness. Likewise, although we have demonstrated that anti–E-selectin treatment effectively blocks acute airway inflammation and late-phase airway obstruction, anti–E-selectin had no effect on chronic airway inflammation.

We have previously demonstrated that pretreatment with anti–ICAM-1 effectively inhibits the influx of newly recruited eosinophils into the airways and the onset of airway hyperresponsiveness (23). The lack of efficacy of anti–ICAM-1 treatment in reducing chronic airway inflammation in the present study may be a consequence of blocking the pathway for clearance of cells from the lungs. Therefore, it is possible to inhibit the influx of newly recruited cells into the lungs with antagonists of ICAM-1 or, alternatively, once cells are present in lung tissue, blocking of ICAM-1 may prevent their clearance from the lungs.

In summary, we have investigated the role of proinflammatory cells, mediators, and adhesion pathways in primate models of acute and chronic lung inflammation. Our studies indicate a divergence among cells, mediators, and mechanisms utilized in the recruitment of cells from the vasculature during the development of acute and chronic lung inflammation.

## ACKNOWLEDGMENT

The authors acknowledge the excellent technical assistance of Ms. Carol A. Torcellini and Mr. Cosmos C. Clarke. We thank Drs. Robert Rothlein and C. Wayne Smith for supplying the monoclonal antibodies to ICAM-1 and E-selectin.

## REFERENCES

1. Guidelines for the diagnosis and treatment of asthma. I. Definition and diagnosis. *J Allergy Clin Immunol* 1991;88:427–38.
2. Nelson HS. *J Allergy Clin Immunol* 1986;77:771–85.
3. Sybert A, Weiss EB. In: Weiss EB, Segal MS, Stein M, eds. *Bronchial asthma: mechanisms and therapeutics*. 2nd ed. Boston: Little, Brown; 1985:808.
4. Springer TA. *Nature* 1990;346:425–34.
5. Dustin ML, Rothlein R, Bhan AK, Dinarello CA, Springer TA. *J Immunol* 1986;137:245–52.
6. Anderson DC, Schmalstieg FC, Finegold MJ, et al. *J Infect Dis* 1985;152:668–89.
7. Anderson DC, Springer TA. *Annu Rev Med* 1987;38:175–94.
8. Kohl S, Springer TA, Schmalstieg FC, Loom LS, Anderson DC. *J Immunol* 1984;133:2972–8.
9. Krensky AM, Sanchez-Madrid F, Robbins E, Nagy J, Springer TA, Burakoff S. *J Immunol* 1983;131:611.
10. Boyd AW, Wawryk SO, Burns GF, Fecondo JV. *Proc Natl Acad Sci USA* 1988;85:3095.
11. Davignon D, Martz E, Reynolds T, Kuhrzinger K, Springer TA. *J Immunol* 1981;127:590.

12. Dougherty GJ, Hogg N. *Eur J Immunol* 1987;17:943.
13. Dougherty GJ, Murdoch S, Hogg N. *Eur J Immunol* 1988;18:35.
14. Haskard D, Cavender D, Beatty P, Springer TA, Ziff M. *J Immunol* 1986;137:2901.
15. Anderson DC, Miller LJ, Schmalstieg FC, Rothlein R, Springer TA. *J Immunol* 1986;137: 15.
16 Smith CW, Rothlein R, Hughes BJ, et al. *J Clin Invest* 1988;82:1746–56.
17. Albelda SM. *Am J Respir Cell Mol Biol* 1991;4:195–203.
18. Kishimoto TK, Larson RS, Corbi AL, Dustin ML, Staunton DE, Springer TA. *Adv Immunol* 1989;46:149–82.
19. Larson RS, Springer TA. *Immunol Rev* 1990;114:181–206.
20. de Fougerolles AR, Stacker SA, Schwarting R, Springer TA. *J Exp Med* 1991;174:253–67.
21. Osborn L, Hession C, Tizard R, et al. *Cell* 1989;59:1203–11.
22. Pober JS, Gimbrone MA, Lapierre LA, et al. *J Immunol* 1986;137:1893–6.
23. Wegner CD, Gundel RH, Reilly P, Haynes N, Letts LG, Rothlein R. *Science* 1990;247: 456–9.
24. Johnston GI, Cook RG, McEver RP. *Cell* 1989;56:1033–44.
25. Larsen E, Celi A, Gilbert GE, et al. *Cell* 1989;59:305–12.
26. Lawrence MB, Springer TA. *Cell* 1991;65:859–73.
27. Hynes RO. *Cell* 1987;48:549–54.
28. Geng J-G, Bevilacqua MP, Moore KL, et al. *Nature* 1990;343:757–60.
29. Luscinskas FW, Brock AF, Arnaout MA, Gimbrone MA. *J Immunol* 1989;142:2257–63.
30. Pober JS, Cotran RS. *Physiol Rev* 1990;70:427–43.
31. Wegner CD, Rothlein R, Gundel RH. *Agents Actions* 1991;34:529–44.
32. Kishimoto TK, Jutila MA, Berg EL, Butcher EC. *Science* 1989;245:1238–41.
33. Laskey LA, Singer MS, Yednock TA, et al. *Cell* 1989;56:1045–55.
34. Siegelman MH, Van de Rijn M, Weissman IL. *Science* 1989;243:1165–72.
35. Watson ML, Kingsmore SF, Johnston GI, et al. *J Exp Med* 1990;172:263–72.
36. Hemler HE. *Annu Rev Immunol* 1990;8:365–400.
37. Brogan RD, Ryley HC, Neale L, Yassa L. *Thorax* 1975;30:72–9.
38. Filley WV, Holley KE, Kephart GM, Gleich GJ. *Lancet* 1982;11–6.
39. Ryley HC, Brogan TD. *Br J Exp Pathol* 1968;49:25–33.
40. Wardlaw AJ, Dunnette S, Gleich GJ, Collins JV, Kay AB. *Am Rev Respir Dis* 1988;137: 62–9.
41. Boushey HA, Holtzman MJ, Sheller JR, Nadel JA. *Am Rev Respir Dis* 1980;121:389–414.
42. McFadden ER. *N Engl J Med* 1975;292:555–9.
43. Wagner EM, Liu MC, Weinmann GG, Permutt S, Bleecker ER. *Am Rev Respir Dis* 1990; 141:584–8.
44. Boulet LP, Cartier A, Thomson NC, Roberts RS, Dolovich J, Hargreave FE. *J Allergy Clin Immunol* 1983;71:399–406.
45. Chan-Young M, Lam S, Koener S. *Am J Med* 1982;72:411–5.
46. Hargreave FE, Ryan G, Thomson NC, O'Byrne PM, Latimer K, Juniper EF, Dolovich J. *J Allergy Clin Immunol* 1981;68:347–55.
47. Ryan G, Latimer K, Dolovich J, Hargreave FE. *Thorax* 1982;37:423–8.
48. Gordon JR, Burd PR, Galli SJ. *Immunol Today* 1990;11:458–64.
49. Gundel RH, Gerritsen ME, Wegner CD. *Am Rev Respir Dis* 1989;140:629–33.
50. Gundel RH, Wegner CD, Torcellini CA, Letts GL. *Am Rev Respir Dis* 1992;146:369–73.
51. Gundel RH, Wegner CD, Letts LG. *Am Rev Respir Dis* 1992;146:369–73.
52. Gundel RH, Kinkade P, Torcellini CA, et al. *Am Rev Respir Dis* 1991;144:76–82.
53. Gundel RH, Torcellini CA, Clarke CC, Desai SN, Lazer ES, Wegner CD. *Adv Prost Throm Leuko Res* 1990;21:457–60.
54. Gundel RH. *Ann NY Acad Sci* 1991;629:205–16.
55. Ward PA, Till GO, Kunkel R, Bearchamp C. *J Clin Invest* 1983;72:789–93.
56. Moy JN, Gleich GJ, Thomas LL. *J Immunol* 1989;143:952–5.
57. Rhorbach MS, Wheatley CL, Slifman NR, Gleich GJ. *J Exp Med* 1990;172:1271–4.
58. Gundel RH, Wegner CD, Torcellini CA, et al. *J Clin Invest* 1991;88:1407–11.
59. Gundel RH, Letts LG, Gleich GJ. *J Clin Invest* 1991;87:1470–3.
60. Gundel RH, Wegner CD, Torcellini CA, Letts LG. *Clin Exp Allergy* 1992;22:569–75.
61. Filley WV, Holley KE, Kephart GM, Gleich GJ. *Lancet* 1982;2:11–6.

62. Ryley HC, Brogan TD. *Br J Exp Pathol* 1968;49:25–33.
63. Brogan RD, Ryley HC, Neale L, Yassa L. *Thorax* 1975;30:72–9.
64. Atkins PC, Norman M, Weiner H, Zweiman B. *Ann Intern Med* 1977;86:415–8.
65. Nagy L, Lee TH, Kay AB. *N Engl J Med* 1982;306:497–501.
66. Buchanan DR, Cromwell O, Kay AB. *Am Rev Respir Dis* 1987;136:1397–1402.
67. Durham SR, Kay AB. *Clin Allergy* 1985;15:411–8.
68. Shaw RJ, Walsh GM, Cromwell O, Mogbel R, Spry CJF, Kay AB. *Nature* 1985;316:150–2.
69. Lee TC, Lenihan DJ, Malone B, Ruddy LL, Wasserman SI. *J Biol Chem* 1984;259:5520–30.

*Advances in Prostaglandin, Thromboxane, and Leukotriene Research*, Vol. 22, edited by S.-E. Dahlén et al. Raven Press, Ltd., New York © 1994

# Clinical and Experimental Studies of Leukotrienes as Mediators of Airway Obstruction in Humans

*§Sven-Erik Dahlén, †Barbro Dahlén, ‡Maria Kumlin, §Thure Björck, †Elisabeth Ihre, and †Olle Zetterström

*Departments of Physiology and Pharmacology, †Thoracic Medicine at Karolinska Hospital, ‡Medical Biochemistry and Biophysics, and §Institute of Environmental Medicine, Karolinska Institutet, S-171 77 Stockholm, Sweden*

At the first Interlaken meeting in 1989, experimental data were presented (1) that gave considerable support to the hypothesis that leukotrienes (LT) were important mediators of asthma and inflammation. For example, it could be demonstrated that cysteinyl leukotrienes ($LTC_4$, $LTD_4$, and $LTE_4$) were the major mediators of IgE-dependent contraction of isolated human bronchi (2). However, at that time there were no reports available that directly proved leukotriene involvement in asthmatic reactions in humans. This chapter summarizes our own further studies, which document that cysteinyl leukotrienes indeed mediate airway obstruction in asthmatics. In addition, some recent data indicating heterogeneity of the receptors for cysteinyl leukotrienes are discussed.

## BRONCHOCONSTRICTION PRODUCED BY INHALATION OF LEUKOTRIENES AND ITS INHIBITION BY POTENT RECEPTOR ANTAGONISTS

In line with their potent action on isolated human bronchi (3), inhalation of $LTC_4$ or $LTD_4$ produced a long-lived bronchoconstrictor response in doses that were 100- to 1,000-fold lower than for histamine or methacholine (4–6). There are also indications that the leukotrienes, in addition to their potency and long duration of action, produce greater airway narrowing than stimuli such as metacholine (7). As will be discussed in other chapters of this volume, asthmatics are generally hyperresponsive to inhaled leukotrienes, but some data suggest that the relative sensitivity to the individual cysteinyl leukotrienes may vary. In particular, $LTE_4$ has been proposed to be specifically important in bronchial hyperresponsiveness (8).

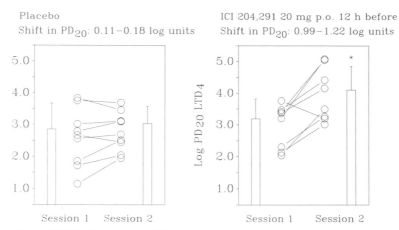

**FIG. 1.** Bronchial challenge with $LTD_4$ was performed twice at an interval of 6 weeks in a group of 16 asthmatics. The $PD_{20}$ (provocative dose causing a 20% decrease in $FEV_1$) for inhaled $LTD_4$ was determined from the dose–response curve at each occasion. **Left:** The excellent repeatability of the challenge in the group ($n = 9$) that received placebo (connected open circles show individual data and bars display group geometric mean $PD_{20}$ values). **Right:** Shows how the leukotriene antagonist ICI-204,219 protects against the $LTD_4$ bronchoconstriction. The average group ($n = 8$) shift in the $PD_{20}$ for $LTD_4$ amounts to about one log order of magnitude. The $LTD_4$ challenge was performed 12 hr after intake of ICI-204,219, i.e., at trough plasma level.

Several of the potent second-generation leukotriene receptor antagonists have now entered the initial clinical stage. The first studies confirmed their ability to inhibit responses to leukotrienes in human subjects (9). The most potent antagonist thus far available, ICI-204,219, has been administered in doses (40 mg) that caused more than a 100-fold displacement of the dose–response curve to inhaled $LTD_4$. We recently observed that a lower dose (20 mg) of ICI-204,219 produced about one log order of magnitude of shift in the $PD_{20}$ for inhaled $LTD_4$ even at 12 hr after dosing (Fig. 1).

## RELEASE OF LEUKOTRIENES DURING ASTHMATIC RESPONSES

Previous studies had shown that $LTE_4$ is the end metabolite of the cysteinyl leukotrienes in human lung (10), and a significant proportion of inhaled $LTD_4$ can be recovered as $LTE_4$ in human urine (11). From animal and human studies it appeared that the fraction, some 10% to 20% of injected $LTE_4$, recovered in urine was fairly constant provided that renal and hepatic function was normal (see also Keppler et al., *this volume*). Therefore, urinary $LTE_4$ was selected as an index to monitor endogenous formation of leukotrienes in humans and a radioimmunoassay (RIA) was used for the measurements (12).

First, HPLC purification confirmed that under basal conditions $LTE_4$ was

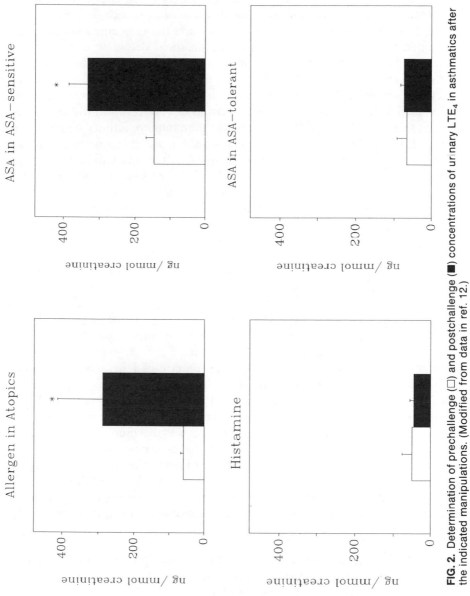

**FIG. 2.** Determination of prechallenge (□) and postchallenge (■) concentrations of urinary LTE$_4$ in asthmatics after the indicated manipulations. (Modified from data in ref. 12.)

the only cysteinyl leukotriene present in significant amounts in hourly collected samples of urine. Second, allergen challenge of atopic asthmatics was followed by the appearance of increased concentrations of immunoreactive $LTE_4$ in the urine (Fig. 2). The elevation of urinary $LTE_4$ occurred within 30 to 60 min after the appearance of a significant airway response [20% drop in $FEV_1$ (forced expiratory volume in 1 sec)], and the concentration of $LTE_4$ remained elevated for 1 to 3 hr after the maximal decrease in pulmonary function. In addition, the increase in immunoreactive $LTE_4$ after challenge consisted almost exclusively of $LTE_4$, as demonstrated by immunoassay of fractions separated by HPLC. In urine samples from subjects who had inhaled high doses of $LTD_4$, some $LTD_4$ could be recovered in the urine, but also in this case the major component of the immunoreactivity consisted of $LTE_4$. It was further observed that significant but variable amounts of $LTE_4$ were lost during the purification of samples. After this validation, it was therefore decided to routinely measure $LTE_4$ by RIA in unpurified urine.

Further studies showed that the increase in urinary $LTE_4$ after allergen challenge appeared to be dose-dependent. Thus, when a group of asthmatics was challenged with both a low and a high dose of allergen, the urinary $LTE_4$ was higher after the high dose (12). To determine whether or not the increase in urinary $LTE_4$ was a consequence of the bronchoconstrictor response, another group of subjects inhaled histamine to produce the same degree of airway obstruction as during the provocations with allergen. However, the bronchoconstriction induced by histamine was not associated with increased urinary $LTE_4$ (Fig. 2), suggesting that the cysteinyl leukotrienes were formed as a consequence of the primary antigen–antibody reaction rather than being secondary to the airflow obstruction.

Interestingly, when urinary $LTE_4$ was determined in aspirin-sensitive asthmatics subjected to inhalation challenge with lysine–aspirin, urinary $LTE_4$ increased after the aspirin-induced bronchoconstriction (Fig. 2). In asthmatics for whom inhalation of aspirin was tolerated, the post-challenge urinary $LTE_4$ remained at basal levels (Fig. 2). Furthermore, when the basal (prechallenge) levels of urinary $LTE_4$ in the aspirin-sensitive asthmatics were compared with those of aspirin-tolerant asthmatics, there was a highly significant elevation of $LTE_4$ among the aspirin-intolerant asthmatics (12) (Fig. 2). As discussed below, these findings in aspirin-sensitive asthmatics suggested that leukotrienes may also be mediators of aspirin-induced airway obstruction.

## INHIBITION OF ALLERGEN-INDUCED AIRWAY OBSTRUCTION IN ASTHMATICS BY DRUGS THAT BLOCK THE ACTION OR FORMATION OF LEUKOTRIENES

Shortly after returning from the first Interlaken meeting in 1989, we conducted a study in which the influence on allergen-induced airway obstruction

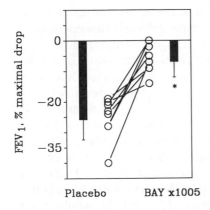

**FIG. 3.** Inhibition of allergen-induced airway obstruction in asthmatics by the leukotriene biosynthesis inhibitor BAY X1005 (750 mg p.o. 4 hr before challenge). The maximal drop in $FEV_1$ after bronchoprovocation with allergen is displayed for the two sessions in all individuals by open circles connected with a line. The group means are shown as bars (error bars indicate SD). The average inhibition of this response by BAY X 1005 was about 75%.

of a single oral dose of the receptor antagonist ICI-204,219 was evaluated in a group of 10 men with atopic asthma. The results were very encouraging and were presented the next year at the International Conference on Prostaglandins and Related Compounds in Florence (13). There was a highly significant and major inhibition of the early airway reaction to inhaled allergen after ingestion of ICI-204,219. Subsequently, Taylor et al. (14) and Rasmussen et al. (15) demonstrated that the late asthmatic reaction may also be inhibited by receptor antagonists of cysteinyl leukotrienes.

More recently, we have studied whether or not inhibition of leukotriene formation may inhibit the allergen-induced airway obstruction in atopic asthmatics. The recently developed inhibitor of five lipoxygenase activation BAY X1005 was used for this study. Before the allergen provocation study, we had documented that this compound inhibited IgE-dependent contractions of isolated human bronchi, as well as allergic inflammation in the hamster cheek pouch (16). When eight subjects were challenged with a single dose of allergen after oral pretreatment with placebo or BAY X1005, there was a uniform and highly significant inhibition of the allergen-induced bronchoconstriction by BAY X1005 (Fig. 3).

The demonstration that either a specific receptor antagonist or a potent biosynthesis inhibitor produced similar and striking inhibition of the allergen-induced airway obstruction in atopic asthmatics, strongly supports the view that cysteinyl leukotrienes are major mediators of this response in humans. As discussed above, it appears that these leukotrienes also contribute to airflow obstruction during the late asthmatic reaction. It can be speculated that the mast cell is the major source of the leukotrienes during the early phase and that the eosinophil may provide the leukotrienes during the late reaction.

## LEUKOTRIENES AS MEDIATORS OF ASPIRIN-INDUCED ASTHMA

After the observations that aspirin-intolerant asthmatics had a basal overproduction of leukotrienes and that the urinary $LTE_4$ increased further in association with the intolerance reaction, the next step was to test whether leukotriene antagonists could influence the aspirin-induced bronchoconstriction. A previous study addressing this issue had produced ambiguous results (17). Eight asthmatics (mean age 45 years) with an average history of asthma and aspirin sensitivity of about 10 years' duration were therefore subjected to bronchial provocation with lysine–aspirin. Baseline aspirin sensitivity was first determined in an open prestudy session by inhalation of cumulative doses of lysine–aspirin to establish $PD_{20}$ (the provocative dose of aspirin decreasing $FEV_1$ by 20%). Rechallenge with lysine–aspirin was performed under double-blind conditions in a randomized crossover design on two different occasions, 1 hr after oral administration of placebo or 750 mg of the cysteinyl leukotriene receptor antagonist MK-0679. The lysine–aspirin challenge was highly reproducible [geometric mean $PD_{20}$ for the whole group being $37 \pm 2$ μmol at the open prestudy day and $34 \pm 2$ μmol at the placebo sessions (mean $\pm$ SD)]. In contrast, after MK-0679 there was a right shift in the dose–response relations for inhaled lysine–aspirin, consistent with the hypothesis that in the presence of the receptor antagonist for leukotrienes higher doses of aspirin were required to trigger formation of leukotrienes sufficient to surmount the competetive antagonist and produce the stipulated airway response. It was in fact documented that the postchallenge increase of urinary $LTE_4$ was substantially elevated after MK-0679. For all eight subjects the mean shift in $PD_{20}$ was more than fourfold. (In the presence of the antagonist, three of the subjects failed to reach a 20% decrease in $FEV_1$ despite inhalation of the highest dose of lysine–aspirin feasible to deliver. This highest dose was used as $PD_{20}$ value in these subjects, and therefore underestimated the magnitude of shift in $PD_{20}$.) In conclusion, the leukotriene antagonist MK-0679 substantially inhibited the airway response to inhalation of lysine–aspirin (18), providing direct evidence that leukotrienes are mediators of aspirin–induced bronchoconstriction.

Further studies showed that a higher dose of the same leukotriene-receptor antagonist, MK-0679, was able to produce a long-lasting improvement in baseline pulmonary function when given to a group of aspirin-sensitive asthmatics (19). The response was significant for the whole group ($n = 8$) and was on average about 80% of the maximal bronchodilatation produced by inhalation of a nebulized solution of the β-stimulant salbutamol. However, the magnitude of the response varied among individuals. Further analysis indicated that the degree of bronchodilatation correlated directly with the severity of their asthma. As an illustration, the baseline pulmonary function in one of the most severe aspirin-sensitive subjects is shown for placebo- and active drug-treated days in Fig. 4. Interestingly, this subject, as well as some of the other best responders, was treated with high doses of inhaled glucocorticosteroids, suggesting that leukotriene antagonists may have anti-asthmatic effects that are additive to those of glucocorticoids.

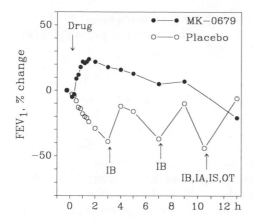

**FIG. 4.** Example of bronchodilator response to a leukotriene antagonist: basal pulmonary function in one aspirin-sensitive asthmatic during 2 study days (placebo or the leukotriene antagonist MK-679). Rescue treatments given on the placebo day as indicated: IB, inhaled β-stimulant; IA, inhaled atropine; IS, inhaled steroid; OT, oral theophylline.

## LEUKOTRIENES AS A FINAL COMMON PATH IN AIRWAY OBSTRUCTION

In parallel with our own studies reported above, the results of other investigators have provided further evidence that many different asthmatic responses can be blunted significantly by drugs that inhibit the action or formation of leukotrienes. Drazen and co-workers reported inhibition of the airway obstruction induced by inhalation of cold, dry air after treatment with the 5-lipoxygenase inhibitor zileuton (20). Pretreatment with leukotriene-receptor antagonists also causes a distinct attenuation of exercise-induced bronchoconstriction (21,22). Taken together, the data available at this time support the conclusion that cysteinyl leukotrienes mediate a major component of the airway obstruction induced by allergens, dry cold air, and exercise, and by aspirin in aspirin-sensitive asthmatics. This leads to the hypothesis that release of leukotrienes is a final common path for different triggers of asthmatic reactions, despite distinct mechanisms being involved in the induction of the responses to these triggers. Such a critical position of leukotrienes in the distal end of different cascades converging into airway obstruction presumably supports the hypothesis that antileukotriene drugs may provide new strategies for the treatment of asthma and airway inflammation. Future studies with antileukotriene drugs in the treatment of asthmatics will define the extent to which this approach will be useful. Obviously, a large number of extensive clinical investigations are required to collect this information.

The results from the initial clinical trials have also generated a number of questions for further basic research into leukotriene mechanisms. As discussed in other chapters of this volume, the enzymes and mechanisms involved in the formation of leukotrienes and the actions of different biosynthetic inhibitors are the subject of considerable attention. Likewise, the nature of the receptors for the leukotrienes is far from being resolved. Therefore, the discussion below addresses issues relating to our present knowledge about the tissue receptors for leukotrienes.

## CLASSIFICATION OF LEUKOTRIENE RECEPTORS

Soon after the discovery of the leukotrienes and the initial studies of the actions of $LTB_4$ and the cysteinyl leukotrienes, it was evident that these two main classes of leukotrienes had distinct activites on certain targets. For example, $LTB_4$ was a potent chemotactic agent with no activity in the classical guinea pig ileum assay, whereas the cysteinyl leukotrienes contracted the latter preparation but had no direct activity in chemotactic assays. Furthermore, the nature of the responses to the leukotrienes (e.g., dose-dependent effects with marked species and tissue variations, presence of specific desensitization, structure–activity requirements) suggested that they acted by binding to specific receptors. The selective antagonism of cysteinyl leukotrienes in many tissues by the antagonist of SRS-A (slow-reacting substance of anaphylaxis) FPL 55712 further supported the idea that there was a specific receptor for each of the two main classes of leukotrienes. In fact, at the Erice NATO meeting in 1982 (23) we provisionally described them as "B-type" and "C-type" LT receptors.

When binding studies were performed, the complexity of the issue increased. For $LTB_4$, high- and low-affinity binding sites were identified in PMN leukocytes, and there appeared to be a functional correlation because the tentative high-affinity receptor mediated chemotaxis, chemokinesis, and leukocyte adherence, whereas the low-affinity site was responsible for enzyme release and production of superoxide anion. For the cysteinyl leukotrienes, distinct binding of radiolabeled $LTC_4$ and $LTD_4$ was observed in several tissues, but the demonstration that liver glutathione transferase could bind $LTC_4$ with a high affinity (24) called into question the relevance of $LTC_4$ binding in many tissues. Another problem with the interpretation of binding data is that at least the initial studies did not take into account the tissue metabolism of leukotrienes. Binding studies with labeled antagonists have been limited, and ICI-198,615 is the only ligand available. Furthermore, high- and low-affinity binding sites have been demonstrated for both the $LTB_4$ receptor and the $LTD_4$ receptor. Sometimes this appears to correlate with distinct functional responses, as for $LTB_4$ in the leukocyte. However, with no strong evidence for agonist or antagonist selectivity at the two sites, it is open to debate if high- and low-affinity sites should be considered as distinct subclasses. In particular, for G-protein–coupled receptors, the two sites may reflect different activity states in the recycling of receptor–G-protein complexes.

From functional studies originally performed in the guinea pig trachea

(25), it was apparent that in several tissues the functional responses to $LTC_4$ could be distinguished from those of $LTD_4$, including differences in sensitivity to FPL 55712 and subsequently developed antagonists. This led to the subclassification of cysteinyl leukotriene receptors into $LTC_4$ and $LTD_4$ receptors. For a while this seemed appropriate, but with time observations accumulated that could not be accommodated within the simple scheme of one receptor each for $LTB_4$, $LTC_4$, and $LTD_4$. Although $LTE_4$ often showed binding to the $LTD_4$ receptor, it was sometimes inhibitory and there was a discrepancy in the results of functional and binding assays.

When the effects of the individual cysteinyl leukotrienes were characterized on human airway smooth muscle, the main target of the clinical development, it was clear that $LTC_4$, $LTD_4$, and $LTE_4$ each acted at one and the same FPL 55712-sensitive receptor (26). In other words, the receptor in human airways was unselective for the three biologically active constituents of SRS-A. With the development of a large number of structurally dissimilar antagonists of cysteinyl leukotrienes, it has been documented that all inhibit $LTD_4$ binding and functional responses to $LTD_4$ in the guinea pig trachea and ileum, as well as the effects of $LTC_4$, $LTD_4$, and $LTE_4$ on human bronchi. However, all of these antagonists fail to block the direct actions of $LTC_4$ in the guinea pig ileum and trachea, in particular when its metabolism to $LTD_4$ is arrested.

The findings are therefore consistent with the presence of a separate receptor for $LTC_4$ and $LTD_4$ in tissues such as guinea pig ileum and trachea but of the same receptor for these two leukotrienes in other preparations, most notably human bronchus. In addition, there is also unequivocal evidence of tissues (e.g., ferret trachea and spleen) in which $LTC_4$ and $LTD_4$ both cause contractions that are unaffected by the presently available antagonists. We have observed the presence of this atypical receptor in sheep trachea (27). In several of these preparations $LTE_4$ behaves as a partial agonist, with ability to selectively inhibit the actions of $LTC_4$ and $LTD_4$.

At this stage, it appears important, first, to recognize that heterogeneity exists among the receptors for cysteinyl leukotrienes and, second, to adopt a classification of the leukotriene receptors that accommodates our present understanding but admits lack of knowledge in certain areas. The agonist-related classification ($LTC_4$ and $LTD_4$ receptors) is inappropriate. It would be more useful to use a classification that is focused on the properties of the receptors, as defined by selective antagonists. Drazen and co-workers suggested "LTR-1" and "LTR-2" for the $LTD_4$ and $LTC_4$ receptors, respectively. Krell et al., at the first Interlaken meeting, proposed that the $LTC_4$ receptor was named $pLT_1$ and the $LTD_4$ receptor(s) $pLT_2$ (prefix "p" for peptide leukotriene). On the basis of differences in functional and binding properties, evidence was also presented by Krell et al. (28) to support the presence of four subtypes of the $pLT_2$ receptor. As an alternative, here we propose that the conventional cysteinyl leukotriene receptors be named $LT_1$

receptors, giving the atypical receptors for cysteinyl leukotrienes the name $LT_2$ and the receptor(s) for $LTB_4$ the name $LT_3$. Thus, all described cysteinyl leukotriene antagonists block the effects of the agonists at the $LT_1$ class of receptors. Although data support (see above) that subclasses exist among the $LT_1$ receptor, the proposed classification is focused on the basic difference that some cysteinyl leukotriene effects are antagonized by the present generation of cysteinyl leukotriene antagonists, whereas other effects are resistant to these antagonists. No selective antagonists of the $LT_2$ receptor have been described thus far. The further subdivision among $LT_1$ receptors is left until more information has accumulated. For the $LT_3$ receptor, a new generation of selective antagonists with increasing potency and bioavailability is presently appearing.

In naming the receptors, another alternative would be to include the distinct differences between the receptors for $LTB_4$ and the cysteinyl leukotrienes in the names. In this context, it should be recognized that peptidoleukotrienes include $LTC_4$ and $LTD_4$ but not $LTE_4$, which contains only the single amino acid cysteine. Therefore, the name cysteinyl leukotrienes must be used to describe $LTC_4$, $LTD_4$, and $LTE_4$ as a group. The simplest abbreviations would be C-LTs or cys-LTs. $LTB_4$ and its metabolites would consequently be collectively named B-LTs. This would lead to the name B-LT receptor for $LTB_4$, and $C-LT_1$ for the conventional and $C-LT_2$ for the atypical receptor for cysteinyl leukotrienes.

Another problem with the present data on leukotriene receptors is that their possible relations to other eicosanoid receptors have generally been tested only to a limited extent. In particular, we know little about the receptors for related lipoxygenase products such as the mono-HETEs (5-HETE, 12-HETE, and 15-HETE), di-HETEs (e.g., 5S,12S-diHETE, 5S,6R-diHETE), tri-HETEs, including lipoxins, and also the many monooxygenase products. Certain interactions are known, e.g., 12R-HETE is a rather potent agonist at the $LTB_4$ receptor, and lipoxin $A_4$ and 5S,6R-diHETE are agonists at some but not all receptors for cysteinyl leukotrienes (29). In fact, some of the receptors here called atypical leukotriene receptors may be receptors for other eicosanoids with crossreactivity for certain leukotrienes.

Gardiner et al. (*this volume*) propose a classification for leukotriene receptors which, as for the prostanoids, is a combination of evidence based on agonist and antagonist properties. Thus, the receptor for $LTB_4$ is named the BL receptor and the family of receptors for cysteinyl leukotrienes are named PL (peptidoleukotriene) receptors. The conventional receptors are then designated PL-1, without further subgroups. On the basis of new evidence indicating that the compound BAY u9773 may inhibit some but not all atypical responses to cysteinyl leukotrienes. Gardiner introduces the names PL-2 and PL-3 for receptors that are sensitive and insensitive, respectively, to this new compound, which is a derivative of $LTE_4$. It should be mentioned that BAY u9773 also is an antagonist at the PL-1 receptor, indicating that it is not selective for the PL-2 but appears to have a broader activity than all other described LT antagonists.

Together, the appearance of these proposals at this meeting strongly supports the idea that it is time to discontinue the use of the preliminary classification of the leukotriene receptors as being specific for $LTB_4$, $LTC_4$, and $LTD_4$. Time will show which particular new classification will be accepted by the scientific community. More important will be to increase the information about the functions of different receptors for leukotrienes, possibly resulting in development of tissue-selective antagonists with enhanced therapeutic value compared with the present generation of antagonists.

## ACKNOWLEDGMENT

The work described was supported by grants from the Swedish Medical Research Council (project 14X-09071, 14X-04342, 03X-5915), the Swedish Association Against Chest and Heart Diseases, the Swedish Association Against Asthma and Allergy (RmA), the Swedish National Board for Laboratory Animals (CFN), the Scientific Council of the Swedish Association Against Use of Experimental Animals in Research, the Institute of Environmental Medicine, the Swedish Environment Protection Board (5324069-3), and Karolinska Institutet.

## REFERENCES

1. Samuelsson B, Dahlén S-E, Fritsch J, Hedqvist P, eds. *Advances in prostaglandin, thromboxane, and leukotriene research,* Vol. 20. New York: Raven Press; 1990.
2. Dahlén S-E, Björck T, Kumlin M, Granström E, Hedqvist P. In: Samuelsson B, Dahlén S-E, Fritsch J, Hedqvist P, eds. *Advances in prostaglandin, thromboxane, and leukotriene research,* Vol. 20. New York: Raven Press; 1990:193–200.
3. Dahlén S-E, Hedqvist P, Hammarström S, Samuelsson B. *Nature* 1980;288:484–6.
4. Holroyde MC, Altounyan REC, Cole M, Dixon M, Elliott EV. *Lancet* 1981;6:17–8.
5. Weiss JW, Drazen JM, Coles N, McFadden ER Jr, et al. *Science* 1982;216:196–8.
6. Barnes NC, Piper PJ, Costello JF. *Thorax* 1984;39:500–4.
7. Bel EH, Van Der Veen H, Kramps JA, Dijkman JH, Sterk PJ. *Am Rev Respir Dis* 1987; 136:979–84.
8. Arm JP, O'Hickey SP, Hawksworth RJ, et al. *Am Rev Respir Dis* 1990;142:1112–8.
9. Smith LJ, Geller S, Ebright L, Glass M, Thyrum PT. *Am Rev Respir Dis* 1990;141:988–92.
10. Kumlin M, Dahlén S-E. *Biochem Biophys Acta* 1990;1044:201–10.
11. Verhagen J, Bel EH, Kijne GM, et al. *Biochem Biophys Res Commun* 1987;148:864–8.
12. Kumlin M, Dahlén B, Björck T, Zetterström O, Granström E, Dahlén S-E: *Am Rev Respir Dis* 1992;146:96–103.
13. Dahlén S-E, Dahlén B, Eliasson E, et al. In: Samuelsson B, Ramwell PW, Paoletti R, Folco GC, Gramström E, eds. *Advances in prostaglandin, thromboxane, and leukotriene research,* Vol. 21. New York: Raven Press; 1991:461–4.
14. Taylor IK, O'Shaoughnessy KM, Fuller RW, Dollery CT. *Lancet* 1991;337:690–4.
15. Rasmussen JB, Eriksson LO, Margolskee DJ, Tagari P, Williams VC, Andersson KE. *J Allergy Clin Immunol* 1992;90:193–201.
16. Hedqvist P, Lindbom L, Palmertz U, Raud J. *Advances in prostaglandin, thromboxane, and leukotriene research,* Vol. 22. New York: Raven Press; 1994:91–9 (this volume).
17. Christie PE, Smith CM, Lee TH. *Am Rev Respir Dis* 1991;144:957–8.

18. Dahlén B, Kumlin M, Margolskee DJ, et al. *Eur Resp J* 1993;6:1018–23.
19. Dahlén B, Margolskee DJ, Zetterström O, Dahlén S-E. *Thorax* 1993;48:1205–10.
20. Israel E, Dermarkarian R, Rosenberg M, et al. *N Engl J Med* 1990;323:1740–4.
21. Manning PJ, Watson RM, Margolskee DJ, Williams VC, Schwartz JI, O'Byrne PM. *N Engl J Med* 1990;323:1736–9.
22. Finnerty JP, Wood-Baker R, Thomson H, Holgate ST. *Am Rev Respir Dis* 1992;145:746–9.
23. Hedqvist P, Dahlén S-E, Björk J. In: Berti F, Folco GC, Velo GP, eds. *Leukotrienes and prostacyclin*. New York: Plenum Press; 1983:81–107.
24. Sun FF, Chau L-Y, Spur B, Corey EJ, Lewis RA, Austen KF. *J Biol Chem* 1986;261:8540–6.
25. Krell RD, Tsai BS, Berdoulay A, Barone M, Giles RE. *Prostaglandins* 1983;25:171–8.
26. Buckner CK, Krell RD, Laravuso RB, Coursin DB, Bernstein PR, Will JA. *J Pharmacol Exp Ther* 1986;237:558–62.
27. Björck T, Harada Y, Dahlén S-E. *Am Rev Respir Dis* 1991;143:A635 (abst).
28. Krell RD, Aharony D, Buckner CK, Kusner EJ. In: Samuelsson B, Dahlén S-E, Fritsch J, Hedqvist P, eds. *Advances in prostaglandin, thromboxane, and leukotriene research*, Vol. 20. New York: Raven Press; 1990:119–26.
29. Dahlén S-E, Serhan CN. In: Crooke ST, Wong A, eds. *Lipoxygenases and their products*. San Diego: Academic Press; 1991:235–75.

*Advances in Prostaglandin, Thromboxane, and Leukotriene Research*, Vol. 22, edited by S.-E. Dahlén et al. Raven Press, Ltd., New York © 1994

# Release of Urinary Leukotriene $E_4$ in Asthmatic Subjects: A Review

I. K. Taylor

*Department of Respiratory Medicine, Chest and Allergy Clinic, St. Mary's Hospital, London W2, 1NY, England*

Among the many inflammatory mediators implicated in asthma, the cysteinyl leukotrienes ($LTC_4$, $LTD_4$, and $LTE_4$), peptidolipid conjugates formed after lipoxygenation of arachidonic acid, have received much attention (1–5). They are generated in vitro after appropriate stimuli, both from lung tissue (6) and from purified inflammatory cells that are of potential relevance in the pathogenesis of asthma, including mast cells (7), monocytes/macrophages (5), and eosinophils (8). The biologic actions of the cysteinyl leukotrienes have been extensively characterized. Within the lung they can impair mucociliary clearance, enhance mucous secretion, and facilitate changes in pulmonary vascular permeability (1–5). Their potent spasmogenic properties on human airway smooth muscle both in vitro and in vivo have similarly been comprehensively documented (9,10), and further evidence suggests they provoke rises in airway reactivity (11,12). These inherent properties, which reproduce many of the functional and histologic features of clinical asthma, have therefore generated considerable interest in the measurement and quantification of cysteinyl leukotrienes in biologic fluids in vivo in human asthmatic subjects.

It is axiomatic that the most suitable place to measure inflammatory mediators is at their putative site of action. The nose is readily accessible to evaluate mediator production, and cysteinyl leukotrienes have been quantified in nasal secretions after local allergen challenge (13,14). The use of fiberoptic bronchoscopy coupled with bronchoalveolar lavage (BAL), now permits similar studies in the lower respiratory tract, and abundant evidence now exists with regard to cellular profiles, their activation status, and secretory products within the asthmatic airway under both basal and challenged conditions (15–17). Although initial reservations over the safety and tolerability of such procedures were expressed, there is now general acceptance of their use in subjects with asthma of various degrees of severity (18), although doubts remain concerning interpretation of BAL solute data (19). Plasma sampling and interpretation of data are less difficult, but plasma concentrations of proinflammatory mediators are, in many cases, exceedingly low, making detection and quantification difficult. Furthermore, invasive sampling may result in ex vivo generation of mediators secondary to activation of inflammatory cells, and repeated measurements are required to give a time-integrated insight into their production.

Biochemical analysis of urine circumvents many of these problems. In the absence of renal synthesis, urinary mediator (or metabolite) levels will reflect plasma levels. Urine collections are easy to perform and are noninvasive, and because urine is essentially free of cells, the potential problem of ex vivo production of mediators is minimized. In humans, $LTE_4$ is the stable bioconversion product of cysteinyl leukotriene metabolism in the lung (20), and many studies (21–25) have now evaluated the metabolism, elimination, and pharmacodynamics of $LTE_4$ excretion into urine after either intravenous infusion of $LTC_4$ (21,22) and $LTE_4$ (23) or inhalation of $LTD_4$ (24,25). These findings, in consensus, have demonstrated the rapid excretion into urine of $LTE_4$, either as an intact molecule or after enzymatic conversion from $LTC_4$ and $LTD_4$, within 4 hr of either systemic or pulmonary administration. In the absence of renal or hepatic dysfunction, measurement of urinary $LTE_4$ excretion can be used to assess endogenous whole-body cysteinyl leukotriene production in vivo in human subjects. To date, this has been utilized both in acute severe asthma and in a wide variety of laboratory-based direct and indirect bronchoconstrictor challenges. The modulatory effects of many anti-asthma therapies on urinary $LTE_4$ excretion have also been evaluated. A consensus of these observations, and the conclusions that can be drawn, form the basis of this review.

## MEASUREMENT OF URINARY LTE₄

The methodology for measurement of urinary $LTE_4$ has been extensively reported (26,27) and will be only briefly discussed here. Quantification is best facilitated by a combination of single-step on-line extraction/reverse-phase HPLC coupled to radioimmunoassay, which minimizes handling steps and consequently increases yields. The incorporation of a chemically identical tritiated internal standard permits accurate definition of endogenous $LTE_4$ in the biologic sample; furthermore, this allows background crossreacting immunoreactive impurities to be defined and quantified.

## CLINICAL STUDIES

Pathogenetic roles for the leukotrienes have been suggested in a wide variety of organ specific pathologies. These include hepatorenal syndromes, myocardial ischemia, and inflammatory conditions of the bowel, skin, and joints. Furthermore, although their pathophysiologic effects have implicated these products in a number of respiratory conditions, my comments are confined to their role in asthma and to a lesser extent, in allergic rhinitis.

There are a number of reports, largely performed in asthmatic patients (but some in normal volunteers), in which parallel observations of airway physiology and urinary $LTE_4$ excretion have been made. Essentially, these studies fall into four major categories. First are those studies in which measurements of urinary $LTE_4$ have been made after administration to the airway of either direct or indirect bronchoconstrictor challenges. The putative role of cysteinyl leukotrienes in each of these challenges, where applicable, is briefly discussed, followed by the experimental data. Second are those studies in which urinary $LTE_4$ has been assessed during disease exacerbations and, third, those in which observations were performed under basal conditions. Finally, studies are discussed in which there have been attempts to pharmacologically modulate urinary $LTE_4$ excretion, either under basal physiologic conditions or after bronchoprovocative stimuli, with a variety of therapeutic agents.

## Urinary $LTE_4$ Excretion after Airway Challenge

### Indirect Challenges

### Allergen Challenge

Activation of mast cells, classically by IgE-dependent mechanisms, results in release of inflammatory mediators such as histamine, prostaglandin $D_2$, and cysteinyl leukotrienes, and it is the end-organ response to these mediators that accounts for many features of the immediate bronchial response to inhaled allergen. A number of studies (25,28–33) have now demonstrated, without exception, elevations in urinary $LTE_4$ excretion during early allergen-evoked bronchoconstriction compared with immediate prechallenge basal data or similarly unchallenged control urine collections: these complement data from BAL analysis (15). Although the magnitude of the increase in urinary $LTE_4$ excretion differs among studies, which may be due at least in part to variable durations of urine collections and dissimilar protocols for allergen administration, the qualitative message is the same and represents an important observation. Interestingly, whereas some of these studies have demonstrated significant correlations between the magnitude of bronchoconstriction during the early response (reported as percent maximal falls in $FEV_1$) and urinary $LTE_4$ excretion (29,30), others have failed to do so (25,28,31). This issue will be addressed later. Indeed, some would argue that given the time-integrated nature of urine collections, similar integrated analysis of the bronchoconstrictor data (such as area under the $FEV_1$ time curve) should be applied.

In contrast to the well-characterized elevation in urinary $LTE_4$ excretion during the first 2 to 3 hr after allergen challenge (25,28–33), comparable elevations during later allergen-evoked bronchoconstrictor responses are equivocal and have proved more difficult to interpret despite the demonstration of these products locally in the lung (34). Whereas the early response to allergen is largely mast-cell mediated, later allergen-evoked bronchoconstriction is characterized by eosinophilic and T lymphocyte infiltration and activation, the concomitant morphologic features of airway inflammation, and the development of heightened airway reactivity. Some studies have reported no significant increase in urinary $LTE_4$ excretion during late-phase bronchoconstriction (29,30) which is particularly convincing when short sequential urine collections have been adopted (30). In another study (25) in which data on late-phase bronchoconstriction were not commented on, the rises in urinary $LTE_4$ evoked by an early response quickly fell toward prechallenge values as the airflow obstruction resolved. In contrast, other workers (28,32) have observed elevated levels of urinary $LTE_4$ at 6 hr after allergen challenge which, despite being associated with significant bronchoconstriction, did not reach statistical significance. Similarly, Westcott et al. (31) found no correlation between the increase in urinary $LTE_4$ excreted during the 12 hr after allergen challenge and the severity of the late (3- to 12-hr) response, although significant elevations in urinary $LTE_4$ (up to 36 hr) were observed in those patients with the most severe late-phase bronchoconstriction. Therefore, it is not clear whether these observations during later allergen-evoked bronchoconstriction represent de novo cysteinyl leukotriene biosynthesis and release, which is *possibly* eosinophil derived, or continued excretion of $LTE_4$ formed some hours previously during the acute response. This issue has still not been clarified, even with the demonstration of significant abrogation of the late allergen-induced bronchoconstriction by potent leukotriene receptor antagonists (35).

### Exercise and Cold Air Challenge

It has long been recognized that exercise is a common stimulus of bronchoconstriction in asthmatic subjects, although the exact pathogenetic sequence of events underlying its causation remains unclear. A number of mechanisms have been proposed, including mast-cell mediator release secondary to respiratory water loss and hyperosmolar provocation and vascular phenomena provoking edema formation within the airway wall. Data relating to the participation of inflammatory mediators in either the maintainance or induction of the bronchoconstriction evoked by exercise are conflicting. Indeed, initial contradictory reports in studies in plasma (36) have been superseded by equivocal evidence in bronchoalveolar lavage (37,38).

Recent studies (39–42) have implicated the cysteinyl leukotrienes in the pathogenesis of both exercise- and cold air-induced asthma. Manning et al. (39), using the highly potent and selective intravenous $LTD_4$-receptor antagonist MK-571, demonstrated marked attenuation of exercise-induced bronchoconstriction, suggesting an important role for $LTD_4$ in the genesis of airflow obstruction that develops in human asthmatic subjects after exercise. A similar observation has been reported with the equally potent oral $LTD_4$-receptor antagonist ICI 204.219 (40). Furthermore, the bronchoconstriction evoked by hyperventilation of cold, dry air (which is believed to share the same mechanism as that after exercise), is ameliorated by both selective inhibition of the 5-lipoxygenase enzyme (41) and by end-organ receptor blockade (42).

To further evaluate the role of cysteinyl leukotrienes in exercise-induced bronchoconstriction, urinary $LTE_4$ has been measured in several studies (32,36,43). In contrast to allergen challenge (32), urinary $LTE_4$ excretion did not change significantly in the 24 hr after exercise. In a complementary study (36), but of different design, exercise-induced bronchoconstriction was not associated with an increased excretion of urinary $LTE_4$ within the 3-hr period of study compared with equibronchoconstricting doses of the direct-acting cholinergic agonist methacholine. By contrast, another study conducted in children showed a small (less than twofold) but significant increase in urinary $LTE_4$ (43). Cold air challenge is not associated with elevations in urinary $LTE_4$ (GW Taylor, unpublished data). Therefore, in contrast to allergen-induced bronchoconstriction, there is little evidence for enhanced cysteinyl leukotriene generation in exercise-induced bronchoconstriction as assessed by urinary $LTE_4$. If local release and subsequent participation of functionally active cysteinyl leukotrienes in the pathways that ultimately lead to bronchoconstriction after exercise challenge do occur, these are of insufficient magnitude to perturb urinary $LTE_4$ excretion.

## PAF Challenge

The role of the ether-linked alkyl phospholipid platelet-activating factor (PAF) in asthma has attracted much attention in recent years, although its precise role in asthma pathogenesis is not clear. In common with other inflammatory mediators, PAF is capable of reproducing many of the functional and histologic features seen in asthma both in vivo and in vitro, including microvascular leakage, bronchoconstriction, and inflammatory cell activation. Despite causing bronchoconstriction after inhalation in humans (44–46), PAF does not possess direct contractile effects on human airway smooth muscle strips in cell-free media in vitro (47), suggesting that some of its function in vivo may be mediated indirectly through the release of secondary mediators. In support of this, generation of leukotrienes in response to PAF has been described from a number of animal preparations and purified human cells in vitro (48).

To evaluate whether the bronchoconstricting effect of inhaled PAF in human asthmatic subjects could be mediated through secondary release of cysteinyl leukotrienes, urinary $LTE_4$ excretion was measured after inhalational challenges with PAF, methacholine, and isotonic saline (48). Saline caused no change in airway physiology, as measured by specific airway conductance (sGaw). In contrast, the bronchoconstriction provoked by PAF (which was matched by methacholine) was rapid in onset, short-lived, and associated with extrapulmonary effects, including facial suffusion and warmth. Urinary $LTE_4$ excretion after inhaled PAF was elevated tenfold above the control challenges in 4-hr urine collections. No correlation, however, was observed between urinary $LTE_4$ excretion and maximal falls in SGaw, or area under the SGaw time curve for the periods 0 to 60 or 0 to 240 min. These data imply that cysteinyl leukotrienes mediate, at least in part, some of the acute bronchoconstricting effects of inhaled PAF in human asthmatic subjects in vivo. Subsequent support for a direct contributory role of the cysteinyl leukotrienes in the airway response to PAF in humans has been demonstrated by the marked abrogatory effect of the selective cysteinyl leukotriene receptor antagonists SKF 104353 (49) and ICI 204,219 (50) on PAF-induced bronchoconstriction. Furthermore, the oral PAF receptor antagonist UK,74505 significantly attenuates PAF-evoked rises in urinary $LTE_4$ (51).

### Aspirin Challenge

A proportion of subjects with asthma are intolerant of aspirin and other nonsteroidal anti-inflammatory drugs, but the etiology of this phenomenon remains unclear. One hypothesis is that inhibition of cyclooxygenase provokes bronchoconstriction via "shunting" of arachidonic acid toward metabolism by cellular lipoxygenases. In support of this, pretreatment of sensitized human bronchus in vitro with indomethacin generates increased $LTC_4$ after immunologic challenge (52). Furthermore, systemic provocations with aspirin in susceptible subjects result in the secretion of inflammatory mediators, including leukotrienes, into nasal lavage fluid (53). Although the capacity of nonsteroidal anti-inflammatory agents to provoke asthma is related both to the dose and to their potency as inhibitors of cyclooxygenase (54), no differences have been demonstrated in vitro in the sensitivity of platelet cyclooxygenase to aspirin inhibition between aspirin-sensitive and aspirin-insensitive asthmatic patients and normal subjects (55).

To test the hypothesis that the bronchoconstriction evoked by aspirin is related to enhanced synthesis and release of cysteinyl leukotrienes, urinary $LTE_4$ excretion has been measured in a number of studies in aspirin-sensitive asthmatic subjects after oral (54,55) or inhalational challenge (25). Christie et al. (54) demonstrated a mean fourfold increase in urinary $LTE_4$ excretion 3 to 6 hr after ingestion of aspirin in sensitive subjects compared to nonsensitive asthmatic controls, which was associated with concomitant airflow obstruction. Similarly, Knapp and co-workers (55) have shown comparable increases in urinary $LTE_4$ during aspirin-evoked bronchoconstriction, which were maximal 3 hr post-ingestion. A further study (25) after bronchial provocation with lysine–acetylsalicylic acid perturbed urinary $LTE_4$ excretion two- to threefold compared to the prechallenge baseline. The magnitude of the increase in urinary $LTE_4$, as demonstrated by Knapp et al. (55), was not correlated with either the dose of aspirin administered, the degree of inhibition of platelet $TXB_2$, or [and in accordance with the study by Christie et al. (54)] the duration or magnitude of airflow obstruction, suggesting that the mechanism of aspirin-induced bronchoconstriction is not directly related to "shunting" of arachidonate metabolism. In support of this, pretreatment with indomethacin in doses that were markedly inhibitory toward cyclooxygenase (30) did not further enhance allergen-evoked bronchoconstriction or urinary $LTE_4$ excretion.

## Adenosine Monophosphate and Sodium Metabisulfite

Both adenosine monophosphate (AMP) and sodium metabisulfite (MBS) mediate indirect bronchoconstriction. The respective mechanisms by which they do so are thought to be via mast-cell degranulation and neurally medicated pathways. Airway responses to both of these spasmogens are attenuated by flurbiprofen, a potent cyclooxygenase inhibitor, suggesting involvement of arachidonate products in their constrictor actions. A recent study by Fuller et al. (56) measured urinary $LTE_4$ after bronchial provocation with AMP, MBS, and methacholine in atopic asthmatic subjects. Although equivalent bronchoconstriction was observed in all three challenges, there was no significant difference in urinary $LTE_4$ excretion.

## Direct Challenges

### Methacholine and Histamine

A number of studies in which urinary $LTE_4$ excretion has been evaluated after indirect bronchial challenges, have incorporated a positive bronchoconstrictor control into their design. Thus, methacholine, the direct-acting cholinergic agonist, has been used for comparative equibronchoconstricting purposes in allergen (31), exercise (36), PAF (48), aspirin (54), and adenosine and metabisulfite (56) challenges. Without exception, despite significant degrees of bronchoconstriction being evoked, methacholine does not significantly perturb urinary $LTE_4$ excretion compared either to "negative" bronchoconstrictor challenges, such as isotonic saline, or to prechallenge basal data. Such data provide information about putative mechanisms by which indirect challenges increase urinary $LTE_4$ excretion, which clearly is not a consequence of bronchial smooth muscle contraction per se. Urinary $LTE_4$ after bronchial challenge with histamine in asthmatic patients has been recently reported (25) and, as with methacholine, does not increase eicosanoid excretion.

## Urinary LTE₄ Excretion During Disease Exacerbations

### Acute Severe Asthma

Given the magnitude of airflow obstruction in acute severe asthma, urinary $LTE_4$ estimations have obvious advantages over more invasive methods of assessing in vivo inflammatory mediator release. Taylor et al. (28) initially observed increases in urinary $LTE_4$ in 24-hr urine collections in patients admitted to hospital with acute severe asthma, although it was noted that there was substantial overlap in this group into the normal range. Furthermore, although urinary $LTE_4$ tended to fall during disease remission, this did not reach statistical significance. Similar observations have been made in another study (26). Drazen et al. (57) have further evaluated the role of cysteinyl leukotrienes in patients presenting acutely with airflow obstruction. These patients received three nebulized doses of salbutamol 20 min apart on arrival in the emergency room, during which time urine for $LTE_4$ estimation was obtained. No other medication was administered, and patients were classified as "responders" or "nonresponders" on the basis of airway reversibility to the administered bronchodilator. Urinary $LTE_4$ excretion was significantly higher in the responders compared with the nonresponders and normal volunteers, although no dynamic assessment of response to treatment using $LTE_4$ was made. Furthermore, given the study design, no evaluation of the possible attenuating effect of $\beta_2$-agonists on endogenous cysteinyl leukotriene release could be made. This study (57), however, provides further strong support for a bronchoconstrictor role of the cysteinyl leukotrienes in acute severe asthma, particularly in those patients in whom bronchoconstriction per se (and by inference, heightened bronchodilator responsiveness) is the major component of the airflow obstruction.

### Allergic Rhinitis

The role of leukotrienes in allergic rhinitis has been extensively reviewed (58). Nasal challenge with antigen has been shown in many studies to provoke local release of cysteinyl leukotrienes; furthermore, their release and the biologic response to nasal allergen challenge are abrogated with 5-lipoxygenase inhibition (59). Although increased levels of $LTC_4$ have been observed in the nasal secretions of children during seasonal exposure to allergen (58), Taylor et al. (28) did not detect any significant elevations in urinary $LTE_4$ excretion in 24-hr urine collections from allergic rhinitis patients studied in and out of the grass pollen season. High, albeit transient, local concentrations of cysteinyl leukotrienes in the nose after appropriate challenge therefore presumably do not perturb whole-body $LTE_4$ excretion, particularly if assessed over long periods. Further, the disparate findings in urinary $LTE_4$ excretion between rhinitis and acute severe asthma may simply reflect reduced inflammatory cell populations in the nose compared to the lower airway, consequent to the smaller mucosal area.

### Urinary LTE₄ Excretion Under Basal Conditions

Recent evidence (15,60–62) suggests that basal airway tone in asthmatic subjects is influenced by endogenous cysteinyl leukotrienes and may be responsible, at least in part, for persistent bronchoconstriction. For example, elevated levels of cysteinyl leukotrienes have been demonstrated in BAL fluid before endobronchial allergen challenge in atopic asthmatic subjects compared with control groups (15). Furthermore, the cysteinyl leukotriene receptor antagonists ICI 204,219 (60) and MK-571 (61), and the hydroxamic acid 5-lipoxygenase inhibitor zileuton (62), have shown significant acute bronchodilatory effects in asthmatics of moderate severity. Although these observations have been supported in prolonged dosing studies in chronic asthma (63,64) and suggest that these agents may be disease-modifying, neither MK-571 nor ICI 204,219 significantly improved baseline pulmonary function before exercise challenge (39,40). This, however, may have been a reflection of the mild nature of the airflow obstruction in the patients studied.

In view of this evidence, baseline observations of urinary $LTE_4$ excretion may also in theory provide useful information. A recent study has reported increased excretion of $LTE_4$ in overnight urine samples in patients with nocturnal asthma (65), which correlated with the magnitude of the morning dip. Several studies have now demonstrated significantly increased (three- to sixfold) basal excretion of urinary $LTE_4$ in aspirin-sensitive asthmatics compared with both aspirin-insensitive asthmatics and normal subjects (25, 54,66). This was further commented on in another study (55) in comparison with other data (30). Interestingly, no relationship was observed between baseline $FEV_1$ and urinary $LTE_4$ excretion in both the aspirin-sensitive and -insensitive asthmatics (25,66), implying that aspirin sensitivity rather than disease severity per se is the explanation for the higher levels of $LTE_4$.

Furthermore, Westcott et al. (31) found no correlation between baseline measurements of $FEV_1$ and urinary $LTE_4$, and others (28,43) have found no difference in urinary $LTE_4$ between asthmatic patients and normal subjects under basal, unchallenged conditions.

Despite the wealth of evidence that airway hyperreactivity to a variety of inhaled spasmogens is a cardinal feature of asthma, the role individual inflammatory mediators may play in generating it is controversial. In asthmatic subjects, inhaled $LTC_4$ potentiates the bronchoconstrictor response to inhaled histamine and $PGD_2$ (67). Arm and colleagues (11) have shown rises in airway reactivity to histamine up to 1 week after a single inhalation of $LTE_4$ in asthmatic but not in normal subjects. The same group reported similar findings over 7 hr with inhaled $LTC_4$ and $LTD_4$ (12). Further support for a direct or indirect role for cysteinyl leukotrienes in the pathogenesis of bronchial hyperreactivity is shown by the abrogatory effect of ICI 204,219 on allergen-evoked hyperresponsiveness (35). Two studies, however (31,66), in which baseline urinary $LTE_4$ excretion and airway reactivity were evaluated showed no relationship. Therefore, with few exceptions, basal urinary $LTE_4$ excretion in the absence of bronchoprovocation or disease exacerbation is not abnormally high. Although the pharmacologic (60–64) and BAL (15) data suggest that in stable, mild-to-moderate asthmatics there are increased local concentrations of cysteinyl leukotrienes in the absence of provocation, this presumably does not lead to a significant increase in whole-body turnover to be reflected in urine. It has been postulated that differences in metabolism and/or clearance of locally generated leukotrienes into urine may differ between normal and asthmatic subjects (66), although a recent study has shown this not to be the case (68).

## Urinary LTE₄ Excretion: Effects of Pharmacologic Modulation

Given the unequivocal demonstration that large increments in urinary $LTE_4$ excretion are observed coincident with allergen-evoked early-phase bronchoconstriction (25,28–33), most but not all of these studies have been designed in this setting.

### Sodium Cromoglycate

Westcott et al. (31) evaluated the attenuating effect of pretreatment with cromoglycate, a putative mast-cell stabilizer, on allergen-evoked rises in urinary $LTE_4$. The drug, administered as two 20-mg nebulizations, abrogated the early response (as demonstrated previously in other studies) but not the late-phase bronchoconstriction after allergen challenge. The elevation in urinary $LTE_4$ excretion in the 12-hr after challenge, however, was not significantly decreased by cromoglycate pretreatment compared to antigen challenge in the absence of the drug. Interestingly, it was noted that in three subjects in whom the drug was markedly bronchoprotective, there was a significant reduction in eicosanoid excretion. This raises an important point that has been addressed by several groups. The tacit assumption that the allergen-evoked rise in urinary $LTE_4$ represents exclusive cysteinyl leukotriene generation within the lung may clearly be an oversimplification. In fact, their precise origin has not been established, and they could arise from extrapulmonary sites. The observation by Westcott et al. (31) suggests that, in some subjects at least, the allergen-provoked elevations in urinary $LTE_4$ do arise from pulmonary mast cells.

## $β_2$-Agonists

$β_2$-Selective agonists are by far the most effective bronchodilators in clinical use. Although reversal of airway smooth-muscle contraction is believed to represent their principal mode of action, considerable in vitro evidence exists suggesting additional properties (69). These include attenuation of inflammatory cell mediator release, including cysteinyl leukotrienes, from pulmonary mast cells and sensitized human lung fragments after immunologic challenge. However, direct in vivo evidence for such effects in human subjects are limited.

In a placebo-controlled comparative study (69), the effect of single-dose inhalation of salbutamol (200 µg) and salmeterol (50 µg), a new long-acting $β_2$ bronchodilator, were evaluated on allergen-evoked bronchoconstriction, airway hyperactivity, and increase in urinary $LTE_4$ excretion in atopic asthmatic subjects. Although clearly separable effects on airway physiology and airway reactivity were demonstrable over the 4-hr period of study by both $β_2$-agonists, neither drug attenuated the allergen-evoked rise in urinary $LTE_4$ compared to placebo. The authors concluded three points. First, the majority of $LTE_4$ reflected in the urine represents systemic as opposed to pulmonary generation, as discussed above. Second, although these $β_2$-agonists are potent inhibitors of cysteinyl leukotriene generation by the lung in vitro (69), this inhibition may not occur to a significant extent after single-dose inhalation in vivo. Finally, although pulmonary mast cells do possess $β_2$-adrenergic receptors, functionally the most important action of inhaled $β_2$-agonists in human asthmatics is relaxation of airway smooth muscle rather than inhibition of mast-cell degranulation.

## 5-Lipoxygenase and Cyclooxygenase Inhibition

The efficacy of 5-lipoxygenase inhibition in allergen-evoked bronchoconstriction, airway reactivity, and leukotriene generation in atopic asthmatics has been recently assessed (70). In this study, a single dose (800 mg) of the oral 5-lipoxygenase inhibitor zileuton (A-64077) was ingested 3 hr before allergen challenge. Both ex vivo generation of $LTB_4$ from calcium iono-phore-stimulated whole blood and in vivo cysteinyl leukotriene generation (urinary $LTE_4$ in a 4-hr collection) were evaluated. Zileuton, although almost completely inhibiting ex vivo generation of $LTB_4$ and significantly reducing (by approximately 50%) the allergen-evoked rises in urinary $LTE_4$ excretion, had no significant abrogatory effect on either early- or late-phase bronchoconstriction or the associated increase in airway reactivity. This may have been simply due to dose- or pharmacokinetic-related factors. Furthermore, differential 5-lipoxygenase inhibition may have been exhibited among cell types either in the peripheral blood or the lung or $LTB_4$, rather than cysteinyl leukotriene, generation more selectively inhibited. Interestingly, treatment differences in the airway response to allergen (although not being significant) correlated more closely with urinary $LTE_4$ excretion than with ex vivo generation of $LTB_4$, suggesting that the former should be used in assessing in vivo 5-lipoxygenase inhibition. However, this study clearly demonstrated that more complete inhibition of 5-lipoxygenase is required in vivo to produce functionally significant protection against allergen-induced bronchoconstriction.

As alluded to earlier, pretreatment with indomethacin in doses that were markedly inhibitory toward cyclooxygenase (30) did not further enhance allergen-evoked bronchoconstriction or urinary $LTE_4$ excretion, tending to refute the hypothesis that inhibition of cyclooxygenase may augment airflow obstruction by shunting of arachidonic acid toward metabolism by cellular lipoxygenases.

### Leukotriene Receptor Antagonists

The development of highly specific and potent end-organ receptor antagonists has facilitated far greater understanding of the role of leukotrienes in asthma. Recent studies have demonstrated their abrogatory effect against aspirin (71), PAF (49,50), and allergen challenges (35), although in none of these studies was urinary $LTE_4$ excretion quantified.

In two further studies of different design in asthmatic subjects, the effect of the leukotriene receptor antagonist ICI 204,219 on allergen-induced $LTE_4$ excretion was assessed. In the first, Kumlin et al. (25) evaluated the effect of ICI 204,219 (ingested as a single 20-mg dose 2 hr before allergen challenge) on allergen $PD_{20}$, the provocative dose required to reduce $FEV_1$ by 20%. On the placebo limb, the mean rise in urinary $LTE_4$, observed within 2 to 3 hr of completion of the challenge, was small (less than twofold). In contrast, after ingestion of ICI 204,219, which permitted inhalation of far greater doses of allergen (administered in half-log increments) to evoke comparable bron-choconstriction, the mean rise in urinary $LTE_4$ over the same time period was four- to fivefold. Although there appeared to be a positive correlation between the increased allergen PD$_{20}$ values and the increased urinary LTE$_4$ excretion after drug administration, suggesting allergen dose-dependent release of leukotrienes, there was no correlation between the amplitude of the fall in FEV$_1$ and urinary excretion of LTE$_4$. The second study by O'Shaughnessy et al. (72), also double-blind and placebo-controlled, evaluated the effects of an inhaled derivative of ICI 204,219 on allergen-induced bronchoconstriction and urinary LTE$_4$ excretion. Drug (1.6 mg) or matched placebo was administered from a metered dose inhaler 30 min before a single allergen inhalation previously shown to reduce FEV$_1$ by 15%. FEV$_1$ was monitored for 10 hr and urine collected over the first 4 hr for LTE$_4$ assessment. As with the oral preparation (35), the early response to allergen (area under the curve, AUC$_{0-2h}$) was significantly inhibited by ICI 204,219 but, in contrast to the earlier study (35), the late response (AUC$_{2-10h}$) was not. Urinary LTE$_4$ in the 4-hr collection after allergen challenge was not significantly different between treatment limbs. Furthermore, correlation of urinary LTE$_4$ and the percent inhibition of the AUC$_{0-2h}$ was not statistically significant.

## PAF Antagonists

Clarification of the role of the cysteinyl leukotrienes as secondary mediators of PAF-induced bronchoconstriction has been evaluated not only by study with leukotriene receptor antagonists but more recently with a selective PAF antagonist (51). PAF is chemotactic for a number of inflammatory cells, and one possible mechanism of PAF-induced bronchoconstriction is through the recruitment of a secondary cell type (or types) to the airway, followed by release of cysteinyl leukotrienes. In humans, the neutrophil in particular has been implicated as the major cell type in mediating PAF-induced bronchoconstriction. O'Connor et al. (51) have recently evaluated the effect of pretreatment with the potent PAF antagonist UK 74505 on airway responses, changes in peripheral blood neutrophil counts, and urinary LTE$_4$ excretion evoked by inhalation of PAF in normal volunteers. UK 74505 abolished PAF-induced bronchoconstriction, the initial transient peripheral blood neutropenia and subsequent rebound neutrophilia, and significantly reduced urinary LTE$_4$ excretion. Although cellular recruitment and eicosanoid production appear to be causally related in the mechanism of PAF-induced bronchoconstriction, it remains to be seen what disease-modifying effects PAF receptor antagonists will have in chronic asthma itself.

## Glucocorticoids

Glucocorticoids (GCs) represent the mainstay of current asthma therapy. They have potent anti-inflammatory properties and consistently reduce heightened bronchial reactivity to a variety of direct and indirect airway challenges. Although extensive in vitro data exist that GCs modulate eicosanoid synthesis both from whole-organ and cell-culture systems, putatively via lipocortin-induced inhibition of phospholipase A$_2$ (PLA$_2$), there is little convincing evidence for a comparable action in vivo. Two recent studies (73,74) looking directly for modulation of cysteinyl leukotriene biosynthesis in response to steroid administration have addressed this. Sebalt et al. (73) administered oral prednisolone (60 mg daily for 1 week) to healthy volunteers and found no change in urinary LTE$_4$ excretion. Similarly, Manso et al. (74) found that prednisolone (30 mg daily for 72 hr), dexamethasone (8 mg daily for 48 hr), or inhaled budesonide (1.6 mg daily for 1 week) had no effect on urinary LTE$_4$ excretion in normal volunteers. Two further studies in asthmatic patients have evaluated the modulating effect of chronically administered inhaled GCs on the allergen-evoked rise in urinary LTE$_4$ excretion. In the first (I. K. Taylor, unpublished data), pretreatment for 1 week with derivatives of budesonide (1.6 mg daily) before allergen challenge attenuated the early bronchoconstrictor response, but urinary LTE$_4$ excretion was not significantly different compared to placebo. In the second (75), pretreatment with inhaled fluticazone dipropionate (1 mg daily for 2 weeks) before allergen challenge, although markedly reducing both baseline airway reactivity and allergen-evoked increases in reactivity and abrogation of both early- and late-phase bronchoconstriction after allergen challenge, had no effect on the increased urinary excretion of LTE$_4$ after allergen challenge. Although these observations could be explained if the proposed inhibitory effect on PLA$_2$ does not occur in vivo in humans at the concentrations of GCs used, or if the enzyme inhibition is too short-lived to facilitate a measurable change in urinary LTE$_4$ excretion, a more likely explanation for the anti-inflammatory effect of these drugs is in an immunomodulatory capacity on cytokine networks between inflammatory cells of relevance, rather than an action directly on the metabolism of arachidonic acid itself.

## CONCLUSIONS

The clinical entity of asthma is now known to comprise a combination of separate but intimately related pathophysiologic processes that include variable airflow obstruction, bronchial hyperreactivity, and airway inflammation. The initiation and propagation of airway inflammation results from the coordinated collaboration of many inflammatory cell types, resident in or recruited to the airway, and their cellular products. It is appropriate in this context, given the abundant literature on the subject, to evaluate the usefulness of urinary LTE$_4$ measurements in clarifying the role of cysteinyl leukotrienes in asthma.

There is little doubt that urine measurements for in vivo assessment of inflammatory mediator release in asthma possess inherent advantages over more invasive means of evaluation, but a number of disadvantages are apparent. Even when the analytical approach can be trusted to generate good-quality data, it is important to interpret the data correctly both in the light of positive and negative findings, particularly when measurements are made distal from the site of mediator production and their putative site of action. Indeed, the nature of urine measurements, by inference an assessment of whole-body production, may not necessarily relate to, or be exclusively derived from, that part of the body at which the physiologic response is observed. Therefore, the unequivocal elevations in urinary $LTE_4$ observed after, for example, allergen challenge may not simplistically represent exclusive cysteinyl leukotriene generation within the lung and must be interpreted with caution particularly in the light of pharmacologic studies that have attempted to modulate this allergen-evoked rise. Similarly, in the case of PAF, the measured increases in urinary $LTE_4$ may equally arise from the systemic vasculature as from the lung parenchyma or airway, particularly given the wide variety of mediator-releasing cells this phospholipid may activate in vitro and also the systemic responses that accompany its inhalation in vivo. The lack of correlation observed in many studies between the magnitude of bronchoconstriction and the evoked elevations in urinary $LTE_4$ after allergen (25,28,31) and PAF challenge (48) and in acute severe asthma (28,57) suggests that although the sensitivity of asthmatic subjects to the generated spasmogens may be very variable, extrapulmonary eicosanoid synthesis cannot be excluded nor, indeed, the role of other products in the inflammatory response.

Although measurement of urinary $LTE_4$ has been useful in delineating increased in vivo production of cysteinyl leukotrienes after selected challenges in the laboratory, in acute severe asthma, and in certain circumstances under basal conditions, absence of increases in urinary $LTE_4$ excretion does not necessarily rule out a mechanistic role for these products in mediating in vivo bronchoconstrictor events, as, for example, in exercise-induced asthma. Many would argue that the best evidence for a mechanistic role of an inflammatory mediator in a physiologic response is pharmacologic inhibition of that response either by selective end-organ receptor antagonism or by inhibition of its synthesis. This raises an important issue relating to interpretation of mechanistic events in vivo, given that apparently conflicting evidence may arise either from pharmacologic modulation of a response or from direct mediator measurements in biological matrices (such as blood, urine, or bronchoalveolar lavage fluid) during the response. High transient local concentrations of cysteinyl leukotrienes in the airway may not result in a significant increase in the whole-body turnover and an increase in their urinary excretion. Therefore, data arising from urinary measurements in these circumstances must be interpreted with caution and further clarification sought, if necessary, with pharmacologic intervention.

## REFERENCES

1. Lewis RA, Austen KF. *J Clin Invest* 1984;73:889–97.
2. Lewis RA, Austen KF, Soberman RJ. *N Engl J Med* 1990;323:645–55.
3. Samuelsson B. *Science* 1983;250:568–75.
4. Barnes PJ, Chung KF, Page CP. *Pharmacol Rev* 1988;40:49–84.
5. Piacentini GL, Kaliner MA. *Am Rev Respir Dis* 1991;143:S96–9.
6. Dahlen S-E, Hansson G, Hedquist P, Bjorck T, Granstrom E, Dahlén B. *Proc Natl Acad Sci USA* 1983;80:1712–6.
7. MacGlashan DW, Schleimer RP, Peters SP, et al. *J Clin Invest* 1982;70:747–51.
8. Weller PF, Lee CW, Foster DW, Corey EJ, Austen KF, Lewis RA. *Proc Natl Acad Sci USA* 1983;80:7626–30.
9. Drazen JM, Austen KF. *Am Rev Respir Dis* 1987;136:985–98.
10. Barnes NC, Piper PJ, Costello JF. *Thorax* 1984;39:500–4.
11. Arm JP, Spur BW, Lee TH. *J Allergy Clin Immunol* 1988;82:654–60.
12. O'Hickey SP, Hawksworth RJ, Fong CY, et al. *Am Rev Respir Dis* 1991;144:1053–7.
13. Creticos PS, Peters SP, Adkinson NF, et al. *N Engl J Med* 1984;310:1626–30.
14. Nacleiro RM, Barody FM, Togias AG. *Am Rev Respir Dis* 1991;143:S91–5.
15. Wenzel SE, Larsen GL, Johnston K, Voelkel NF, Westcott JY. *Am Rev Respir Dis* 1990;142:112–9.
16. Murray JJ, Tonnel AG, Brash AR, et al. *N Engl J Med* 1986;315:800–4.
17. Casale TB, Wood D, Richerson HB, et al. *J Clin Invest* 1987;79:1197–1203.
18. Vyve TM, Chanez P, Bousquet J, et al. *Am Rev Respir Dis* 1992;146:116–21.
19. Walters EH, Gardiner PV. *Thorax* 1991;46:613–8.
20. Kumlin M, Dahlén S-E. *Biochim Biophy Acta* 1990;1044:201–10.
21. Orning L, Kaijser L, Hammarstrom S. *Biochem Biophy Res Commun* 1985;130:214–20.
22. Maltby NH, Taylor GW, Ritter JM, Moore KM, Fuller RW, Dollery CT. *J Allergy Clin Immunol* 1990;85:3–9.
23. Sala A, Voekel NF, Maclouf J, Murphy RC. *J Biol Chem* 1990;265:21771–8.
24. Verhagen J, Bel E, Kijne GM, et al. *Biochem Biophy Res Commun* 1987;148:846–8.
25. Kumlin M, Dahlén B, Bjorck T, Zetterstrom O, Granstrom E, Dahlén SE. *Am Rev Respir Dis* 1992;146:96–103.
26. Westcott JY, Johnston K, Batt RA, Wenzel SE, Voelkel NF. *J Appl Physiol* 1990;68:2640–8.
27. Richmond R, Turner NC, Maltby N, et al. *J Chromatogr* 1987;417:241–51.
28. Taylor GW, Taylor IK, Black P, et al. *Lancet* 1989;1:584–7.
29. Manning PJ, Rokach J, Malo J-L, et al. *J Allergy Clin Immunol* 1990;86:211–20.
30. Sladek K, Dworski R, Fitzgerald GA, et al. *Am Rev Respir Dis* 1990;141:1441–5.
31. Westcott JY, Smith HR, Wenzel SE, et al. *Am Rev Respir Dis* 1991;143:1322–8.
32. Smith CM, Christie PE, Hawksworth RJ, Thien F, Lee TH. *Am Rev Respir Dis* 1991;144:1411–3.
33. Tagari P, Rasmussen JB, Delorme D, et al. *Eicosanoids* 1990;3:75–80.
34. Diaz P, Gonzalez C, Galleguillos FR, et al. *Am Rev Respir Dis* 1989;139:1383–9.
35. Taylor IK, O'Shaughnessy KM, Fuller RW, Dollery CT. *Lancet* 1991;337:690–4.
36. Taylor IK, Wellings R, Taylor GW, Fuller RW. *J Appl Physiol* 1992;73:743–8.
37. Broide DH, Eisman S, Ramdell JW, Ferguson P, Schwartz LB, Wasserman S. *Am Rev Respir Dis* 1990;141:563–8.
38. Pliss LB, Ingenito EP, Ingram RH Jr, Pichurko B. *Am Rev Respir Dis* 1990;142:73–8.
39. Manning PJ, Watson RM, Margolskee DJ, Williams VC, Schwartz JI, O'Bryne PJ. *N Engl J Med* 1990;323:1736–9.
40. Finnerty JP, Wood-Baker R, Thomson H, Holgate ST. *Am Rev Respir Dis* 1992;145:746–9.
41. Israel E, Dermarkarian R, Rosenberg M, et al. *N Engl J Med* 1990;323:1740–4.
42. Israel E, Juniper EF, Callaghan JT, et al. *Am Rev Respir Dis* 1989;140:1348–53.
43. Kikawa Y, Miyanomae T, Inoue Y, et al. *J Allergy Clin Immunol* 1992;89:1111–9.
44. Cuss FM, Dixon CMS, Barnes PJ. *Lancet* 1986;2:189–92.
45. Rubin AE, Smith LJ, Patterson R. Am Rev Respir Dis 1987;136:1145–51.
46. Smith LJ, Rubin AE, Patterson R. *Am Rev Respir Dis* 1988;137:1015–9.
47. Schellenberg RR. *Am Rev Respir Dis* 1987;136:S28–31.

48. Taylor IK, Ward PS, Taylor GW, Dollery CT, Fuller RW. *J Appl Physiol* 1991;71:1396–1402.
49. Spencer DA, Evans JM, Green SE, Piper PJ, Costello JF. *Thorax* 1991;46:441–5.
50. Kidney JC, Ridge S, Chung KF, Barnes PJ. *Am Rev Respir Dis* 1991;143:A811(abst).
51. O'Connor BJ, Uden S, Carty TJ, Eskra JD, Barnes PJ, Chung KF. *Am Rev Respir Dis* [*in press*].
52. Undem BJ, Pickett WC, Lichtenstein LM, Adams GK. *Am Rev Respir Dis* 1987;136: 1183–7.
53. Ferreri NR, Howland WC, Stevenson DD, Spiegelberg HL. *Am Rev Respir Dis* 1988;137: 847–54.
54. Christie PE, Tagari P, Ford-Hutchinson AW, et al. *Am Rev Respir Dis* 1991;143:1025–9.
55. Knapp HR, Sladek K, Fitzgerald GA. *J Lab Clin Med* 1992;119:48–51.
56. Fuller RW, Taylor GW, O'Connor BJ. *Am Rev Respir Dis* 1990;145:A290(Abstract).
57. Drazen JM, O'Brien J, Sparrow D, et al. *Am Rev Respir Dis* 1992;146:104–8.
58. Nacleiro RM, Baroody FM, Togias AG. *Am Rev Respir Dis* 1991;143:S91–5.
59. Knapp HR. *N Engl J Med* 1990;323:1735–8.
60. Hui KP, Barnes NC. *Lancet* 1991;337:1062–3.
61. Gaddy J, Bush RK, Margolskee D, Williams VC, Busse W. *J Allergy Clin Immunol* 1990; 85:197A[Abstract].
62. Israel E, Rubin P, Pearlman H, Cohn J. Drazen J. *Am Rev Respir Dis* 1992;145:A16 [Abstract].
63. Spector SL, Glass M, Minkwitz MC. *Am Rev Respir Dis* 1992;145:A16[Abstract].
64. Margolskee D, Bodman S, Dockhom R, et al. *J Allergy Clin Immunol* 1991;87: 309A[Abstract].
65. Bellia V, Cuttitta G, Mirabella A, et al. *Am Rev Respir Dis* 1992;145:A16(Abstract).
66. Smith CM, Hawksworth RJ, Thien FCK, Christie PE, Lee TH. *Eur Respir J* 1992;5:693–9.
67. Phillips GD, Holgate ST. *J Appl Physiol* 1989;66:304–12.
68. Westcott JY, Voekel NF, Wenzel SE. *Am Rev Respir Dis* 1992;145:A22[Abstract].
69. Taylor IK, O'Shaughnessy KM, Choudry NB, Adachi M, Palmer JBD, Fuller RW. *J Allergy Clin Immunol* 1992;89:575–83.
70. Hui KP, Taylor IK, Taylor GW, et al. *Thorax* 1991;46:184–9.
71. Christie PE, Smith CM, Lee TH. *Am Rev Respir Dis* 1991;144:957–8.
72. O'Shaughnessy KM, Taylor IK, O'Connor BJ, O'Connell F, Thomson H, Dollery CT. *Am Rev Respir Dis* 1993;147:1431–5.
73. Sebaldt R, Sheller JR, Oates JA, Roberts LJ II, Fitzgerald GA. *Proc Natl Acad Sci USA* 1990;87:6974–8.
74. Manso G, Baker AJ, Taylor IK, Fuller RW. *Eur Respir J* 1992;5:712–6.
75. O'Shaughnessy KM, Wellings R, Gillies, Fuller RW. *Am Rev Respir Dis* 1993;147:1472–6.

*Advances in Prostaglandin, Thromboxane,*
*and Leukotriene Research,* Vol. 22, edited by
S.-E. Dahlén et al. Raven Press, Ltd., New York © 1994

# Aspirin-Induced Asthma: An Update and Novel Findings

Andrew Szczeklik

*Department of Medicine, Copernicus Academy of Medicine,*
*31-006 Cracow, Poland*

In 1902, 3 years after its introduction into therapy, aspirin was implicated as the cause of an anaphylactic reaction in an article by Hirschberg (1) of the Polish city of Poznan. He presented the first case report of acute angioedema/urticaria occurring shortly after the ingestion of aspirin. The reaction subsided in 3 days and the patient survived. Reports of anaphylactic reactions to aspirin soon followed; violent, acute bronchospasm was first published by Cooke in 1919 (2). The association of aspirin sensitivity, asthma, and nasal polyps was described by Widal and colleagues in 1922 (3). This clinical entity, later named aspirin triad, was popularized by the studies of Samter and Beers (4) who, in the late 1960s, presented a perceptive description of the clinical course of the syndrome.

Adverse reactions to aspirin and other nonsteroidal anti-inflammatory drugs (NSAIDs) may have different clinical presentations and different pathogeneses (5–7). Here we discuss one of them. It affects asthmatics and, indeed, constitutes a special, common type of asthma, called aspirin-induced asthma.

## DEFINITION AND MAIN CLINICAL FEATURES

Aspirin-induced asthma (AIA) is a clear-cut clinical syndrome with a distinct clinical picture (6–10). Precipitation of asthma attacks by aspirin and other NSAIDs is the hallmark of the syndrome. It affects about 10% of adults with asthma but is rare in asthmatic children. The majority of patients have a negative family history.

Although the onset of symptoms before puberty or after the age of 60 has been well documented, in most patients the first symptoms appear during the third or fourth decade. The typical patient starts to experience intense vasomotor rhinitis characterized by intermittent and profuse watery rhinorrhea. Over a period of months, chronic nasal congestion appears and physical examination reveals nasal polyps. Bronchial asthma and intolerance to aspirin develop during subsequent stages of the illness. The intolerance presents as a unique picture: within an hour after ingestion of aspirin an acute asthma attack develops, often accompanied by rhinorrhea, conjunctival irritation, and scarlet flushing of the head and neck. These reactions are dangerous; indeed, a single therapeutic dose of aspirin or other anticyclooxygenase agent can provoke violent bronchospasm, shock, unconsciousness, and respiratory arrest.

Asthma runs a protracted course, despite the avoidance of aspirin and crossreactive drugs. Blood eosinophil count is elevated and eosinophils are present in upper respiratory tract mucosa. The distribution pattern of serum IgG subclasses is characterized by a marked rise in $IgG_4$ (11). Skin tests with common aeroallergens are often negative, and those with aspirin are always negative.

Major offenders that precipitate bronchoconstriction include: indomethacin, mefenanic, flufenamic, and cyclofenamic acids, ibuprofen, fenoprofen, ketoprofen, naproxen, diclofenac sodium, piroxicam, sulindac, tiaprofenic acid, aminopyrine, noramidopyrine, sulfinpyrazone, phenylbutazone, zomepirac, tolmetin, diflunisal, and fenflumizole. All of these drugs are contraindicated in patients with AIA. Not all of them produce adverse symptoms with the same frequency. This depends both on the drug's anticyclooxygenase potency and dosage and on individual sensitivity. If necessary, patients with AIA can safely take sodium salicylate, salicylamide, choline magnesium trisalicylate, dextropropoxyphene, benzydamine, guacetisal (guaiacolic ester of acetylsalicylic acid), and chloroquine. The majority of patients also tolerate paracetamol well (10,12). Tartrazine, a yellow azo dye used for coloring drinks, foods, drugs, and cosmetics, very rarely triggers adverse reactions (13).

## PATHOGENESIS

### The Cyclooxygenase Theory of Aspirin-Induced Asthma

Many concepts advanced to explain the pathogenesis of AIA have been recently reviewed (6–10). The idea that the attacks might result from the specific inhibition in the respiratory tract of a single enzyme, i.e., cyclooxygenase (14), has been most discussed. It stimulated a number of hypotheses on the mechanism of bronchoconstriction. All of these hypotheses operate within the framework of the cyclooxygenase theory. Therefore, their major assumption, now rather firmly established, is that inhibition of cyclooxygenase triggers specific biochemical reactions that lead to overt asthma attacks.

In the early 1970s, allergic mechanisms as an explanation for aspirin intolerance were vigorously pursued. Contrary to these concepts, the cyclooxygenase theory proposed that precipitation of asthma attacks by aspirin is not based on antigen–antibody reactions but stems from the pharmacologic action of the drug. The original observations (5,14) that the drug intolerance could be predicted on the basis of its in vitro inhibition of cyclooxygenase have been consistently reaffirmed during the ensuing years (15). Evidence in favor of the cyclooxygenase theory (16) can be summarized by the finding that analgesics with anticyclooxygenase activity invariably precipitate bronchoconstriction in aspirin-sensitive asthmatic patients. Analgesics that do not affect cyclooxygenase do not provoke bronchospasm. There is a positive correlation between the potency of analgesics to inhibit cyclooxygenase in vitro and their potency to induce asthma attacks in aspirin-sensitive patients. After aspirin desensitization, crossdesensitization with other analgesics that inhibit cyclooxygenase also occurs.

Therefore, the inhibition of bronchial cyclooxygenase by aspirin-like drugs appears to set off a chain of reactions that lead to asthma attacks in aspirin-intolerant patients. What follows at the biochemical level remains largely unknown.

## Participation of Leukotrienes

### Diversion of Arachidonic Acid Metabolism to the 5-Lipoxygenase Pathway

When leukotrienes were discovered, it became an attractive hypothesis that arachidonic acid could be diverted from the cyclooxygenase pathway to the 5-lipoxygenase pathway when the cyclooxygenase was inhibited (17). The definition of leukotrienes suggested that they would provide potent mediation of neutrophil influx into the tissue via the action of leukotriene $B_4$ ($LTB_4$) and potent stimulation of bronchoconstriction, mucosal permeability, and mucous secretion by the action of the cysteinyl leukotrienes, leukotriene $C_4$ ($LTC_4$), leukotriene $D_4$ ($LTD_4$), and leukotriene $E_4$ ($LTE_4$). The explanation for aspirin-induced asthma then postulated that it was simply caused by shunting of arachidonic acid from the generation of prostaglandins to the biosynthesis of leukotrienes. It has been also suggested that the biosynthesis of leukotrienes could be enhanced by the overproduction of 12-HETE (18) or by removal of inhibiting control of $PGE_2$ (19). Both possibilities are a logical consequence of cyclooxygenase pathway inhibition.

There is some experimental support for the concept of a shift in arachidonic acid metabolism. In a guinea pig model of antigen-induced anaphylaxis, pretreatment of animals with indomethacin led to augmentation of the pulmonary mechanical response to intravenous antigen, accompanied by increased generation of $LTB_4$ (20). In antigen-challenged sheep lung in vivo, cyclooxygenase inhibition enhanced leukotriene production (21). Pretreatment of passively sensitized human airways with indomethacin resulted in an increased release of leukotrienes from human bronchi in response to both antigen and anti-IgE stimulation (22). However, others (23) have found that in normal human parenchyma an anti-IgE challenge in the presence of indomethacin does not produce a shift toward leukotriene formation. Sladek et al. (24) observed that $LTE_4$ urinary excretion was elevated in atopic asthmatics after challenge with allergen. When these authors had pretreated the patients with indomethacin and repeated the allergen challenge, they noted that levels of urinary 11-dehydro-$TXB_2$ decreased, but pulmonary function and $LTE_4$ values showed no further changes. Therefore, Sladek et al. failed to obtain evidence that inhibition of cyclooxygenase in vivo would alter leukotriene release, already augmented by allergic stimulation.

### Aspirin-Induced Release of Leukotrienes

Aspirin-induced nasal reactions involve increased vascular permeability, glandular secretion, and possibly mast-cell activation (25). Three groups studied the release of leukotrienes into the nasal cavity after aspirin administration to patients with AIA. Ortolani et al. (26) noted an increase in mean $LTC_4$ concentrations in nasal washings from seven aspirin-sensitive asthmatics after aspirin provocation by nasal spray. However, the clinical symptoms occurred within 1 or 2 min of the aspirin challenge, whereas the $LTC_4$ increase was observed 60 min later. Ferreri et al. (27) used oral aspirin to provoke clinical symptoms in five aspirin-intolerant patients. During the aspirin-provoked reactions, $LTC_4$ increased in three patients. In two of five patients a fall in $PGE_2$ preceded the appearance of clinical symptoms. In the control subjects, ingestion of higher doses of aspirin (650 mg) resulted in a distinct fall in $PGE_2$ without the release of $LTC_4$. One hour after local instillation of aspirin in aspirin-sensitive asthmatics, Picado et al. (28) detected significant levels of peptidoleukotrienes and depression of $PGE_2$; 15-HETE remained unchanged in nasal washings.

In human blood, $LTC_4$ is rapidly converted enzymatically to $LTD_4$ and then to $LTE_4$, which is excreted in the urine. Therefore, measurement of urinary $LTE_4$ concentration may act as a marker for systemic release of cysteinyl leukotrienes. Within the last year, four research groups have measured urinary $LTE_4$ in patients with AIA after oral (29–31) or inhaled (32) aspirin challenge. The results were very similar. The baseline $LTE_4$ in the urine of aspirin-sensitive asthmatic subjects was significantly greater than that of asthmatic subjects without aspirin intolerance (Fig. 1). Furthermore, there was a three- to sevenfold increase in the urinary $LTE_4$ concentrations after aspirin provocation in AIA subjects, and 11-dehydro-$TXB_2$ became gradually depressed (Fig. 2). The intensity of both $LTE_4$ and 11-dehydro-$TXB_2$ responses depended on the dose of aspirin used (30). Peak $LTE_4$ levels were not correlated with a maximal fall in $FEV_1$. There was no

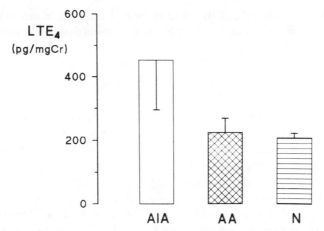

**FIG. 1.** Basal urinary LTE$_4$ excretion in aspirin-sensitive asthmatics (AIA, $n$ = 10), atopic asthmatics (AA, $n$ = 10), and healthy controls (N, $n$ = 10).

significant change in urinary LTE$_4$ in aspirin-sensitive subjects after placebo challenge or in the control asthmatic subjects without aspirin intolerance after provocation with aspirin or placebo (29). The finding that urinary excretion of LTE$_4$ is not raised after methacholine-induced bronchoconstriction in subjects sensitive to aspirin suggests that the enhanced secretion of LTE$_4$ was not a nonspecific sequela of bronchoconstriction. Interestingly, one group (30) measured serum tryptase and blood eosinophil count and

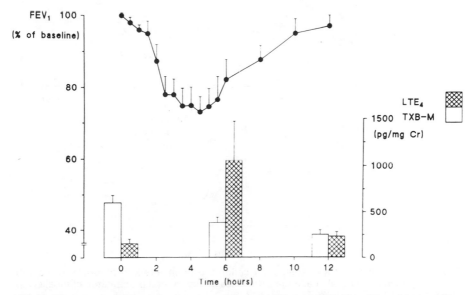

**FIG. 2.** Changes in FEV$_1$ and urinary excretion of LTE$_4$ and TXB-M in 12 aspirin-sensitive asthmatics after oral challenge with threshold doses of aspirin.

observed in AIA patients, at the time of peak $LTE_4$ excretion, a significant fall in blood eosinophil count and a tendency toward an elevation in serum eosinophil cationic protein.

### Cellular Source of Leukotrienes

It is not clear in which cells of the respiratory tract alterations in arachidonic acid metabolism might occur. Leukocytes, especially eosinophils, present in large amounts in nasal and bronchial tissue of aspirin-sensitive asthmatics could be considered as a source of leukotrienes. Goetzel et al. (33) suggested a generalized abnormality of the regulation of arachidonic acid oxidative pathways in peripheral blood leukocytes of patients with AIA. Two studies failed to support this idea. Nizankowska et al. (34) studied the production by polymorphonuclear leukocytes of 5-hydroperoxyeicosatetraenoic acid (5-HETE) and $LTB_4$ in 10 aspirin-sensitive asthmatics and 10 matched healthy controls. The blood cells were obtained before administration of the threshold doses of aspirin and during the aspirin-induced reactions. Initial levels of eicosanoids determined did not differ between the two groups and remained unchanged after aspirin challenge. Tsuda et al. (35) measured the production of $LTB_4$ and $LTC_4$ in peripheral blood leukocytes

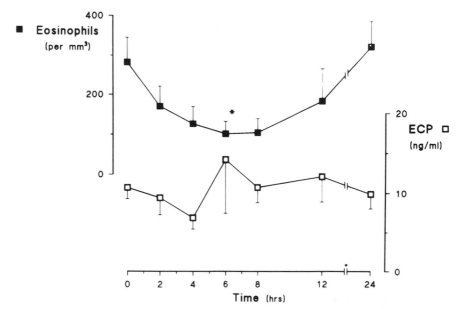

**FIG. 3.** Eosinophil count and eosinophil cationic protein levels in blood of 10 aspirin-sensitive patients after oral challenge with doses of aspirin that precipitated clinical symptoms (*$p < 0.05$).

stimulated by the calcium ionophore A 23187. They compared four groups (controls, AIA, atopic, and intrinsic asthma) before and after indomethacin challenge. All three asthmatic groups produced more $LTC_4$ than did the healthy controls, but there was no difference between aspirin-intolerant patients and patients with atopic or intrinsic asthma. $LTB_4$, $PGE_2$, and $TXB_2$ production was similar in all four groups. Indomethacin did not affect leukotriene generation in any of the groups studied.

In some patients with AIA, aspirin challenge is associated with a rise in serum tryptase (36,37). This phenomenon was observed in patients with extrapulmonary symptoms, i.e., skin and gastrointestinal reactions accompanying bronchial obstruction. At the same time, there was a fall in blood eosinophil count and a tendency to an elevation of serum eosinophil cationic protein (Fig. 3). Therefore, in some patients mast cells and eosinophils may be the source of leukotrienes and other mediators responsible for clinical symptoms.

### Airway Responsiveness to Leukotrienes

The concept of arachidonic acid shunting requires the additional assumption that the airways of aspirin-intolerant patients are more sensitive to leukotrienes than are those of other patients with asthma (38). If not, all asthmatic patients would react with bronchoconstriction in response to aspirin-like drugs. Several research groups have addressed this problem. Vaghi et al. (39) measured the bronchial response to $LTC_4$ in 10 aspirin-sensitive asthmatics compared with 10 controls. They were unable to find any significant difference. Bianco (40) reported similar findings. Sakakibara et al. (41) studied airway responsiveness to methacholine, histamine, and $LTD_4$ in 12 patients with AIA, 13 patients with extrinsic asthma, and 12 patients with intrinsic asthma. There were no significant differences either in concentrations of any of the agents producing a 20% fall in $FEV_1$ or in the slope of $FEV_1$ changes among the groups studied. The only positive finding was somewhat delayed recovery in $FEV_1$ after challenge with $LTD_4$ in the aspirin-intolerant group compared with the others.

These three studies do not support the concept of increased bronchial reactivity to $LTC_4$ or $LTD_4$. However, the findings of Arm et al. (42) suggest a selective increase in airway responsiveness of $LTE_4$. They measured a 35% fall in the specific airway conductance ($PD_{35}$) after histamine and $LTE_4$ inhalation in five subjects with aspirin-induced asthma and in 15 asthmatic patients without aspirin sensitivity. The airways of aspirin-intolerant patients had a significant 13-fold increase in responsiveness to $LTE_4$ relative to histamine compared with asthmatics without aspirin sensitivity. Hyperresponsiveness to $LTE_4$ became abolished after aspirin desensitization.

### Leukotriene Inhibitors

Are cysteinyl leukotrienes specific mediators for AIA? A rise in urinary $LTE_4$ was observed in clinical reaction precipitated not only by aspirin but also by allergens (24). Interesting, preliminary studies demonstrated that both allergen and aspirin-provoked bronchoconstriction can be attenuated or prevented by new leukotriene antagonists (17,43,44). The potent broncho-constrictor cysteinyl leukotrienes could act as one of the final mediators, their release being triggered by specific stimuli, different in various types of asthma.

### Mast-Cell Activation

Mast-cell activation in AIA has been a matter of controversy. These cells may be the source of the arachidonic acid products with bronchoconstrictor leukotrienes and histamine. Some authors have reported a rise in plasma histamine levels and mast-cell–associated neutrophil chemotactic activity after aspirin challenge in AIA patients. Others provided data pointing to lack of mast-cell activation (9). However, in two recently published studies, el-evation of serum tryptase levels, a specific marker of mast-cell activation, during aspirin-provoked asthma attacks was reported in some AIA patients (36,37). Mean serum tryptase level increased significantly within 4 hr of aspirin ingestion, preceding by 2 hr the peak excretion of urine $LTE_4$ (37). In contrast, inhalation challenge with lysine–aspirin, resulting in comparable bronchoconstriction, did not produce any alteration in serum tryptase levels

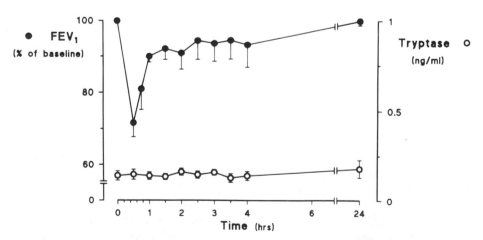

**FIG. 4.** Lack of changes in tryptase levels in seven aspirin-sensitive asthmatics after in-haled provocation test with lysine–aspirin. Four of these patients responded on another occasion to an oral aspirin provocation test with a rise in serum tryptase.

(Fig. 4). Oral but not inhalation challenge was associated with such nonrespiratory symptoms as flushing, rhinorrhea, headache, and conjunctival irritation. Tryptase therefore could be released from degranulating mast cells of skin, nose, bowel tissue, and cerebral vessels.

## Platelet Involvement

During the last few years, attention has been focused on the possible participation of platelets in the pathogenesis of bronchial asthma. In patients with AIA, aspirin challenge may lead to activation of peripheral blood platelets that parallels the time course of bronchospastic reaction. In contrast to platelet activation, the detection of endogenous PAF release has not been a consistent finding. Aspirin-induced bronchoconstriction appears not to be based on the contracting properties of PAF (45).

Capron et al. (46) reported that platelets from patients with aspirin-induced asthma react abnormally in vitro to aspirin and other cyclooxygenase inhibitors by generating cytocidal molecules that can kill parasitic larvae. Aspirin-like drugs had no similar effect on platelets from normal donors or allergic asthmatics. This abnormality appears to be associated with the inhibiting properties of the analgesics on the cyclooxygenase pathway, which leads to a defect in the binding of prostaglandin endoperoxide $PGH_2$ to its receptors on the platelet membrane. Others, however, found that in vitro platelet activation precipitated by aspirin is not a reliable indicator of in vivo sensitivity (47). A recent study reported low glutathione peroxidase activity in patients with AIA (47).

Bonne et al. (48) observed that the ratio of cyclooxygenase to lipoxygenase products is similar in platelets of patients with AIA compared with controls. Nizankowska et al. (34) measured 12-HETE production by platelets in 10 aspirin-sensitive asthmatics and 10 matched healthy controls before and after administration of threshold doses of aspirin. Initial levels of 12-HETE did not differ between the two groups. After aspirin challenge, 12-HETE rose to similar levels in both groups. These data do not support the concept that there is a generalized abnormality in arachidonic acid oxidative pathways in platelets of aspirin-sensitive asthmatics. The lack of a protective effect of prostacyclin infusion on aspirin challenge also raises doubts about participation of platelets in the discussed reactions (49).

## Viral Infection

Viruses have been implicated in the pathogenesis of asthma (50), including aspirin intolerance, although in the latter case no explanation was offered as to how virus infection might be linked with a cyclooxygenase-dependent mechanism. Such an explanation has been provided by a recent hypothesis

(51). The hypothesis postulates that aspirin-induced asthma results from chronic viral infection. In response to a virus, specific cytotoxic lymphocytes are produced. Their activity is suppressed by $PGE_2$ produced by pulmonary alveolar macrophages. Anticyclooxygenase analgesics block $PGE_2$ production and allow cytotoxic lymphocytes to attack and kill their target cells, i.e., virus-infected cells of the respiratory tract. During this reaction, toxic oxygen intermediates, lysosomal enzymes, and mediators are released, which precipitate attacks of asthma. These acute attacks can be prevented by avoidance of all drugs with anticyclooxygenase activity. However, asthma continues to run a protracted course because of chronic viral infection.

The hypothesis is based on the following concepts: First, the clinical course of aspirin-induced asthma is reminiscent of viral infection. Second, the latency or semi-latency of viruses is being increasingly recognized (50). In humans, a notable example is Epstein–Barr virus, which causes infection that persists for life and is subject to reactivations. Interestingly, some of the clinical manifestations of acute Epstein–Barr virus infection, such as Guillain–Barre syndrome, hepatitis, and suppression of hematopoesis, may be caused by secondary immune responses to latently infected lymphocytes. Third, cytotoxic T lymphocytes form a part of the human immune system in the respiratory tract. They increase in numbers in response to viral infections and are highly specific. Fourth, lung macrophages produce $PGE_2$, which suppresses the immunologic response, including cytotoxic activity of lymphocytes. This inhibition can be overcome by anticyclooxygenase analgesics, which deprive macrophages of $PGE_2$. Finally, viral infection of pulmonary alveolar macrophages causes increased production of $PGE_2$ and 5-lipoxygenase pathway metabolites (52).

## DIAGNOSIS

Although a patient's clinical history might raise the suspicion of AIA, the diagnosis can be established with certainty only by aspirin challenge. There are no in vitro tests suitable for routine clinical diagnosis, although a search for them continues (46,47,53,54).

There are three types of provocation tests, depending on the route of aspirin administration: oral, inhaled, and nasal. Oral challenge tests are most commonly performed. In inhalation challenge tests an aerosol of lysine–acetylsalicylatic is administered. Inhalation challenge is faster than the oral challenge, but symptoms evaluated are restricted only to the bronchopulmonary tract. The methods of performing both tests have lately been summarized (8–10,55,56). There has been some recent interest in nasal provocation testing (57–59). Although such testing is an attractive research model, its diagnostic value is limited by its low sensitivity. Patriarca et al. (59)

reported that this test was positive in only 38% of documented aspirin-intolerant patients.

Glucocorticosteroids attenuate aspirin-precipitated reactions (60). A clinician attempting to establish a diagnosis of aspirin idiosyncrasy with challenge tests should be aware of the possibility of false-negative results related to corticotherapy. This might be particularly relevant in patients with a mild degree of idiosyncrasy (threshold dose of aspirin greater than 200 mg). On the other hand, adverse reactions precipitated by aspirin in intolerant patients treated with steroids might be expected to become more accentuated once steroids are discontinued.

In the majority of patients, once it develops aspirin intolerance remains for the rest of the patient's life. Repeated aspirin challenges are therefore positive, although some variability in intensity and spectrum of symptoms occurs. However, in an occasional patient a positive aspirin challenge might become negative after a period of a few years.

AIA should be clearly differentiated from other forms of aspirin intolerance. For example, urticaria aggravated by aspirin is something quite different from AIA, and the two syndromes very rarely occur in the same patient (7–10).

In summary, diagnosis of aspirin-induced asthma should pose no difficulties to a perceptive physician. Once the diagnosis is made, the patient should be given a detailed list of drugs known to be major offenders, as well as a list of safe alternatives.

## PREVENTION AND TREATMENT

Patients with AIA should avoid aspirin, all products containing it, and other analgesics that inhibit cyclooxygenase. They are left with two options. If necessary, they can safely take, even for prolonged periods, certain agents that do not inhibit cyclooxygenase, such as choline magnesium trisalicylate, dextropropoxyphene, azapropazone, and benzydamine. Most patients also tolerate paracetamol, at a dose not exceeding 1,000 mg daily. Alternatively, they can undergo desensitization.

Desensitization can be achieved by giving four to eight incremental doses of aspirin every 2 to 3 hr under careful observation. The procedure takes 2 days. It usually starts with a dose that produces mild adverse symptoms and ends with 600 mg aspirin, which is then well-tolerated. The state of aspirin tolerance (refractory period) lasts for 2 to 5 days, but in most patients it can be extended over months if aspirin is administered regularly at a daily dose of 600 mg. At the same time, patients can take other anticyclooxygenase drugs without any adverse effects. Refractoriness to aspirin after indomethacin administration has also been observed. Desensitization is possible in most but not all aspirin-intolerant patients with asthma.

Some patients note improvement in their underlying chronic respiratory symptoms after aspirin desensitization and during maintenance of the desensitized state (61). Recently, Sweet et al. (62) published results of a long-term study on aspirin desensitization in 107 AIA patients. The on-aspirin treatment appeared to improve clinical course of aspirin-sensitive rhinosinusitis/asthma and allowed a reduction of systemic corticosteroids. The significant improvements in multiple objective and subjective parameters in the aspirin treatment patients and the deterioration in these parameters after stopping of aspirin administration suggested that long-term aspirin treatment may prevent or retard ongoing inflammation in the nose, sinuses, and bronchial tree. At present, desensitization is reserved for severe cases of asthma. Relapse of nasal polyposis can be prevented by chronic daily treatment with intranasal lysine–acetylsalicylate (63).

Despite being desensitized to aspirin, all patients remain asthmatic. Patients maintained on aspirin in a desensitized state still develop asthmatic relapses from all of their previous provoking factors, except for aspirin-like drugs.

The mechanism of desensitization is unknown. One possible explanation is that during the period necessary for replacement of irreversibly inhibited cyclooxygenase, the original regulatory mechanisms are removed and the functional balance in the bronchi is based on a prostanoid-independent regulatory system. Hypersensitivity to aspirin would then reoccur with the return of the tissue's capacity to generate prostaglandins after aspirin withdrawal. The exact time of cyclooxygenase blockade by aspirin-like drugs in the bronchi is unknown. It is conceivable that this time might expand even to a few days, as several NSAIDs are capable of inhibiting the message expression of the cyclooxygenase gene and consequently the de novo enzyme synthesis (64). According to Arm et al. (42), desensitization leads to reduction of airways responsiveness to inhaled $LTE_4$ in AIA patients, and it might therefore depend on downregulation of leukotriene receptors.

Whether desensitized or not, most patients with aspirin-induced asthma require regular therapy to control symptoms of their disease. The therapy does not differ from that of other types of asthma. Hydrocortisone (65) and other hemisuccinate salts (66) should be avoided because they might precipitate bronchoconstriction. Long-term treatment with systemic corticosteroids is necessary in at least half of these patients.

## REFERENCES

1. Hirschberg VGS. *Dtsch Med Wochenschr* 1902;28:416 as cited in *Allergy Proc* 1990;11:
   249–50.
2. Cooke RA *JAMA* 1991;73:759.
3. Widal MF, Abrami P, Lermeyez J. *Presse Med* 1992;30:189.
4. Samter M, Beers RF Jr. *Ann Intern Med* 1968;68:975–83.

5. Szczeklik A, Gryglewski RJ, Czerniawska-Mysik G. *J Allergy Clin Immunol* 1977;60:276–84.
6. Szczeklik A. *Drugs* 1986;32(suppl 4):148–63.
7. Hoigne RV, Szczeklik A. In: Borda IT, Koff RS, eds. *NSAIDs, a profile of adverse effects.* Philadelphia: Hanley & Belfus; 1992:157–84.
8. Stevenson DD. *J Allergy Clin Immunol* 1984;74:617–22.
9. Szczeklik A, Virchow C, Schmitz-Schumann M. In: Page CP, Barnes PJ, eds. *Pharmacology of asthma.* Berlin: Springer-Verlag; 1991:291–314.
10. Szczeklik A, Nizankowska E. In: Charpin J, Vervloet D, eds. *Allergologie* Paris: Flammarion; 1992:762–78.
11. Szczeklik A, Schmitz-Schumann M, Nizankowska E, Milewski M, Roehlig F, Virchow C. *Clin Exp Allergy* 1992;22:283–8.
12. Settipane GA, Stevenson DD. *J Allergy Clin Immunol* 1989;84:26–33.
13. Virchow C, Szczeklik A, Bianco S, et al. *Respiration* 1988;53:20–3.
14. Szczeklik A, Gryglewski RJ, Czerniawska-Mysik G. *Br Med J* 1975;1:67–9.
15. Stevenson DD, Lewis RA. *J Allergy Clin Immunol* 1987;80:788–90.
16. Szczeklik A. *Eur Resp J* 1990;3:588–93.
17. Lee TH. *Am Rev Respir Dis* 1992;145:S34–6.
18. McLouf F, Fruteau de Laclos B, Borgeat P. *Proc Natl Acad Sci USA* 1982;79:6042–6.
19. Kuehl FA, Dougherty HW, Ham EA. *Biochem Pharmacol* 1984;33:1–5.
20. Lee TH, Israel E, Drazen JM. *J Immunol* 1986;136:2575–82.
21. Dworski R, Sheller JR, Wickersham NE. *Am Rev Respir Dis* 1989;139:46–51.
22. Underm BJ, Pickett WC, Lichenstein LM, Adams GK III. *Am Rev Respir Dis* 1987;136:1183–7.
23. Vigano T, Toia A, Crivellari MT, Galli G, Mezzetti M, Folco GC. *Eicosanoids* 1988;1:73–7.
24. Sladek K, Dworski R, FitzGerald GA, et al. *Am Rev Respir Dis* 1990;141:1441–5.
25. Kowalski ML, Wojciechowska B, Sliwinska-Kowalska M. *J Allergy Clin Immunol* 1991;87:216[Abstract].
26. Ortolani C, Mirone C, Fontana A. *Ann Allergy* 1987;59:106–12.
27. Ferreri NR, Howland WC, Stevenson DD, Spiegelberg HL. *Am Rev Respir Dis* 1988;137:847–54.
28. Picado C, Ramis I, Rosello J, et al. *Am Rev Respir Dis* 1992;145:65–9.
29. Christie PE, Tagari P, Ford-Hutchinson AW, Charlesson S, Chee P, Arm JP. *Am Rev Respir Dis* 1991;143:1025–9.
30. Sladek K, Szczeklik A. *Am Rev Respir Dis* 1992;145:A17.
31. Knapp HR, Sladek K, FitzGerald GA. *J Lab Clin Med* 1992;119:48–51.
32. Dahlén B, Kumlin M, Johansson H, Larsson C. Zetterstrom O, Granstrom E, Dahlén S-E. *Am Rev Respir Dis* 1991;143:A599.
33. Goetzel EJ, Valacer DJ, Payan DG, Wong MYS. *J Allergy Clin Immunol* 1986;77:693–8.
34. Nizankowska E, Michalska Z, Wandzilak M, Radomski M, Marcinkiewicz E, Gryglewski RJ. *Eicosanoids* 1988;1:45–8.
35. Tsuda M, Sakakibara H, Kamidaira T, Saga T, Suetsugu S, Umeda H. *N Engl Region Allergy Proc* 1988;9:437[Abstract].
36. Bosso JV, Schwartz LB, Stevenson DD. *J Allergy Clin Immunol* 1991;88:830–7.
37. Sladek K, Szczeklik A. *J Allergy Clin Immunol* 1992;89:233[Abstract].
38. Szczeklik A. Gryglewski RJ. *Drugs* 1983;25:533–43.
39. Vaghi A, Robuschi M, Simone P, Bianco S. *SEP 4th Congress* Milano-Stresa 1985;171[Abstract].
40. Bianco S. In: Charpin J, ed. *Allergologie* Paris: Flammarion; 1986:683–700.
41. Sakakibara H, Suetsugu S, Saga T. *J Jpn Thorac Soc* 1988;26:612–9.
42. Arm JP, O'Hickey SP, Spur BW, Lee TW. *Am Rev Respir Dis* 1989;140:148–53.
43. Christie PE, Smith CM, Lee TH. *Am Rev Respir Dis* 1991;144:957–8.
44. Dahlén B, Kumlin M, Johansson H, et al. *Am Rev Respir Dis* 1992;145:A15.
45. Schmitz-Schumann M, Menz G, Schaufele A. *Agents Actions* 1987;21(suppl):215–24.
46. Capron A, Ameisen JC, Joseph M, Auriault C, Tonnel AB, Caen J. *Int Arch Allergy Appl Immunol* 1985;77:107–14.
47. Paerson DJ, Suarez-Mendez VJ. *Clin Exp Allergy* 1990;20:157–63.
48. Bonne C, Moneret-Vautrin D-A, Wayoff M, et al. *Ann Allergy* 1985;54:158–60.

49. Nizankowska E, Czerniawska-Mysik G, Szczeklik A. *Eur J Respir Dis* 1986;69:363–8.
50. Hogg JC. *Am Rev Respir Dis* 1992;145:S7–9.
51. Szczeklik A. *Clin Allergy* 1988;18:15–20.
52. Laegried WW, Taylor SM, Leid RW, et al. *J Leukocyte Biol* 1989;45:283–92.
53. Williams WR, Pawlowicz A, Davies BH. *J Allergy Clin Immunol* 1990;86:445–51.
54. Williams WR, Pawlowicz A, Davies BH. *Int Arch Allergy Appl Immunol* 1991;95:303–8.
55. Dahlén B, Zetterstrom O. *Eur Respir J* 1990;3:527–34.
56. Philips GD, Foord R, Holgate ST. *J Allergy Clin Immunol* 1989;84:232–41.
57. Schapowal A, Schmitz-Schuman M, Szczeklik A, Bruijnzeel P, Hansel T, Virchow C. *Atemw Lungenkrankh Jahrgang* 1990;16(suppl 1):S1–5.
58. Pawlowicz A, Williams WR, Davies BH. *Allergy* 1991;46:405–9.
59. Patriarca G, Nucera E, DiRienzo V, Schiavino D, Pellegrino S, Fais G. *Ann Allergy* 1991; 67:60–2.
60. Nizankowska E, Szczeklik A. *Ann Allergy* 1989;63:159–62.
61. Kowalski ML, Grzelewska-Rzymowska I, Rozniecki J, Szmidt M. *Allergy* 1984;39:171–8.
62. Sweet JM, Stevenson DD, Simon RA, Mathison DA. *J Allergy Clin Immunol* 1990;85:59–69.
63. Patriarca G, Bellioni P, Nucera E, et al. *Ann Allergy* 1991;67:588–92.
64. Sanduja R, Sanduja S, Wu KK. *Thromb Haemost* 1991;65:782[Abstract].
65. Szczeklik A, Nizankowska E, Czerniawska-Mysik G, Sek S. *J Allergy Clin Immunol* 1985; 76:530–6.
66. Taniguchi M, Sato A. *N Engl Region Allergy Proc* 1988;9:388[Abstract].

*Advances in Prostaglandin, Thromboxane,*
*and Leukotriene Research*, Vol. 22, edited by
S.-E. Dahlén et al. Raven Press, Ltd., New York © 1994

# Summary: Leukotrienes as Mediators of Asthma in Humans But Not Always in Experimental Animals

William A. Taylor and *Giancarlo Folco

*Research Department, Bayer plc, Stoke Poges, Buckinghamshire SL2 4LY,
England; and *Institute of Pharmacological Sciences, University of Milan, Center
for Cardiopulmonary Pharmacology, 20133 Milan, Italy*

In the study of asthma, the question of whether or not animal models are relevant to the human disease still remains and is further highlighted when one considers that the lung is an exceedingly complex organ composed of many cell types with a wide variety of functions.

Several selective antagonists of leukotrienes (LTs) and thromboxanes (TXs) have been tested in asthmatic patients and in various animal models of asthma. As a consequence, it is now possible to draw preliminary conclusions regarding the usefulness of animal models in assessing the therapeutic potential of substances known to inhibit eicosanoids. Notable advances in analytical and biochemical techniques have had a significant impact on current eicosanoid research and have allowed better prediction of the efficacy of this type of drug in asthma.

The principal animal models of asthma are those that involve antigen challenge in guinea pigs, sheep, or monkeys; these allow ready comparison with the effects of antigen provocation in asthmatic patients. Even though its inadequacies have long been recognized, the antigen-induced immediate asthma-like reaction (IAR) in guinea pigs is now the standard, time-honored model of asthma. To improve this model it is usually modified by pretreating the test animals with a cocktail of drugs including an antihistamine, a β-receptor blocker and, when an LT inhibitor is to be tested, a cyclooxygenase inhibitor. Under these conditions, the potent TX antagonist BAY u3405 at doses of greater than 600 μg/kg inhibited the IAR in the guinea pig model by 50% or more. In humans, the same antagonist at 50 mg p.o. failed to shift the dose–response curve significantly to allergen even though it markedly shifted the curve to $PGD_2$. In the guinea pig, the potent LT antagonist ICI 204,219, even at 58 mg/kg, failed to inhibit the antigen-induced guinea pig IAR (1) whereas in atopic volunteers, substantial inhibition was achieved with a dose of only 40 mg per person (2). It therefore appears that the guinea pig model overrated the TX antagonist and underrated the LT antagonist with respect to their activity in human subjects.

In addition to the IAR, the occurrence of a late allergen-induced reaction (LAR) in guinea pigs has been reported. This LAR occurs 2 hr or more after antigen exposure (3). However, many groups have failed to achieve a reproducible functional LAR response in this species. The induction of pulmonary eosinophilia, however, does appear to be consistent (4). Furthermore, if guinea pigs are exposed to inhaled antigen on many and frequent occasions (in the absence of antihistamine) they develop pulmonary edema, goblet-cell hyperplasia, and mucous plugging, all reminiscent of severe asthma in humans (5). Such a condition may provide a good model for future testing of respiratory drugs with anti-inflammatory activity.

The sheep model (established by the Miami group) involves the selection of dual-responding animals (i.e., those with both an IAR and an LAR); these animals are then regularly challenged with *Ascaris suum* extracts to which they are naturally sensitive. This model therefore includes a consistent late reaction but one that is smaller than the LAR observed in human subjects.

BAY u3405, at a high i.v. infusion dose (2 mg/kg/hr), inhibited the sheep IAR and LAR by 52% and 64%, respectively (6), but at a lower infusion dose (which still achieved plasma levels higher than those reached in humans in the study referred to above) little inhibition was seen. Whether or not higher doses of BAY u3405 in humans will achieve the marked inhibition observed in the sheep remains to be seen. In reference to this point, GR 32191, another TX antagonist, slightly inhibited the early reaction in human subjects but actually enhanced the intensity of the late reaction (7).

The potent LT antagonist MK 571, given as an i.v. infusion at 25 μg/kg/min, inhibited the IAR and the LAR in the sheep model by 57% and 87%, respectively (8), and in humans a comparable dose (160 mg bolus plus 0.6 mg/min i.v.) inhibited the IAR and LAR by 88% and 66%, respectively (9).

It therefore appears that at the doses investigated in humans, the sheep model predicted with reasonable accuracy the human response to both the TX and LT antagonists. However, MK 571 was more effective on the late than on the early reaction in sheep; this pattern was also seen in other studies with LT antagonists (5). This contrasts with the results in human subjects, in whom the early reaction appears to be more sensitive to inhibition by MK 571.

There are too few reported data from studies with eicosanoid receptor antagonists to allow accurate comparison of the monkey model of allergen-induced asthma with that in humans. We know that MK 571, at 0.5 mg/kg p.o. given 2 hr before to *Ascaris* antigen to conscious squirrel monkeys, inhibited the immediate antigen-induced increase in airway resistance by approximately 70% and the decrease in lung compliance by 100% (10). In humans, the only comparable study is one that used an i.v. infusion of 37.5 mg MK 571 per patient (10 mg bolus and 0.06 mg/min i.v.). Here the IAR was suppressed by 45% and the LAR by 31% (9). Obviously this comparison should not be overinterpreted, but the data do suggest that the monkey model of IAR may be somewhat more sensitive to inhibition by LT antagonists than is the human subject.

Some squirrel monkeys have been shown to exhibit substantial late-phase responses to *Ascaris* antigen. Studies with the LT-synthesis inhibitor L-651,392 have shown that 5 mg/kg p.o. will reduce both this LAR and the IAR (11). The model of asthma in the cynomolgus monkey also depends on a natural sensitivity to *Ascaris suum*. The LAR in this model was reduced by the LT-synthesis inhibitor BI-L-239, given as an aerosol at 10 mg/ml, but the IAR was not inhibited (12). Similarity with respect to the timing and intensity of the LARs in monkeys compared with those in humans makes such a model important in trying to understand the LAR in human subjects, and further evaluation of these models is likely to prove fruitful.

The evidence to date therefore suggests that some animal models can be used successfully to predict activity of eicosanoid inhibitors in allergen challenge studies in humans. However, other models may be misleading unless careful account is taken of the special sensitivity or insensitivity of the model to the particular type of inhibitor under test, yet because of the lack of comparative data even this conclusion remains preliminary. The next year or two should see a clearer picture emerge as several new, potent, and selective LT antagonists and synthesis inhibitors will be tested in human subjects. It should also be recognized that the response of allergic asthmatics to experimentally administered allergen is probably not identical to clinical asthma. Indeed, even if the various mediator substances involved in the two situations are the same, their relative contributions may not be, except, of course, in the probably rare event of induction of asthma by environmental exposure to a single high dose of allergen.

The study of cysteinyl leukotrienes in asthma, their measurement and quantification in biologic fluids in asthmatic patients, and the related effort toward achieving more potent and selective therapy is complicated by the unique way in which these autacoids are produced and transported to their target cells; they are synthesized by specific cells within a tissue and act within its microenvironment.

The difficulty in sampling for the synthesis of leukotrienes has focused attention on the possibility of identifying urinary metabolites that might serve as convenient index for leukotriene production in humans, in much the same way as several metabolites of prostaglandins are measured to indicate the synthesis of these biologically active cyclooxygenase products of arachidonic acid (13). Measurement of urinary $LTE_4$ has been widely used to assess whole-body cysteinyl leukotriene production in vivo in human subjects (14). However, the timing of the urine collection might be critical in that, after airway challenge, excretion of $LTE_4$ occurs rapidly (within 2 hr). Collection of urine samples after this time interval may lead to excessive dilution of $LTE_4$ and thus hampers detection of any changes in the urinary level. An alternative would be to measure the major metabolites of $LTE_4$, which have recently been structurally characterized (15). This would not only eliminate the potential problems associated with kidney $LTE_4$ production and elimination but might better reflect total body production of cysteinyl leukotrienes. This may be particularly important in seeking a better understanding of the role of cysteinyl leukotrienes in the pathogenesis of the late asthmatic response. The recent demonstration of significant inhibition of late allergen-induced bronchoconstriction by potent leukotriene receptor antagonists (2) has provided important evidence to support a definitive role for peptidoleukotrienes in causing this response. However, to date no significant increase in urinary $LTE_4$ excretion during late-phase bronchoconstriction has been convincingly documented (see Taylor, *this volume*). It may be that $\beta$-oxidation metabolites, such as $14\text{-COOH-LTE}_3$ and $16\text{-COOH-}\Delta^{13}\text{-LTE}_4$, are more predominant in urine during the late asthmatic response; however, no methodology is presently available with the necessary sensitivity, specificity, and accuracy to measure these metabolites.

The experimental evidence from eicosanoid research, accumulated over the past 20 years, clearly indicates that there is a strong rationale for measurement of major enzymatic derivatives of biologically active prostanoids (e.g., $TXA_2$, $PGI_2$) to reflect changes in their production in humans (16). This may be particularly relevant in the study of aspirin-induced asthma, a syndrome characterized by a distinct clinical picture (17), in which cysteinyl leukotrienes might be involved and for which no animal or in vitro models are available.

"Unexplicable idiosyncrasy" to acetylsalicylic acid (ASA) was first reported in 1902 (18) and since then has been confirmed in a large number of case reports (19). Several pathomechanisms have been proposed for ASA intolerance (20). Since the signs and symptoms of ASA-induced intolerance are identical to those of immediate-type allergic reactions, research has focused on immunologic mechanisms. However, there is a lack of convincing evidence for the presence of reaginic antibodies responsible for immediate-type allergic reactions. Other mechanisms, such as abnormal chemoreceptor reactivity, acetylation of autologous proteins, or direct activation of the complement system by ASA, have been proposed, but none of them has been generally accepted.

Since the elucidation of the mechanism of action of ASA and the observation 7 years later that arachidonic acid could be metabolized, via the 5-lipoxygenase pathway to powerful bronchoconstrictor proinflammatory mediators (such as leukotrienes), intolerance to the drug has been consistently reported to be a direct consequence of its inhibition of cyclooxygenase (21). More recent evidence on increased urinary $LTE_4$ levels after aspirin-provoked bronchoconstriction and inhibition of symptoms by leukotriene antagonists (22) supports the concept that leukotrienes may be responsible for the clinical symptoms. Shunting of arachidonic acid metabolism and/or increased sensitivity of the airways to $LTE_4$ in ASA-intolerant patients have been proposed as mechanisms that may account for the observed hyperreactivity.

Another explanation for acquired sensitivity to ASA, which is also linked to its mechanism of action, comes from the involvement of environmental factors, and viruses are likely candidates (23). ASA may inhibit the formation of an immunosuppressive prostanoid, e.g., $PGE_2$, and thus induce cytotoxic lymphocytes to kill virus-infected cells within the airways. During this reaction, release of lysosomal enzymes and mediators from the virus-infected cells would trigger the clinical symptomatology of asthma. This hypothesis is strongly supported by the fact that a relationship exists between inhibition of prostaglandin biosynthesis by analgesics and induction of asthma attacks in ASA-sensitive patients (21). A large number of structurally unrelated chemicals and drugs that inhibit the prostaglandin biosynthesis elicit the intolerance syndrome in ASA-sensitive individuals. This issue, however, is further complicated by the fact that there exist many other drug hypersensitivities, which may be confused with intolerance to ASA and related drugs (20).

Undoubtedly there is a need for simple in vitro systems to allow better definition of the mechanisms of ASA-induced asthma and of the precise role played by arachidonic acid metabolites. This is particularly important in light of the fact that there is a tendency to present only arguments in favor of the cyclooxygenase theory of ASA-induced asthma, and arguments against it appear to be disregarded.

## REFERENCES

1. Malo PE, Bell RL, Shaughnessy T, et al. *Eighth International Conference on Prostaglandins and Related Compounds.* Montreal; 1992:42.
2. Taylor IK, O'Shaughnessy KM, Fuller RW, Dollery CT. *Lancet* 1991;337:690–4.
3. Hutson PA, Church MK, Clay TP, Miller P, Holgate ST. *Am Rev Respir Dis* 1988;137: 548–57.
4. Foster A, Chan CC. *Int Arch Allergy Appl Immunol* 1991;96:279–84.
5. Ahmed A, Cortes A, Sielczak MW, Abraham WM. *Am Rev Respir Dis* 1992;145:A288 (Abstract).
6. Abraham WM, Ahmed A, Cortes A, Sielczak MW. *Am Rev Respir Dis* 1992;145:A291 (Abstract).
7. Twentyman OP, Holgate ST. *Thorax* 1990;45:798–9.
8. Abraham WM, Stevenson JS. *Fed Proc* 1988;2:A1057 (Abstract).
9. Rasmussen JB, Eriksson L-O, Margolskee DJ, Tagari P, Williams VC, Andersson KE. *J Allergy Clin Immunol* 1992;90:193–201.
10. Jones TR, Zamboni R, Beeley M, et al. *Can J Physiol Pharmacol* 1989;67:17–28.
11. McFarlane CS, Hamel R, Ford-Hutchinson AW. *Agents Actions* 1987;22:63–8.
12. Gundel RH, Torcellini CA, Clarke CC, Desai S, Lazer ES, Wegner CD. *Adv Prostaglandin Thromboxane Leukot Res* 1990;21:457–60.
13. Patrono C, Ciabattoni G, Patrignani P. In: FitzGerald GA, Patrono C, eds. *Platelets and vascular occlusion.* New York: Raven Press; 1989:193–201.
14. Manning PJ, Rokach J, Malo JL, et al. *J Allergy Clin Immunol* 1990;86:211–20.

15. Sala A, Voelkel N, Maclouf J, Murphy RC. *J Biol Chem* 1990;265:21771–8.
16. Ciabattoni G, Maclouf J, Catella GA, FitzGerald GA, Patrono C. *Biochim Biophys Acta* 1987;918:293–300.
17. Stevenson DD. *J Allergy Clin Immunol* 1984;74:617–22.
18. Hirschberg H. *Dtsch Med Wochenschr* 1902;1:416.
19. Stevenson DD, Mathison DA. *J Allergy Clin Immunol* 1975;55:127–35.
20. Schlumberger HD. *PAR. Pseudo allergic reactions. Involvement of drugs and chemicals.* Basel: Karger; 1980:125–203.
21. Szczeklik A, Gryglewski RJ, Czerniawska-Mysik. *Br Med J* 1975;1:67–9.
22. Dahlén B, Kumlin M, Johansson H, et al. *Am Rev Respir Dis* 1992;145:A15 (Abstract).
23. Szczeklik A. *Clin Allergy* 1988;18:15–20.

# 4. Leukotrienes as Inflammatory Mediators in Bronchial Asthma

Advances in Prostaglandin, Thromboxane,
and Leukotriene Research, Vol. 22, edited by
S.-E. Dahlén et al. Raven Press, Ltd., New York © 1994

# Bronchial Provocation with Leukotrienes and Other Stimuli

P. M. O'Byrne, E. Ädelroth, and P. J. Manning

*Asthma Research Group and Department of Medicine, McMaster University,
Hamilton, Ontario, L8N 3Z5 Canada*

Asthma is a disease characterized by variable airflow obstruction and airway hyperresponsiveness to a variety of chemical bronchoconstrictor stimuli and physical stimuli, such as exercise and hyperventilation of cold, dry air (1). Airway hyperresponsiveness means that asthmatics require less of a bronchoconstrictor agonist to induce airway narrowing than normal subjects. The severity of airway hyperresponsiveness is correlated with the severity of asthma (2) and with the amount of treatment needed to optimally control symptoms of asthma (3). More recently, it has been recognized that both variable airflow obstruction and airway hyperresponsiveness occur as a consequence of inflammatory and structural changes in the airway wall (4).

Airway hyperresponsiveness can be stable for many years in some asthmatics (5). However, several stimuli can increase airway responsiveness acutely, and this is associated with worsening symptoms of asthma. These stimuli include inhalation of allergen (6) and occupational sensitizing agents (7) by sensitized subjects, upper respiratory viral infections (8), and inhalation of the atmospheric pollutant ozone (9). Allergen inhalation is the most relevant of these inducers of airway hyperresponsiveness and clinical asthma and is the stimulus most carefully studied in humans.

Allergen-induced asthma appears to be caused by the release of chemical mediators from cells within the airway (10,11), leading to airway narrowing resulting from airway smooth-muscle contraction, mucosal edema, and release of secretions. The degree of smooth-muscle contraction depends on the degree of underlying airway hyperresponsiveness. The relative importance of different mediators in causing each of these events has recently been clarified.

The importance of slow-reacting substance of anaphylaxis (SRS-A) in the events that occur after immunologic challenge of the lungs was identified in the early 1940s (12). Later, Brocklehurst (13) demonstrated that SRS-A was released from lung segments from an asthmatic subject when these segments were exposed to allergen. SRS-A was suggested to be an important mediator in causing symptoms after exposure to allergen in sensitized subjects, mainly because it was a potent airway smooth-muscle constrictor with a much longer duration of action than other smooth-muscle constrictors, such as histamine. SRS-A is now known to consist of the cysteinyl leukotrienes (LT) $LTC_4$, $LTD_4$, and $LTE_4$. The cysteinyl leukotrienes are now known to be released after allergen inhalation (10,11), after aspirin challenge (14), and in asthmatic patients with airflow obstruction (15).

## INHALED CYSTEINYL LEUKOTRIENES IN HUMAN SUBJECTS

The cysteinyl leukotrienes were initially demonstrated to be very potent constrictors of human airway smooth muscle in vitro (16,17). The availability of $LTC_4$, $LTD_4$, and $LTE_4$ also made possible the opportunity to study the effects of inhaling these substances on airway function in human subjects. The first report of the effects of inhaled $LTC_4$ and $LTD_4$ was published in 1981 by Holroyde et al. (18), who demonstrated that these mediators caused bronchoconstriction in normal human subjects. Subsequently, inhaled $LTC_4$ and $LTD_4$ have been demonstrated to be potent bronchoconstrictors in both normal and asthmatic subjects (18–23) (Fig. 1), being up to 10,000 times more potent than methacholine in some normal subjects (23). The cysteinyl leukotrienes also have a longer duration of action than inhaled histamine (21). The bronchoconstrictor effects of inhaled $LTD_4$ are usually resolved within 1 to 2 hr and are not followed by the development of a second (late) phase bronchoconstrictor response (24) as occurs after allergen inhalation in many allergic asthmatic subjects (25).

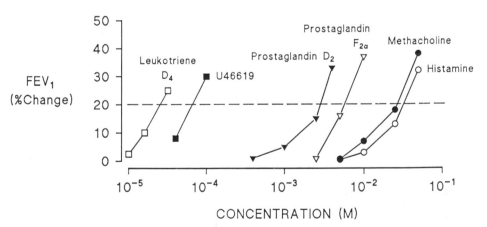

**FIG. 1.** Airway responses to a variety of inhaled bronchoconstrictor mediators in one asthmatic subject. The relative potency of the mediators differ, with the cysteinyl leukotrienes and the thromboxane mimetic U46619 being the most potent studied to date in human subjects.

LTC$_4$ and LTD$_4$ appear to have unique characteristics as bronchocon-strictors in asthmatic subjects. Airway hyperresponsiveness in asthmatic subjects is nonspecific. Therefore, an asthmatic subject who is hyperrespon-sive to inhaled histamine will be hyperresponsive to inhaled methacholine (26), prostaglandins D$_2$ (27) and F$_{2a}$ (28), and to exercise (29) and isocapnic hyperventilation (30). However, the relationships between the airway re-sponsiveness to inhaled histamine or methacholine and LTC$_4$ and LTD$_4$ are more complex. As has been described, inhaled LTC$_4$ and LTD$_4$ cause air-way narrowing in normal subjects (18–20). These investigators have usually needed to use very sensitive indices of airway caliber to measure airway narrowing after inhalation of cysteinyl leukotrienes. In normal subjects, LTC$_4$ and LTD$_4$ were between 1,000 and 6,000 times more potent in causing bronchoconstriction than was histamine. In asthmatic subjects, the concen-trations of LTC$_4$ and LTD$_4$ needed to reduce airway narrowing are less than in normals subjects, thus confirming that asthmatic subjects have airway hyperresponsiveness to the inhaled leukotrienes, which is consistent with other agonists. However, the degree of this difference between asthmatics and normals is much less than for other bronchoconstrictors. For example, Griffin et al. (31) demonstrated that mild asthmatics required 1/140 the con-centration of histamine than normals to induce similar degrees of airway narrowing, and they required only one-third the concentration of LTD$_4$. Similar results have been reported by Bisgaard et al. (32) and Adelroth et al. (23), who documented that asthmatics required one–fifty-fifth the concen-tration of methacholine than normals to induce the same degrees of bron-choconstriction, but only one-fourth the concentration of LTC$_4$ and one-eleventh the concentration of LTD$_4$. In addition, Adelroth et al. (23) reported that the relative potency of LTC$_4$ and LTD$_4$ compared with meth-acholine was closely related to the level of airway hyperresponsiveness (Fig. 2). This is not true for other bronchoconstrictors, such as histamine (23) and

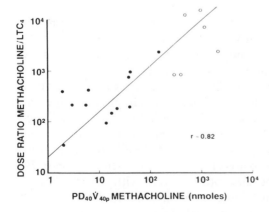

**FIG. 2.** Relationship between airway responsiveness to methacholine, as indicated by the dose causing a 40% fall in V40p (PD40V40p) and the rela-tive potency of LTC$_4$ compared with methacholine, as indicated by the dose ratio of methacholine to LTC$_4$. There is a linear relationship between these two variables ($r = 0.82$; $p < 0.001$), indicating that the relative po-tency of LTC$_4$ compared with meth-acholine was least in the subjects most responsive to methacholine. (From ref. 23 with permission.)

$PGF_{2a}$ (28). Therefore, although asthmatics are hyperresponsive to both $LTC_4$ and $LTD_4$, both leukotrienes are less potent bronchoconstrictors, compared with histamine and methacholine, in asthmatic compared to normal subjects.

## LEUKOTRIENE TACHYPHYLAXIS IN ASTHMATIC SUBJECTS

The reasons for the difference in relative potency of $LTC_4$ and $LTD_4$ in asthmatic subjects are not yet known. Possible explanations include a different site of action of $LTC_4$ and $LTD_4$ on the airways of asthmatics and normal subjects. For example, $LTD_4$ contracts guinea pig lung parenchyma while having little effect on more central airways (33). Therefore, more central deposition of $LTC_4$ or $LTD_4$ in asthmatic airways and more peripheral deposition in normal airways may make these bronchoconstrictors appear less potent in asthmatic subjects. Another explanation might be that the presence of leukotrienes in asthmatic airways may be responsible for the airway hyperresponsiveness to methacholine. Alternatively, downregulation of leukotriene receptors in asthmatic airways may occur, owing to the presence of endogenous leukotrienes or the presence of another substance that specifically antagonizes leukotriene receptors. Until recently, no evidence existed that would support any of these hypotheses.

We (34) and others (35) have previously demonstrated that tachyphylaxis exists to the bronchoconstrictor effects of inhaled histamine in stable asthmatic subjects and to inhaled methacholine in normal but not in asthmatic subjects (36). An important role for inhibitory prostaglandins in causing these effects was initially suggested by studies demonstrating that histamine-stimulated $PGE_2$ release attenuates airway smooth-muscle constrictor responses to histamine in vitro (37). After this observation, tachyphylaxis to other bronchoconstrictor mediators, such as histamine in asthmatics (34) and methacholine in normal subjects (36), was shown to be attenuated by the cyclooxygenase inhibitors indomethacin and flurbiprofen. In addition, pretreatment with oral $PGE_1$ significantly improves airway responsiveness to both inhaled histamine and methacholine (38), and inhaled $PGE_2$ attenuates allergen-induced early and late asthmatic responses (39).

The release of inhibitory prostaglandins is not a nonspecific effect of bronchoconstriction in asthmatic subjects, because tachyphylaxis does not occur if similar degrees of bronchoconstriction are induced by inhaled acetylcholine (40). However, once released by histamine, inhibitory prostaglandins can reduce airway responsiveness to acetylcholine (40) and exercise (41). In addition, histamine tachyphylaxis occurs through stimulation of $H_2$-receptors in asthmatic airways, because pretreatment with the $H_2$-receptor antagonist cimetidine prevents histamine tachyphylaxis in asthmatic subjects (42). This suggests that inhibitory prostaglandin release occurs through stimulation of airway $H_2$-receptors. The cell(s) of origin of this prostanoid is not yet known, but the probable source is a structural cell in the airway epithelium or smooth muscle. This has been suggested by a recent study from our laboratory, which has shown histamine-stimulated $PGE_2$ release from canine trachealis smooth muscle and its inhibition by $H_2$-receptor antagonists (43).

Tachyphylaxis has been shown to occur in response to repeated stimulation with inhaled $LTD_4$ in normal subjects (44) but has never been demonstrated in asthmatics. These studies raised the question of whether tachyphylaxis exists to inhaled $LTD_4$ in asthmatic subjects and, if so, whether this effect is mediated through inhibitory prostaglandin release. This question was addressed in 14 stable asthmatic subjects who did not require anything other than intermittently inhaled $\beta_2$-agonists to control their asthma. Two inhalation challenges with inhaled $LTD_4$ were performed 1 hr apart and the results were expressed as the provocation concentration of $LTD_4$ that caused a fall in the forced expired volume in 1 sec ($FEV_1$) by 20% ($PC_{20}$). Inhaled $LTD_4$ caused bronchoconstriction and tachyphylaxis in all subjects. The mean initial $LTD_4$ $PC_{20}$ was 0.31 µg/ml, which increased to an $LTD_4$ $PC_{20}$ of 0.96 µg/ml 1 hr later. This effect was attenuated by pretreatment with the cyclooxygenase inhibitor flurbiprofen. These studies demonstrated that $LTD_4$ tachyphylaxis does exist in asthmatic subjects and is mediated through $LTD_4$-stimulated inhibitory prostaglandin release. These studies may also provide an explanation for the reduced relative potency of $LTD_4$ in asthmatic subjects because of recent studies showing that $LTD_4$ antagonists are bronchodilators in asthmatic subjects. Therefore, endogenous cysteinyl leukotrienes are released in asthmatic airways at times when a challenge with exercise has not occurred. This endogenous release of leukotrienes may result in tachyphylaxis to the effects of exogenous inhaled $LTD_4$, an effect that does not occur with cholinergic agonists, such as methacholine, in asthmatics (36). This means that asthmatic, but not normal subjects, would have a lower relative potency of $LTD_4$ compared to methacholine. This explanation is presently under investigation.

## ROLE OF CYSTEINYL LEUKOTRIENES IN EXERCISE BRONCHOCONSTRICTION AND REFRACTORINESS IN ASTHMA

Exercise is another important stimulus that causes airway narrowing in asthmatics. Efforts to measure $LTD_4$ release in bronchoalveolar lavage fluid (BAL) after exercise have not been successful (45). However, this result may reflect a lack of sensitivity of BAL to measure the levels of $LTD_4$ released and causing bronchoconstriction in the airways. Increases in urinary $LTE_4$, the metabolite of $LTD_4$, after exercise have been demonstrated in one (46) but not in another study (47). However, a central role for the cysteinyl leukotrienes in causing exercise-induced bronchoconstriction is suggested by the observation that a number of different LTD$_4$-receptor antagonists markedly reduce exercise bronchoconstriction (48–50) (Fig. 3). These studies have indicated that LTD$_4$ antagonists can inhibit exercise-induced bronchoconstriction by a mean of between 50% and 70%. Indeed, in some asthmatic subjects they completely inhibit the response.

Repeated exercise challenges in asthmatic subjects, at intervals of up to 4 hr, usually results in less bronchoconstriction after the second compared with the initial exercise challenge (51). This has been termed *exercise refractoriness*. We (52) and others (53) have demonstrated that this effect is abolished by pretreatment with indomethacin. This, again, suggested that inhibitory prostaglandins released as a consequence of exercise could modify bronchoconstrictor responses in asthmatics. An initial hypothesis to explain these events in asthmatic airways after exercise was that histamine released after exercise causes bronchoconstriction but also provides partial protection against subsequent exercise-induced bronchoconstriction via

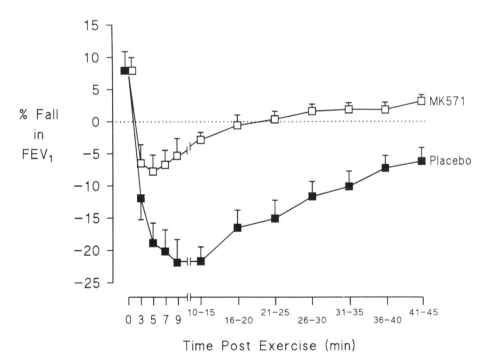

**FIG. 3.** The % change in FEV$_1$ (mean ± SEM) over time post exercise after treatment with placebo (solid squares) or MK-571 (open squares). Measurements were made in all subjects immediately after exercise, then at 3 min and every 2 min until the FEV$_1$ began to improve. Treatment with MK-571 significantly reduced the maximal fall in FEV$_1$ after exercise ($p < 0.001$) and shortened the recovery time ($p < 0.001$). (From ref. 48 with permission.)

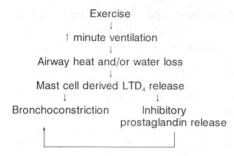

Exercise
↓
↑ minute ventilation
↓
Airway heat and/or water loss
↓
Mast cell derived $LTD_4$ release
↓                    ↓
Bronchoconstriction    Inhibitory
↑                prostaglandin release

**FIG. 4.** Hypothesis to explain the development of exercise refractoriness in asthmatic subjects. Exercise causes bronchoconstriction through the release of cysteinyl leukotrienes, which, in turn, causes inhibitory prostaglandin release that inhibits the subsequent bronchoconstrictor responses to the leukotrienes.

$PGE_2$ released by stimulation of histamine $H_2$-receptors. However, several recent studies have suggested that this hypothesis is incorrect. First, the marked attenuation of exercise-induced bronchoconstriction by pretreatment with $LTD_4$-receptor antagonists (48–50) indicates that $LTD_4$, rather than histamine, is the main mediator responsible for exercise-induced bronchoconstriction. Second, we have been unable to prevent exercise refractoriness by pretreatment with the $H_2$-receptor antagonists cimetidine and ranitidine, which effectively prevent histamine tachyphylaxis (54). Therefore, histamine-stimulated inhibitory prostaglandin release does not appear to be the cause of exercise refractoriness.

These studies raise the possibility that exercise refractoriness is caused by leukotriene-stimulated inhibitory prostaglandin release (leukotriene tachyphylaxis). This possibility has recently been tested in a study in asthmatic subjects who develop exercise-induced bronchoconstriction and refractoriness. The study demonstrated that there is an interdependence between the cyclooxygenase and lipooxygenase pathways of arachidonate metabolism in causing exercise bronchoconstriction and refractoriness in asthmatic subjects. This hypothesis (Fig. 4) is supported by the fact that the results of this study demonstrated that: exercise refractoriness and $LTD_4$ tachyphylaxis exist in the same subjects and the magnitude of the protection afforded by exercise correlates with that afforded by $LTD_4$; crossrefractoriness exists between exercise and $LTD_4$; and all of these effects are attenuated by cyclooxygenase inhibition, suggesting that the release of inhibitory prostaglandins is the common mechanism that affords protection after each of these stimuli.

## CONCLUSIONS

The leukotrienes $LTC_4$ and $LTD_4$ are important causes of bronchoconstriction in asthmatic subjects and may have an important role in the pathogenesis of airway hyperresponsiveness. Inhaled $LTC_4$ and $LTD_4$ are the most potent bronchoconstrictors yet studied in human subjects. Previously, because of the difficulty in measuring these mediators at their site of action in the airways, the evidence implicating them in this disease process was indirect. More direct evidence became available when potent and specific leukotriene antagonists were used in studies in asthmatic subjects. These studies have supported an important role for leukotrienes in the clinical manifestations of exercise-, allergen-, and aspirin-induced asthma. In addition, leukotriene release is in part responsible for spontaneous bronchoconstriction in asthma. Our recent studies suggest that the cysteinyl leukotrienes can also cause the release of inhibitory prostaglandins in asthmatic airways. This results in the development of $LTD_4$ tachyphylaxis, which may be the cause of the previously demonstrated reduced relative potency of the cysteinyl leukotrienes in asthmatics compared to normal subjects. In addition, cysteinyl leukotriene-stimulated inhibitory prostaglandin release is also the probable cause of exercise refractoriness in asthmatic subjects.

## REFERENCES

1. Hargreave FE, Ryan G, Thomson NC, et al. *J Allergy Clin Immunol* 1981;68:347–55.
2. Cockcroft DW, Killian DN, Mellon JJA, Hargreave FE. *Clin Allergy* 1977;7:235–43.
3. Juniper EF, Frith PA, Hargreave FE. *Thorax* 1981;36:575–9.
4. O'Byrne PM, Adelroth E. In: Goldie RG, ed. *Immunopharmacology of epithelial barriers.* London: Academic Press; 1994:147–57.
5. Juniper EF, Frith PA, Hargreave FE. *Thorax* 1982;37:288–91.
6. Cockcroft DW, Ruffin RE, Dolovich J, Hargreave FE. *Clin Allergy* 1977;7:503–13.
7. Chan-Yeung M, Lam S. *Am Rev Respir Dis* 1986;133:686–703.
8. Empey DW, Laitinen LA, Jacobs L, Gold WM, Nadel JA. *Am Rev Respir Dis* 1976;113:131–9.
9. Golden JA, Nadel JA, Boushey HA. *Am Rev Respir Dis* 1978;118:287–94.
10. Manning PJ, Rokach J, Malo JL, et al. *J Allergy Clin Immunol* 1990;86:211–20.
11. Taylor GW, Black P, Turner N, et al. *Lancet* 1989;1:584–7.
12. Kellaway CH, Trethewie ER. *Q J Exp Physiol* 1940;30:121–45.
13. Brocklehurst WE. *J Physiol* 1960;151:416–35.
14. Kumlin M, Dahlén B, Bjorck T, Zetterstrom O, Granstrom E, Dahlén S-E. *Am Rev Respir Dis* 1992;146:96–103.
15. Drazen JM, O'Brien J, Sparrow D, et al. *Am Rev Respir Dis* 1992;146:104–8.
16. Dahlen SE, Hedqvist P, Hammarstrom S, Samuelsson B. *Nature* 1980;288:484–6.
17. Dahlén SE, Hansson G, Hedqvist P, Bjorck T, Gramstrom E, Dahlén B. *Proc Natl Acad Sci USA* 1983;80:1712–6.
18. Holroyde MC, Altounyan REC, Cole M, Dixon M, Elliott EV. *Lancet* 1981;2:17–8.
19. Weiss JW, Drazen JM, Coles N, et al. *Science* 1982;216:196–8.
20. Weiss JW, Drazen JM, McFadden ER Jr, et al. *JAMA* 1983;249:2814–7.
21. Barnes NC, Piper PJ, Costello JF. *Thorax* 1984;39:500–4.
22. Smith LJ, Greenberger PA, Patterson R, Krell RD, Bernstein PR. *Am Rev Respir Dis* 1985;131:368–72.
23. Adelroth E, Morris MM, Hargreave FE, O'Byrne PM. *N Engl J Med* 1986;315:480–4.
24. Higgins DA, O'Byrne PM. *J Allergy Clin Immunol* 1987;79:141A (abst).
25. O'Byrne PM, Dolovich J, Hargreave FE. *Am Rev Respir Dis* 1987;136:740–51.
26. Juniper EF, Frith PA, Dunnett C, Cockcroft DW, Hargreave FE. *Thorax* 1978;33:705–10.
27. Hardy CC, Robinson C, Tattersfield AE, Holgate ST. *N Engl J Med* 1984;311:209–13.
28. Thomson NC, Roberts R, Bandouvakis J, Newball H, Hargreave FE. *J Allergy Clin Immunol* 1981;68:392–8.
29. Anderton RC, Cuff MT, Frith PA, et al. *J Allergy Clin Immunol* 1979;63:315–20.

30. O'Byrne PM, Ryan G, Morris M, et al. *Am Rev Respir Dis* 1982;125:281–5.
31. Griffin M, Weiss JW, Leitch AG, et al. *N Engl J Med* 1983;308:436–9.
32. Bisgaard H, Groth S, Madsen F. *Br Med J* 1985;290:1468–71.
33. Lewis RA, Austen KF, Drazen JM, Clark DA, Corey EJ. *Proc Natl Acad Sci USA* 1980; 77:3710–4.
34. Manning PJ, Jones GL, O'Byrne PM. *J Appl Physiol* 1987;63:1572–7.
35. Connolly MJ, Hendricks DJ. *Thorax* 1985;40:216–7.
36. Stevens WH, Manning PJ, O'Byrne PM. *J Appl Physiol* 1990;69:875–9.
37. Anderson WH, Krzanowski JJ, Polson JB, Szentivanyi A. *Biochem Pharmacol* 1979;28: 2223–6.
38. Manning PJ, Lane CG, O'Byrne PM. *Pulmonary Pharmacol* 1989;2:121–4.
39. Pavard ID, Wong C, Williams A, et al. *Am Rev Respir Dis* 1992;145:A54.
40. Manning PJ, O'Byrne PM. *Am Rev Respir Dis* 1988;137:1323–5.
41. Hamilec CM, Manning PJ, O'Byrne PM. *Am Rev Respir Dis* 1988;138:794–8.
42. Jackson PA, Manning PJ, O'Byrne PM. *Am Rev Respir Dis* 1988;138:784–8.
43. Manning PM, Jones GL, Lane CG, O'Byrne PM. *Am Rev Respir Dis* 1988;137:373A.
44. Kern R, Smith LJ, Patterson R, Krell RD, Bernstein PR. *Am Rev Respir Dis* 1986;133: 1124–6.
45. Broide DH, Eisman E, Ramsdell JW, Ferguson P, Schwartz LB, Wasserman SI. *Am Rev Respir Dis* 1990;141:563–8.
46. Kikawa Y, Miyanomae T, Inoue Y, et al. *J Allergy Clin Immunol* 1992;89:1111–9.
47. Taylor IK, Wellings R, Taylor GW, Fuller RW. *Am Rev Respir Dis* 1992;145:A15.
48. Manning PJ, Watson RM, Margolskee DJ, et al. *N Engl J Med* 1990;323:1736–9.
49. Finnerty JP, Wood-Baker R, Thomson H, Holgate ST. *Am Rev Respir Dis* 1992;145:746–9.
50. Robuschi M, Riva E, Fuccella LM, et al. *Am Rev Respir Dis* 1992;145:1285–8.
51. Edmunds AT, Tooley M, Godfrey S. *Am Rev Resp Dis* 1978;117:247–54.
52. O'Byrne PM, Jones GL. *Am Rev Respir Dis* 1986;134:69–72.
53. Margolskee DJ, Bigby BG, Boushey HA. *Am Rev Respir Dis* 1988;137:842–6.
54. Manning PJ, Watson RL, O'Byrne PM. *J Allergy Clin Immunol* 1992;88:125–6.

Advances in Prostaglandin, Thromboxane,
and Leukotriene Research, Vol. 22, edited by
S.-E. Dahlén et al. Raven Press, Ltd., New York © 1994

# Influence of Leukotriene Antagonists on Baseline Pulmonary Function and Asthmatic Responses

N. C. Barnes and L. Kuitert

*London Chest Hospital, London E2 9JX, England*

After the discovery of the slow-reacting substances of anaphylaxis (SRS-A) as mediators of allergic reactions, it seemed likely that they would be important mediators in asthma. Research into these mediators was hindered by difficulty in elucidating their chemical structure. The elucidation of the structure of the SRS-A as a group of peptidolipids now known as the leukotrienes led to an explosion of research in this area. A massive effort by the pharmaceutical industry has led to the synthesis of a range of receptor antagonists for the cysteinyl leukotrienes. A variety of these have now been tested in human subjects in studies ranging from simple tests of their potency against the effect of inhaled leukotrienes, through models of clinical asthma such as antigen- and exercise-induced bronchospasm, to medium-term studies in clinical asthma. Sufficient numbers of compounds have now been studied for their effect in models of asthma for us to be reasonably confident of their actions, although there are still gaps in our knowledge. The difficulty and expense of longer-term studies in clinical asthma has meant that our knowledge of the role of these drugs in the treatment of chronic asthma is more limited.

## EFFECT OF LEUKOTRIENE ANTAGONISTS ON LEUKOTRIENE-INDUCED BRONCHOCONSTRICTION

To interpret the results of studies of leukotriene antagonists in clinical models of asthma and in chronic asthma, it is useful to have a clear idea of the potency of these drugs in human subjects. The ability to perform reproducible challenge tests with inhaled leukotrienes (1), both in normal and asthmatic subjects, allows measurement of the potency of leukotriene antagonists in humans. Measurement of the potency of leukotriene antagonists by performing challenge tests with inhaled leukotrienes has become almost a routine part of their evaluation. The first antagonists to be reported were

FPL-55712 and FPL-59257, which were synthesized before the structure of leukotrienes had been discovered. Only very limited studies of these drugs were performed, but they were shown to have some slight effect on bronchospasm caused by inhaled leukotrienes (2).

The first group of leukotriene antagonists to be studied extensively was the acetophenone derivatives, whose structure was based on that of FPL-55712. Two of these drugs, L649,923 (3) and LY171,883 (4), were active by the oral route of administration, whereas L648,051 (5) was active by inhalation. At an oral dose of 1 g, L649,923 caused an almost fourfold shift to the right of the dose–response curve to inhaled $LTD_4$ (6), whereas LY171,883 caused an approximately sixfold shift at a dose of 400 mg (7) (Table 1). L648,051 was active only by the inhaled route, so that dose–response curves to this drug were not constructed, but at the highest dose of 12 mg it was able to block just over 50% of the bronchoconstriction caused by a single inhalation of $LTD_4$ (8). The relative lack of potency of these early drugs, together with disappointing results against antigen challenge (9,10) and their gastrointestinal (6,9) and hepatic side effects, led to their abandonment.

Drugs of chemical structures completely different from the acetophenone derivatives have now been synthesized and tested. Both in vitro and in human studies they have shown much greater potency than the acetophenone derivatives. SK&F 104353 (11) is a cysteinyl leukotriene analogue active via the inhaled route of administration. It almost totally blocks the effect of a single dose of inhaled $LTD_4$ and has a duration of action of at least 4 hr (12,13). ICI204,219 is an indazoline (14), the most potent leukotriene antagonist yet studied in human subjects. It causes an approximately 100-fold shift in the dose–response curve to inhaled $LTD_4$ when given orally at a dose of 40 mg (15). ICI204,219 is also active by the inhaled route of administration. MK-571 is active when given intravenously, orally, or by inhalation (16) and causes an at least 40-fold shift in the $LTD_4$ dose–response curve (17). Other reported compounds include RG12525 (18), although this agent is less potent than some of the other more recent drugs (19).

**TABLE 1.** *Potency of $LTD_4$ antagonists in vitro and in human subjects*

| Compound | Potency $(K_i, \mu M)^a$ | Right shift of $LTD_4$ dose–response curve | | Dose, route[b] |
|---|---|---|---|---|
| L649,923 | 8.9 | 3.8 | Normal | 1 g, O |
| L648,051 | 6.2 | ~4 | Normal | 1.2 mg, inh |
| LY171,883 | 22.9 | 4.6–6.1 | Asthmatic | 400 mg, O |
| SK&F 104,353 | 0.04 | 12.3 | Asthmatic | 800 μg, inh |
| | | ~10 | Normal | 800 μg, inh |
| ICI204,219 | 0.003 | 117 | Normal | 40 mg, O |
| RG12525 | 0.003 | 7.5 | Asthmatic | 800 mg, O |
| MK-571 | 0.009 | 44 | Asthmatic | 28 mg, i.v. |
| | | 84 | Asthmatic | 277 mg, i.v. |

[a] Determined by [³H]$LTD_4$ binding assay.
[b] Route of administration: O, oral; inh., inhaled; i.v., intravenous.

Studies of putative leukotriene antagonists for their effects against inhaled $LTD_4$ have been a useful step in their evaluation. There has been a reasonable correlation between their efficacy in vitro and their effects in vivo in humans. Their potency against inhaled $LTD_4$ challenge has correlated with their ability to block responses to more clinically relevant challenges, such as antigen and exercise challenge.

## EFFECT ON HISTAMINE AND METHACHOLINE CHALLENGE

The demonstration that a drug can block the effects of inhaled leukotrienes does not mean that it is doing so by acting as a leukotriene antagonist. Functional antagonists, such as $\beta_2$-agonists or anticholinergic agents, also cause a shift to the right of the inhaled $LTD_4$ dose–response curve. To demonstrate that any putative compound is causing a shift of the $LTD_4$ dose–response curve by acting as a receptor antagonist rather than as a functional antagonist, most evaluations of such drugs have included methacholine or histamine challenge to rule out any nonspecific action. None of the leukotriene antagonists thus far reported has shown any effect on histamine- or methacholine-induced bronchoconstriction in normal subjects (6–8, 12). This suggests that they are in fact selective leukotriene antagonists.

## RESPONSE TO ANTIGEN INHALATION

The inhalation of an antigen to which an atopic asthmatic is sensitive usually leads to one of two responses. The first pattern is an isolated early response. This consists of an episode of bronchospasm occurring within about 10 min of antigen inhalation, which then recovers over the subsequent hour. The second type of response is the dual response. The early episode of bronchoconstriction is followed approximately 4 to 6 hr later by a further episode of bronchospasm that lasts for several hours. In some subjects after a late asthmatic response, there is an increase of nonspecific bronchial hyperresponsiveness and a worsening of asthma that may last for several weeks. The pathogenesis of the early and late asthmatic responses appears to be different. The early asthmatic response is caused by the generation and release of chemical mediators, whereas the late asthmatic response is caused by a combination of increased airway inflammation owing to the influx of inflammatory cells and the release of mediators.

Investigation into the effect of new anti-asthmatic drugs on the response to inhaled antigen has frequently been part of their evaluation. Studies of the acetophenone derivatives for their effects on inhaled antigen were rather disappointing. L649,923 (9) and LY171,883 (10) had small but statistically significant effects on the early response to inhaled antigen but no significant effect on the late response (Table 2). L648,051 at a dose of 800 μg by

**TABLE 2.** *Effect of LTD$_4$-antagonist administration on the response to allergen, cold air, or exercise*

| Compound | % Inhibition of bronchoconstriction to allergen | | % Inhibition of bronchoconstriction to cold air or exercise |
|---|---|---|---|
| | EAR[a] (dose, route[c]) | LAR[b] | |
| L649,923 | 27% (1 g, O) | None | ND |
| L648,051 | 18% (6 mg, inh) | None | ND |
| SK&F 104,353 | 70% (1.2 mg, inh) | ~50% | 31% (800 µg, inh) Exercise |
| ICI204,219 | 80% (400 mg, O) | 50% | 40% (20 mg, O) Exercise |
| MK-571 | 62% (450 mg i.v.) | 50% | 70% (165 mg, i.v.) |
| LY171883 | 35% (400 mg, O) | None | Some protection (cold air) (600 mg b.i.d., 2 wk) |

[a] EAR, early asthmatic response.
[b] LAR, late asthmatic response.
[c] Route of administration: O, oral; inh, inhaled; i.v., intravenous; ND, not done.

inhalation had a trivial effect on the early response and no effect on the late response (20). SK&F 104353 has a significant blocking effect on the early asthmatic response, together with some effect on the late response (21). It is of interest that in a study with SK&F 104353 in combination with the potent H$_1$-histamine antagonist terfenadine, the combination of the two drugs completely blocked the early asthmatic response (21). This is in keeping with studies of histamine antagonists, which showed that they block approximately 50% of the early asthmatic response and seem particularly potent during the first part of the early response (22). There are also studies of isolated sensitized human lung tissue showing that the combination of leukotriene antagonist and histamine antagonist completely prevented antigen-induced contraction of bronchial smooth muscle (23).

The clearest evidence for the effect of leukotriene antagonists on antigen-induced bronchoconstriction has come from studies of ICI204,219 (24–26) and MK-571 (27,28). These studies have shown between 70% and 80% blockade of the early asthmatic response and an approximately 50% blockade of the late asthmatic response. The blockade of the early asthmatic response seen with these drugs is likely to be the maximum achievable with a leukotriene antagonist. Whether any further activity than the 50% blockade thus far achieved against the late asthmatic response is possible with higher doses of the drugs, more potent drugs, or longer acting drugs is not clear.

One of the most intriguing observations made in the study of ICI204,219 was that the increase in nonspecific bronchial hyperresponsiveness that can occur after a late asthmatic response was partially inhibited (24). It is not yet clear whether this improvement was due to the difference in baseline lung function at the time the methacholine challenge test was performed or represented a true decrease in airway inflammation caused by the leukotriene antagonist. The late asthmatic response has been considered by many to be a model for chronic asthma, and it has been argued that drugs that affect the late asthmatic response are anti-inflammatory and have beneficial effects in chronic asthma. This hypothesis has been questioned after it was shown that the long-acting $\beta_2$-agonist salmeterol can block the late asthmatic response (29), and yet biopsy studies have shown no effect of $\beta_2$-agonists on airway inflammation in chronic asthma (30). The relationship of the late asthmatic response to chronic asthma therefore remains unclear. However, the ability of leukotriene antagonists to block the late asthmatic response has led some to believe that these agents will have an anti-inflammatory effect in chronic asthma.

## COLD AIR AND EXERCISE-INDUCED BRONCHOSPASM

There is considerable controversy over the exact mechanism of exercise-induced and cold air-induced bronchospasm. However, the response to pharmacologic manipulation of the two stimuli is very similar, and in terms of leukotriene antagonists they can be considered together. LY171,883 gives some protection against cold air-induced asthma (31). MK-571 at an i.v. dose of 160 mg provides approximately 80% protection against exercise-induced bronchospasm (32). At an oral dose of 20 mg, ICI204,219 blocked about 50% of the response to exercise in eight asthmatic patients (33). At a dose of 800 $\mu$g by inhalation, SK&F 104353 was equipotent with 20 $\mu$g of disodium cromoglycate in attenuating exercise-induced bronchoconstriction by about one-third in 18 patients with mild asthma (34). The lesser degree of attenuation of exercise-induced bronchoconstriction by SK&F 104353 than by MK-571 may be due to a difference in potency. It has been shown that potent $H_1$-antagonists can partially attenuate cold air- and exercise-induced bronchoconstriction (35). It is likely that the mechanisms of exercise- and cold air-induced bronchoconstriction are very similar to those of the early response to antigen challenge and that histamine and cysteinyl leukotrienes are the main mediators.

## BASELINE AIRWAY FUNCTION

In normal subjects a degree of baseline airway tone is maintained by vagal activity, which can be reversed with anticholinergics, such as ipratropium bromide, or by functional antagonists, such as salbutamol. Studies in normal subjects with a variety of leukotriene antagonists have failed to show any alteration in lung function (6–8,12), indicating, as would be expected, that cysteinyl leukotrienes do not play any role in the maintenance of baseline airway tone in normal subjects. In asthmatic subjects, apart from the baseline vagal tone shown in normal subjects, there is an additional variable degree of resting airflow obstruction. The degree of resting airway tone varies from very slight in mild asthmatics to very marked in severe chronic asthmatics. The cause of this impaired airway function is probably multifactorial and may include irreversible structural changes to the lung caused, for example, by the subepithelial fibrosis, the thickening of the airway wall due to inflammation and edema, and the acutely reversible bronchospasm resulting from the presence of inflammatory mediators. There is evidence for some histamine tone in the airways in asthmatics, as $H_1$-antagonists cause a minor degree of bronchodilatation (36). However, this acute bronchodilatation demonstrates tachyphylaxis if histamine antagonists are administered chronically.

Several studies have addressed the questions of whether there is any leukotriene tone in the airways in asthmatics and whether leukotriene antagonists may act acutely as bronchodilators. The first such study was per-

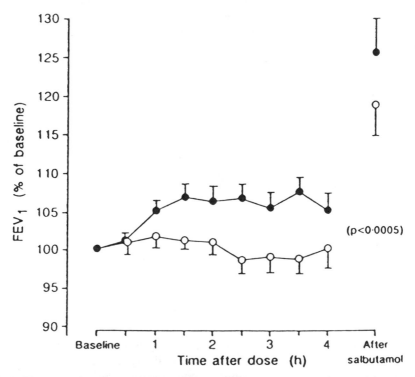

**FIG. 1.** $FEV_1$ for 4 hr after ICI204,219 (●) or placebo (○) and after nebulized salbutamol. (From ref. 38 with permission.)

formed with the weak inhaled leukotriene antagonist L648,051. At a dose of 1.6 mg it was given to a group of wheezy asthmatics, and there was a small improvement in both specific airway conductance and flow at low lung volumes, which just failed to reach statistical significance (37). This study was repeated with the more potent oral leukotriene antagonist ICI204,219 (38). Chronic asthmatics with impaired lung function and a resting $FEV_1$ of less than 70% of predicted level were studied. Nine of the 10 subjects who completed the study were taking inhaled corticosteroids. When ICI204,219 at an oral dose of 20 mg was given, bronchodilatation ensued which was apparent within 30 min and reached a maximum at 1 hr, thereafter remaining stable for the following 3 hr (Fig. 1). At the end of the study, inhalation of a large dose of salbutamol caused further bronchodilatation, but noteworthy was the fact that the bronchodilatation caused by the leukotriene antagonist and the $\beta_2$-agonist was additive. This study indicates that there is leukotriene tone in the airways of asthmatics and that this leukotriene tone is present even when inhaled steroids are being used. This, together with the additive bronchodilatation with $\beta_2$-agonists, provides considerable hope that leukotriene antagonists will be a useful therapy in chronic asthma. Other studies have confirmed this bronchodilatation with leukotriene antagonists. Both MK-571 (39) and its active enantiomer verlukast (MK0679) (40) have been shown to cause bronchodilatation that is additive to that of inhaled $\beta_2$-agonists (Fig. 2). In a study of $LTD_4$-induced bronchoconstriction in asth-

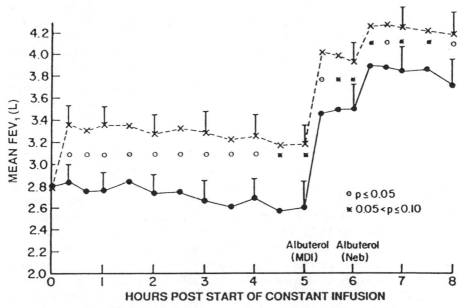

**FIG. 2.** $FEV_1$ after intravenous MK-571 (×) or placebo (●) and after subsequent inhaled and nebulized albuterol (salbutamol) (38).

matics, SK&F 104353 also exhibited some minor bronchodilatory activity (13).

The mechanism of the additive bronchodilatory activity of leukotriene antagonists and $\beta_2$-agonists is unclear. One possibility is that both cause relaxation of bronchial smooth muscle and that the portion of bronchospasm relieved by a leukotriene antagonist is not amenable to relaxation by $\beta_2$-agonists. This seems unlikely because leukotriene-induced bronchoconstriction is rapidly reversed with even a small dose of a $\beta_2$-agonist. The second possibility is that the leukotriene antagonists reverse airway narrowing caused by mechanisms other than smooth-muscle constriction, such as reversing airway edema or inflammation. This mechanism also seems unlikely, because the bronchodilatation produced by leukotriene antagonists is rapid in onset and is much more suggestive of an alteration in smooth-muscle tone (Figs. 1 and 2). Upregulation of $\beta_2$-receptors by leukotriene antagonists is another possibility. Unfortunately, there has been a paucity of in vitro animal work and in vivo work to investigate the interaction between leukotriene antagonists and $\beta_2$-agonists, and the mechanism of this response therefore remains unclear.

## BRONCHIAL HYPERRESPONSIVENESS

A number of studies have investigated the question of whether or not leukotrienes can increase bronchial hyperresponsiveness. It seems clear that leukotrienes cannot induce airway hyperresponsiveness to histamine and methacholine in normal subjects (41,42), but in asthmatic subjects there has been a suggestion that the cysteinyl leukotrienes can increase airway hyperresponsiveness (42). Two studies have suggested that inhaled leukotrienes may increase bronchial responsiveness to inhaled prostanoids (43,44). There are considerable methodological problems with these studies, and therefore it is useful to reverse the experimental situation and investigate whether a leukotriene antagonist can decrease airway responsiveness. Several studies that have investigated the potency of leukotriene antagonists in asthmatics have used histamine or methacholine challenge as a nonspecific control to prove that a leukotriene antagonist is not acting as a functional antagonist. None of these has shown any change in responsiveness to histamine or methacholine. We have specifically investigated whether the inhaled leukotriene antagonist SK&F 104353 can decrease airway hyperresponsiveness to either histamine or $PGD_2$ (45). Despite its use in a dose that effectively blocks antigen challenge and causes bronchodilatation, there was no effect on either histamine or $PGD_2$ responsiveness in a group of eight asthmatic subjects. The study by Taylor et al. of the effect of ICI204,219 on antigen-induced bronchoconstriction showed that the drug appeared to attenuate the increase in bronchial hyperresponsiveness that occurs after a late asthmatic response. However, it is not clear whether this attenuation of bronchial hyperresponsiveness is caused by an improvement in baseline airway function or by a true decrease in bronchial hyperresponsiveness.

Comprehensive studies have not been performed to determine conclusively whether leukotriene antagonists can alter bronchial hyperresponsiveness. The weight of evidence thus far suggests that when acutely administered they cannot alter baseline hyperresponsiveness but that there they may be able to block an increase in hyperresponsiveness. It is not known if, when chronically administered, they will be able to alter bronchial hyperresponsiveness.

## CONCLUSION

Leukotriene-receptor antagonists have proven effective in a variety of controlled clinical models of asthma, including antigen-, cold air-, and exercise-induced asthma. They have also been shown to cause acute bronchodilatation in the presence of inhaled steroids, and this bronchodilatation is additive to that of $\beta_2$-agonists. These results, taken together, are very favorable and suggest that leukotriene antagonists should be a useful addition to therapy for chronic asthma.

## REFERENCES

1. Barnes NC, Zakrzewski JT, Piper PJ, Costello JF. Br J Clin Pharmacol 1985;20:554P.
2. Holyroyde MC, Altounyan REC, Cole M, Dixon M, Elliot EV. Lancet 1981;2:17–8.
3. Jones TR, Young R, Champion E, et al. Can J Physiol Pharmacol 1986;64:1068–75.
4. Fleisch JH, Rinkema LE, Haisch KD, et al. J Pharmacol Exp Ther 1985;233:148–57.
5. Jones TR, Guindon Y, Young R, et al. Can J Physiol Pharmacol 1986;64:1535–42.
6. Barnes NC, Piper PJ, Costello JF. J Allergy Clin Immunol 1987;79:816–21.
7. Phillips GD, Rafferty P, Robinson C, Holgate ST. J Pharmacol Exp Ther 1988;245:732–8.
8. Evans JM, Barnes NC, Zakrzewski JT, et al. Br J Clin Pharmacol 1989;28:125–35.
9. Britton JR, Hanley SP, Tattersfield AE. J Allergy Clin Immunol 1987;79:811–6.
10. Fuller RW, Black PN, Dollery CT. Br J Clin Pharmacol 1988;25:626P.
11. Hay WP, Muccitelli RM, Tucker SS, et al. J Pharmacol Exp Ther 1987;243:474–84.
12. Evans JM, Piper PJ, Costello JF. In: Samuelsson B, Paoletti R, Ramwell P, eds. Advances in prostaglandin, thromboxane, and leukotriene research, Vol. 21A. New York: Raven Press; 1990:469–72.
13. Joos GF, Kips JC, Pauwels RA, Van der Straeten ME. Pulmonary Pharmacol 1991;4:37–42.
14. Krell RD, Aharony D, Buckner CK, et al. Am Rev Respir Dis 1990;141:978–87.
15. Smith LJ, Geller J, Elbright L, Glass M, Thyrum PT. Am Rev Respir Dis 1990;141:988–92.
16. Jones TR, Zamboni R, Belley M, et al. Can J Physiol Pharmacol 1988;67:17–28.
17. Kips J, Joos G, De Lepelaire I, et al. Am Rev Respir Dis 1991;144:617–21.
18. Carnathan GW, Sweeney D, Travis J, van Inwegen RC. Agents Actions 1989;27:316–8.
19. Wahedna I, Wisniewski AS, Tattersfield AE. Br J Clin Pharmacol 1991;32:512–5.
20. Rasmussen JB, Eriksson L-O, Andersson KE. Allergy 1991;46:266–73.
21. Eiser N, Hayhurst M, Denman W. Am Rev Respir Dis 1989;139(Suppl):A462(abst).
22. Rafferty P, Beasley R, Holgate ST. Am Rev Respir Dis 1987;136:369–73.
23. Wasserman MA, Torphy TJ, Hay DWP, et al. In: Samuelsson B, Paoletti R, Ramwell PW, eds. Advances in prostaglandin, thromboxane, and leukotriene research, Vol. 17A. New York: Raven Press; 1987:532–5.

24. Taylor IK, O'Shaughnessy KM, Fuller RW, Dollery CT. *Lancet* 1991;337:690–3.
25. Dahlen S-E, Dahlen B, Eliasson E, et al. In: Samuelsson B, Paoletti R, Ramwell P, eds. *Advances in prostaglandin, thromboxane, and leukotriene research,* Vol. 21A. New York: Raven Press; 1991:461–4.
26. Findlay SR, Barden JM, Easley CB, Glass M. *J Allergy Clin Immunol* 1992;89:1040–5.
27. Hendeles L, Davidson D, Blake K, Haman E, Cooper R, Margolskee D. *J Allergy Clin Immunol* 1990;85:197[Abstract].
28. Rasmussen JB, Margolskee DJ, Eriksson L-O, Williams VC, Andersson K-E. *Ann NY Acad Sci* 1991;29:436.
29. Twentyman OP, Finnerty JP, Harris A, Palmer J, Holgate ST. *Lancet* 1990;336:1338–42.
30. Jeffery PK, Godfrey RW, Adelroth E, Nelson F, Rogers A, Johansson S-A. *Am Rev Respir Dis* 1992;145:890–9.
31. Israel E, Juniper EF, Callaghan JT, et al. *Am Rev Respir Dis* 1989;140:1348–53.
32. Manning PJ, Watson RM, Margolskee DJ, Williams VC, Schwartz JI, O'Byrne PM. *N Engl J Med* 1990;323:1736–9.
33. Finnerty JP, Wood-Baker R, Thomson H, Holgate ST. *Am Rev Respir Dis* 1992;145:746–9.
34. Robuschi M, Riva E, Fuccella LM, et al. *Am Rev Respir Dis* 1992;145:1285–8.
35. Patel KR. *Br Med J* 1984;288:1496–7.
36. Brik A, Tashkin DP, Gong JH, Dauphinee B, Lee E. *J Allergy Clin Immunol* 1987;80:51–6.
37. Evans J, Barnes NC, Piper PJ, Costello JF. *Br J Clin Pharmacol* 1988;25:112P–13P[Abstract].
38. Hui KP, Barnes NC. *Lancet* 1991;337:1062–3.
39. Gaddy JN, Margolskee DJ, Bush RE, Williams VC, Busse WW. *Am Rev Respir Dis* 1992;146:358–63.
40. Lammers J-WJ, Van Daele P, Van den Elshout FMJ, et al. *Pulmonary Pharmacol* 1992;5:121–5.
41. Barnes NC, Evans J, Zakrzewski J, Piper P, Costello JF. *Ann NY Acad Sci* 1988;524:369–78.
42. Arm JP, Spur BW, Lee TM. *J Allergy Clin Immunol* 1988;182:654–60.
43. Barnes NC, Watson A, Kouloris N, Piper PJ, Costello JF. *Thorax* 1984;39:697[Abstract].
44. Phillips GD, Holgate ST. *J Appl Physiol* 1989;66:304–12.
45. Hui KP, Barnes NC. *Am Rev Respir Dis* 1991;143(pt 2):A636[Abstract].

Advances in Prostaglandin, Thromboxane,
and Leukotriene Research, Vol. 22, edited by
S.-E. Dahlén et al. Raven Press, Ltd., New York © 1994

# Evidence for a Specific Role of Leukotriene $E_4$ in Asthma and Airway Hyperresponsiveness

Jonathan P. Arm and Tak H. Lee

*Department of Allergy and Allied Respiratory Disorders, Guy's Hospital, London
SE1 9RT, England*

## SYNTHESIS AND ACTIONS OF THE CYSTEINYL LEUKOTRIENES

### Synthesis

The cysteinyl leukotrienes (LT) $LTC_4$, $LTD_4$, and $LTE_4$ are lipid mediators formed from oxidative metabolism of arachidonic acid by the lipoxygenase enzyme cascade (1). In contrast to mediators such as histamine, which are preformed and stored in granules, leukotrienes are newly synthesized on cell activation. Arachidonic acid, released from membrane phospholipids by the action of phospholipase $A_2$, is metabolized by 5-lipoxygenase to generate the unstable intermediate 5$S$-hydroperoxy-6-*trans*-8,11,14-*cis*-eicosatetraenoic acid (5-HPETE), which is reduced to 5$S$-hydroxy-6-*trans*-8,11,14-*cis*-eicosatetraenoic acid (5-HETE) or is converted to an epoxide, 5,6-oxido-7,9-*trans*-11,14-*cis*-eicosatetraenoic acid ($LTA_4$). $LTA_4$ is processed by an epoxide hydrolase to 5$S$,12$R$-dihydroxy-6,14-*cis*-8,10-*trans*-eicosatetraenoic acid ($LTB_4$) or by a glutathione S-transferase to 5$S$-hydroxy-6$R$-S-glutathionyl-7,9-*trans*-11,14-*cis*-eicosatetraenoic acid ($LTC_4$). $LTC_4$ is cleaved by γ-glutamyl-transpeptidase to 5$S$-hydroxy-6$R$-S-cysteinyl -glycyl-7,9-*trans*-11,14-*cis*-eicosatetraenoic acid ($LTD_4$), which is cleaved by a dipeptidase to 5$S$-hydroxy-6$R$-S-cysteinyl-7,9-*trans*-11,14-*cis*-eicosatetraenoic acid ($LTE_4$).

### Cellular Sources

The distribution and action of 5-lipoxygenase are limited, and different cells demonstrate specificity in their metabolism of arachidonic acid. Peripheral blood neutrophils and monocytes preferentially generate $LTB_4$, whereas eosinophils preferentially generate $LTC_4$ (2–4). Monocytes and macrophages have the capacity to generate both $LTB_4$ and $LTC_4$ (5–7).

Human mast cells isolated from both skin and lung generate $LTC_4$ in response to IgE-mediated stimulation, both in vivo (8) and in vitro (9–11), although $PGD_2$ is the major eicosanoid released from human mast cells in an approximate 10-fold molar excess compared with $LTC_4$ (12). $LTA_4$ hydrolase is widely distributed. Therefore, $LTA_4$ can be metabolized within its cell of origin or can be released for metabolism by other cells. Such transcellular metabolism may lead to the generation of $LTC_4$ by platelets (13,14), endothelial cells (15), and mast cells (16).

In addition to their generation by inflammatory cells, the cysteinyl leukotrienes may be synthesized and metabolized by lung tissue. Using radiolabeled leukotrienes, the conversion of $LTA_4$ to $LTB_4$, $LTC_4$, $LTD_4$, and $LTE_4$ was demonstrated in guinea pig lung (17). Lung parenchyma from human, ferret, and guinea pig converted [³H]$LTC_4$ to [³H]$LTD_4$ and [³H]$LTE_4$ (18). After 30 min, $LTD_4$ was the predominant leukotriene recovered from human and guinea pig lung parenchyma and $LTE_4$ was the major leukotriene recovered from ferret lung. The conversion of $LTC_4$ to $LTD_4$ and $LTE_4$ by human lung parenchyma and bronchus was confirmed by Conroy et al. (19). The half-life of $LTC_4$ incubated with human lung parenchyma and bronchus was 4 min and 7 min, respectively. By 60 min, 63% and 46% of $LTC_4$ was converted to $LTE_4$ by human lung parenchyma and bronchus, respectively.

## Biologic Activity

Cysteinyl leukotrienes are potent spasmogenic agents on nonvascular smooth muscle. They also enhance mucous secretion, constrict arterioles, and enhance venopermeability. Bronchial mucosal explants respond in tissue culture by enhanced mucous secretion to as little as $10^{-9}$ $M$ $LTC_4$ (20,21). Augmented postcapillary venular permeability was demonstrated for dermal vascular beds of the guinea pig responding to locally injected $LTC_4$, $LTD_4$, and $LTE_4$ in concentrations as low as $10^{-7}$ $M$ (22,23) and was confirmed by the leakage of intravascular dye into the tissue of the hamster cheek pouch after topical application of each leukotriene (24). Intradermal administration of $LTC_4$, $LTD_4$, and $LTE_4$ in normal human subjects produces a local wheal and flare response, in which the wheal, representing enhanced venopermeability, is sustained for 2 to 4 hr (25,26). The cysteinyl leukotrienes are potent contractile agonists for bronchial smooth muscle both in vitro and in vivo (see below).

## CYSTEINYL LEUKOTRIENES IN BRONCHIAL ASTHMA

### Release of Leukotrienes in Asthma

Physical, chemical, and immunologic methods have been employed to detect leukotrienes in bronchoalveolar lavage (BAL) fluid of asthmatic subjects at rest and after bronchial challenge. With the use of fast atom bombardment mass spectroscopy to analyze the BAL fluid of asthmatic and normal subjects, $LTE_4$ was the predominant leukotriene recovered, being detected in the BAL fluid of 15 out of 17 asthmatic subjects (27). $LTD_4$ was detected in two subjects and 20-hydroxy $LTB_4$ in 12 subjects with asthma. Leukotrienes were not detected in the BAL fluid of healthy subjects. In further studies, radioimmunoassay (RIA), with or without HPLC, has been used to analyze BAL fluid of asthmatic individuals (28–30). Significant amounts of $LTC_4$ and $LTB_4$ were detected in BAL fluid of symptomatic asthmatic subjects compared with normal controls (28). In the study of Crea and colleages (30), $LTE_4$ was the predominant cysteinyl leukotriene recovered in BAL fluid of both normal and asthmatic subjects. Leukotrienes have been detected in BAL fluid after local endobronchial challenge with allergen (29) and after isocapnic hyperventilation (31). As assessed by HPLC, the predominant cysteinyl leukotriene in lavage fluid of atopic asthmatics before allergen challenge was $LTC_4$, with lesser amounts of $LTD_4$ and $LTE_4$. After allergen challenge, mean $LTC_4$ levels rose from 64 pg/ml of lavage fluid to 616 pg/ml (29). Leukotrienes were undetectable in nonatopic controls before and after allergen challenge. After asthma provoked by isocapnic hyperventilation, BAL concentrations of $LTB_4$ and immunoreactive cysteinyl leukotrienes rose from baseline levels of 10 pg/ml and 46 pg/ml, respectively, to 121 pg/ml and 251 pg/ml, respectively (31). The relative concentrations of the various leukotrienes recovered in BAL fluid vary among studies and may depend on the selection of subjects and the methods used to process and analyze BAL fluid. It is clear, however, that $LTE_4$ is present in the BAL fluid of asthmatic subjects, consistent with the hypothesis that $LTC_4$ and $LTD_4$ may be metabolized to $LTE_4$ within the airways in vivo.

Automated reversed-phase HPLC with RIA has been used to analyze leukotrienes in complex biologic fluids (32). In humans, $LTC_4$ is converted enzymatically in blood to $LTD_4$ and $LTE_4$, which are excreted in the urine (33). After infusion of radiolabeled $LTC_4$, 12% to 20% appeared in the urine. Four to six percent of the total administered dose was excreted as $LTE_4$, most of which appeared in the first 4 hr (34). Measurement of urinary $LTE_4$ concentration has therefore been used as a marker of systemic release of cysteinyl leukotrienes. Urinary $LTE_4$ levels increase during acute severe asthma (35,36) and at 3 hr after antigen challenge of asthmatic subjects (35,37,38). No increases in urinary $LTE_4$ were observed during the development of the late asthmatic response 3 to 7 hr after challenge (38). Smith et al. (37) also demonstrated release of urinary leukotrienes after allergen challenge, although urinary $LTE_4$ did not rise after exercise-induced asthma (EIA) despite a similar fall in $FEV_1$. In contrast, an increase in urinary $LTE_4$ was demonstrated after EIA in 8 of 13 children (39). The release of leukotrienes after aspirin challenge is discussed below.

## Potency

LTC$_4$ and LTD$_4$ are potent constrictors of human airways in vitro and in vivo, being approximately 1,000-fold more potent than histamine on a molar basis in contracting isolated human bronchi in vitro (40). Other investigators have confirmed the potent contractile properties of LTC$_4$ and LTD$_4$ in vitro (41) and in vivo (42–44). In normal subjects, LTC$_4$ was 600- to 9,500-fold more potent than histamine and LTD$_4$ was 6,000-fold more potent than histamine on a molar basis (43). Although LTC$_4$ and LTD$_4$ have similar potencies in human airways, in vivo they have a different time course of contraction. Maximal bronchoconstriction occurs 10 to 15 min after inhalation of LTC$_4$ and 2 min after inhalation of LTD$_4$ (43).

In asthmatic subjects the cysteinyl leukotrienes are also potent bronchoconstrictors. LTD$_4$ was reported to be 140-fold more potent than histamine in eliciting a 30% fall in $\dot{V}_{30}P$ in asthmatic subjects (45), in contrast to the data in normal subjects in whom LTD$_4$ was 6,000-fold more potent than histamine (43). A comparison between these two groups of subjects revealed that the asthmatic subjects were only one-third more responsive to LTD$_4$ than the normal subjects despite an approximate 100-fold hyperresponsiveness to inhaled histamine. Barnes et al. (46) demonstrated a correlation between airway responses to histamine and LTD$_4$ and confirmed the relative lack of hyperresponsiveness to LTC$_4$ and LTD$_4$ in asthmatic subjects. Adelroth et al. (47) similarly showed a correlation between the airway responsiveness to methacholine and the airway responsiveness to LTC$_4$ and LTD$_4$. A correlation was also observed between airway responsiveness to methacholine and the relative responsiveness to LTC$_4$ and LTD$_4$. Therefore, the subjects with the most responsive airways demonstrated the lowest relative responsiveness to LTC$_4$ and LTD$_4$ compared with methacholine (47). The study by Smith et al. (48) contrasts with these results, reporting that a group of asthmatic subjects, who were 35-fold more responsive to methacholine than normal controls, were 100-fold more responsive to LTD$_4$.

There are more limited data on the bronchoconstrictor properties of LTE$_4$. Using $\dot{V}_{30}$ as an index of airway bronchoconstriction, Davidson et al. (49) demonstrated that LTE$_4$ is 39-fold more potent than histamine in normal subjects and 14-fold more potent than histamine in asthmatic subjects. However, using airway-specific conductance (sGaw) as an index of bronchoconstriction, the relative potency of LTE$_4$ compared with that of histamine and methacholine was two to three times greater in asthmatic than in normal subjects (50). The discrepancies between these studies may be due to patient selection or to the parameter of airway caliber used to monitor the bronchoconstrictor response. It is notable that in Davidson's study a 30% fall in $\dot{V}_{30}P$ in response to LTE$_4$ was accompanied by a 2.6% fall in FEV$_1$ in normal subjects but a 15% fall in FEV$_1$ in asthmatic subjects. In contrast, a 30% fall in $\dot{V}_{30}P$ induced by histamine was accompanied by comparable falls in $FEV_1$ in both groups of subjects (49). Therefore, the relative hyperresponsiveness to $LTE_4$ observed by O'Hickey and colleagues (50) may be selective for the central airways.

The relative hyperresponsiveness of the airways of asthmatic subjects to $LTE_4$ is in contrast to the data for $LTC_4$ and $LTD_4$ (see above). Because of the inherent difficulties in comparing studies performed in different subjects using different methodologies, we compared the potency of $LTC_4$, $LTD_4$, and $LTE_4$ to one another and to both histamine and methacholine in normal and asthmatic individuals (51). The airways of asthmatic subjects were 14-fold, 15-fold, 6-fold, 9-fold, and 219-fold more responsive than the airways of normal subjects to histamine, methacholine, $LTC_4$, $LTD_4$, and $LTE_4$, respectively. Although $LTC_4$ and $LTD_4$ were 90- to 500-fold more potent than $LTE_4$ in constricting the airways of normal subjects, they were only 1.1- to 13-fold more potent than $LTE_4$ in asthmatic subjects (Fig. 1). The cumulative data therefore suggest that the airways of asthmatic subjects are relatively unresponsive to $LTC_4$ and $LTD_4$ but have a marked hyperresponsiveness to $LTE_4$.

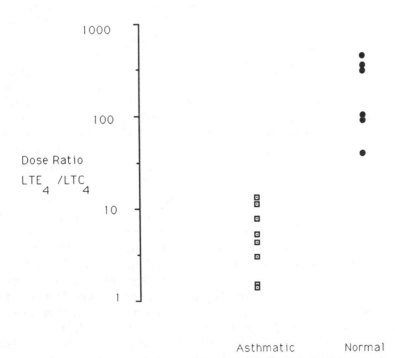

**FIG. 1.** The potency of $LTE_4$ compared to $LTC_4$ in eight asthmatic and six normal subjects. Dose ratio, dose of $LTE_4$ causing a 35% fall in sGaw divided by the dose of $LTC_4$ causing a 35% fall in sGaw.

These data are consistent with the existence of a separate $LTE_4$ receptor in human airways, which is selectively upregulated in asthmatic subjects. Experimental data in guinea pigs support the suggestion that there is heterogeneity of receptors for the cysteinyl leukotrienes. In the guinea pig, $LTC_4$, $LTD_4$, and $LTE_4$ are potent contractile agonists for tracheal spirals and parenchymal strips, eliciting equivalent contractions in a molar ratio of 1:1:0.1 and 1:0.05:3, respectively (22,41,52). This reversal of potency ratios for $LTD_4$ and $LTE_4$ with airway smooth muscle from the same species suggests that there are separate receptors for each. Furthermore, whereas $LTC_4$ and $LTE_4$ elicit monophasic contraction in guinea pig peripheral airway strips, $LTD_4$ evokes a biphasic response (23). Exposure of guinea pig tracheal smooth muscle, but not lung parenchymal strips, to $LTE_4$ produces a hyperresponsiveness to subsequent stimulation with histamine, an effect that was not produced by $LTC_4$ or $LTD_4$ (41). Furthermore, preincubation of the tracheal spirals with indomethacin or a TP receptor antagonist prevented the histamine-induced hyperresponsiveness without altering the contractile response (41,53). Evidence of separate receptors for the cysteinyl leukotrienes also comes from radioligand binding studies in guinea pig lung. The activity and binding of $LTC_4$ are insensitive to the actions of FPL 55712, which is a selective $LTD_4/LTE_4$ antagonist (54,55). The binding of $LTD_4$ and $LTE_4$ to guinea pig lung membranes is antagonized by $Na^+$ ions and GTP analogues and is enhanced by divalent cations (56). In contrast, the binding of $LTC_4$ to guinea pig lung membranes is independent of these compounds. Studies by Cheng and Townley (57) demonstrated biphasic dissociation kinetics for $LTD_4$, and Scatchard analysis suggested the existence of both low- and high-affinity receptors for $LTD_4$. Studies of the antagonism of $[^3H]LTD_4$ and $[^3H]LTE_4$ action on guinea pig trachea by FPL 55712 demonstrated a bimodal distribution of dissociation constants for $LTD_4$ (58). Further analysis suggested that there were two distinct receptors for $LTD_4$ and that $LTE_4$ bound to the high-affinity $LTD_4$ receptor. The ability of $LTD_4$ to elicit further contraction of guinea pig trachea after a maximally effective concentration of $LTE_4$, but not vice versa (59), and the observation that, in the presence of salbutamol, $LTE_4$ shifted the dose–response curve for $LTD_4$ to the right (59), suggest that $LTE_4$ may be a partial agonist at the $LTD_4$ receptor. Binding studies showed that the binding of $[^3H]LTE_4$ was completely reversed by an excess of $LTD_4$ but that the reverse was not seen (60). The density and affinity of binding sites for $LTE_4$ were lower than for $LTD_4$. The binding of $LTE_4$ was also more sensitive to $Na^+$, divalent cations, and GTP analogues, thereby providing further evidence that $LTE_4$ binds to a subset of $LTD_4$ receptors (60). The differences in the rank order of relative contractile potencies for the cysteinyl leukotrienes in various tissues, the differences in the time courses of spasmogenic responses to the three compounds in the same tissues, the distinct effect of $LTE_4$ in producing hyperresponsiveness, and the results of binding studies cannot be explained by interaction of these agonists for a single population of receptors, even if different affinities for each leukotriene are postulated. Therefore, physiologic studies of the cysteinyl leukotriene subclasses in guinea pig tissues indicate that there may be different recognition mechanisms and, in view of the stereochemical requirement for agonist action, suggest the involvement of two or more distinct receptors.

In human lung, binding of [$^3$H]LTD$_4$ is also sensitive to guanine nucleotides and the concentration of Na$^+$ and divalent cations (61). In contrast to the results in guinea pig tissues, a study conducted in the presence of bioconversion inhibitors on intralobar airways isolated from human subjects undergoing surgery for carcinoma of the bronchus did not reveal evidence for multiple leukotriene receptors (62). FPL 55712 was an effective competitive inhibitor of contractions mediated by all three cysteinyl leukotrienes, with similar PA$_2$ values calculated for each agonist. SK&F 104353 is also a selective LTD$_4$/LTE$_4$ antagonist in guinea pig lung but antagonizes the actions of LTC$_4$, LTD$_4$, and LTE$_4$ in isolated human bronchi (63). However, it should be emphasized that data from human tissue are very limited. Furthermore, the effect of underlying disease on the expression of the different leukotriene receptors has not been studied and data are not available for asthmatic lung.

## Leukotrienes and Airway Hyperresponsiveness

The in vitro observation that slow-reacting substance of anaphylaxis (SRS-A) enhanced the contractile response of guinea pig ileum to histamine (64) suggested that the cysteinyl leukotrienes might contribute to the pathogenesis of airway hyperresponsiveness in asthma. This is supported by in vitro studies with guinea pig pulmonary tissue. Pretreatment of guinea pig tracheal spirals with 10 to 23 n$M$ LTE$_4$, but not LTC$_4$ or LTD$_4$, enhanced the subsequent contractile response to histamine (41). Although LTE$_4$ elicited a similar contractile response in parenchymal strips, there was no enhancement in the response to histamine. Pretreatment of tracheal spirals with indomethacin had no effect on the contractile response to LTE$_4$ but abolished the LTE$_4$-induced histamine hyperresponsiveness. Further studies have shown that LTE$_4$-induced hyperresponsiveness of guinea pig tracheal spirals is selective for histamine and is not seen for carbachol or substance P (53). LTE$_4$-induced hyperresponsiveness is blocked not only by indomethacin but also by the TP-receptor antagonist GR32191, atropine, and tetrodotoxin (53). Preincubation of tracheal spirals with LTE$_4$ also potentiated the contractile response to electrical field stimulation. These results suggest that LTE$_4$ augments the contractile response of guinea pig tracheal spirals to histamine by facilitating cholinergic neurotransmission and is mediated via the secondary generation of prostanoids acting at the TP receptor. Treatment of human bronchus with 4.8 n$M$ $LTE_4$ produced a fourfold leftward displacement of the histamine dose–response curve (53). This effect was blocked by 1 $\mu M$ atropine or 10 $\mu M$ GR32191, suggesting a mechanism similar to that defined for guinea pig trachea.

In vivo studies support a role for the cysteinyl leukotrienes in enhancing airway hyperresponsiveness in asthma. Inhalation of a bronchoconstricting dose of $LTD_4$ in normal subjects produced an approximately twofold increase in airway methacholine responsiveness (65). In a further study, inhalation of a dose of $LTD_4$ that gave a mean 57% fall in sGaw led to a significant increase in the airway response to methacholine in six of eight normal subjects (66). In these six subjects the maximal effect on methacholine responsiveness was observed at day 7, and persisted for 2 to 3 weeks in five individuals, comparable to the change in methacholine responsiveness observed after inhalation of platelet activating factor (PAF) in the same individuals (66). In normal subjects, inhalation of a bronchoconstricting dose of $LTD_4$ did not significantly enhance the airway response to exercise (67), and a subthreshold dose of $LTD_4$ had no effect on the airway response to histamine, although it increased the sensitivity of the airways to inhaled $PGF_{2\alpha}$ by approximately sevenfold (46).

Normal and asthmatic airway responses in vivo differ by their sensitivity to a wide range of pharmacologic and nonpharmacologic agents (68) and by the presence of maximal airway narrowing to histamine and methacholine in nonasthmatic subjects (69,70). Bel and colleagues (71) investigated the effect of $LTD_4$ on the position of the dose–response curve to methacholine and the degree of maximal airway narrowing in normal subjects. The degree of maximal airway narrowing was consistently greater in response to $LTD_4$ than to methacholine. After administration of $LTD_4$ there was no change in the position of the dose–response curve to methacholine; however, the maximal airway response to methacholine increased. Pretreatment with inhaled corticosteroids diminished the maximal response to $LTD_4$ and also abolished the $LTD_4$-induced increase in maximal airway narrowing to methacholine (72). The authors suggested that the greater maximal airway narrowing caused by $LTD_4$ was due to changes in vascular permeability leading to edema of the mucosa and possibly increased mucous production. Persistence of the mucosal changes may account for the subsequent increase in maximal airway narrowing to methacholine.

Studies in asthmatic subjects have been more limited. Inhalation of bronchoconstricting doses of $LTC_4$ did not enhance the airway response to inhalation of ultrasonically nebulized distilled water (73). Because $LTC_4$ and $LTD_4$ may be metabolized within the airways to $LTE_4$ (17–19), and because $LTE_4$ may persist longer at the site of contraction (74), our initial studies focused on the effects of this mediator. Preinhalation of a bronchoconstricting dose of $LTE_4$ in asthmatic subjects increased histamine responsiveness by approximately threefold (75) (Fig. 2). Changes in airway histamine responsiveness were maximal at 4 to 7 hr after inhalation of $LTE_4$ and had returned to baseline values by 1 week. Methacholine inhalation, which led to a similar decrease in sGaw as $LTE_4$, did not elicit any change in histamine hyperresponsiveness. Subsequent work has shown that bronchoconstricting doses of $LTC_4$ and $LTD_4$ elicit a comparable increase in airway responsiveness to histamine in asthmatic individuals (76). In the absence of specific inhibitors of the bioconversion of $LTC_4$ and $LTD_4$ to $LTE_4$, it is not possible to determine whether the ability of $LTC_4$ and $LTD_4$ to augment histamine hyperresponsiveness is dependent on their bioconversion to $LTE_4$. None of the cysteinyl leukotrienes increased the airway responses to histamine in normal subjects, although each mediator was administered in a dose that elicited a mean 35% fall in sGaw (75,76). In addition to the capacity of inhaled leukotrienes to enhance subsequent airway responses to histamine in subjects with asthma, there is evidence that $LTC_4$ may interact synergistically with histamine and $PGD_2$ in the acute bronchoconstrictor response (77).

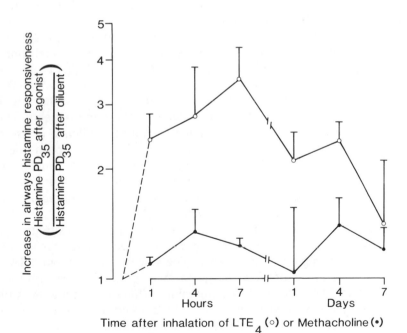

**FIG. 2.** The change in airway responsiveness to histamine in four asthmatic subjects after inhalation of a bronchoconstricting dose of methacholine (closed circles) or $LTE_4$ (open circles). (Reprinted from ref. 75 with permission.)

## Aspirin-Induced Asthma

A proportion of subjects with asthma are intolerant of aspirin. In these subjects, ingestion of aspirin is followed within 1 to 2 hr by the onset of bronchospasm that may be accompanied by rhinitis and/or urticaria (78–80). Many of these individuals have troublesome asthma controlled only by the use of inhaled or oral corticosteroids, often with a severe perennial rhinosinusitis. The role of cyclooxygenase inhibition in AIA is suggested by the observation that aspirin-sensitive subjects also react adversely to other inhibitors of this enzyme (81,82), the potency of these drugs in causing asthma being related to their potencies as inhibitors of cyclooxygenase, and by the observation of crossdesensitization among these drugs (83).

The mechanism by which inhibition of cyclooxygenase leads to the occurrence of asthma, rhinitis, and/or urticaria is unclear. It has been suggested that individuals with AIA are overdependent on bronchodilator prostanoids (84,85), although there are limited data to support this. An alternative hypothesis for the pathogenesis of AIA is that inhibition of cyclooxygenase leads to a shunting of arachidonate metabolism, with the increased generation of bronchoconstrictor leukotrienes. Several investigators have reported release of cysteinyl leukotrienes into the nasal lavage fluid of subjects after aspirin-induced asthma and rhinitis (86–88). There were no changes in leukotriene levels in nasal washings of subjects with AIA who had been desensitized, in aspirin-tolerant asthmatics, and in normal controls after ingestion of 650 mg aspirin. Increased excretion of LTE$_4$ in the urine has also been demonstrated after aspirin-induced asthma (89–91). After oral aspirin challenge, there was a three- to fourfold increase in urinary LTE$_4$, which was not observed after placebo challenge in the same subjects. There was no increase in urinary LTE$_4$ after methacholine challenge in aspirin-sensitive subjects, nor after aspirin or placebo challenge in aspirin-tolerant asthmatics. An interesting observation was that of increased urinary LTE$_4$ concentrations in subjects with AIA, compared with aspirin-tolerant asthmatics, before challenge (89,91). This is consistent with an upregulation of arachidonate metabolism in aspirin-sensitive subjects.

An additional mechanism of AIA might be an increased sensitivity of the airways to leukotrienes released after aspirin challenge. Airway responses to histamine were comparable between subjects with and without AIA. In contrast, the mean dose of LTE$_4$ causing a 35% fall in sGaw was 0.17 nmol in subjects with AIA compared to 2.8 nmol in asthmatics without AIA (92). Therefore, subjects with AIA demonstrated a marked hyperresponsiveness of the airways to LTE$_4$ compared with normal individuals. After oral desensitization to aspirin there was a mean 20-fold decrease in the sensitivity of the airways to LTE$_4$ but not to histamine (Fig. 3). These data suggest that increased sensitivity of the airways to LTE$_4$ may be an important part of the

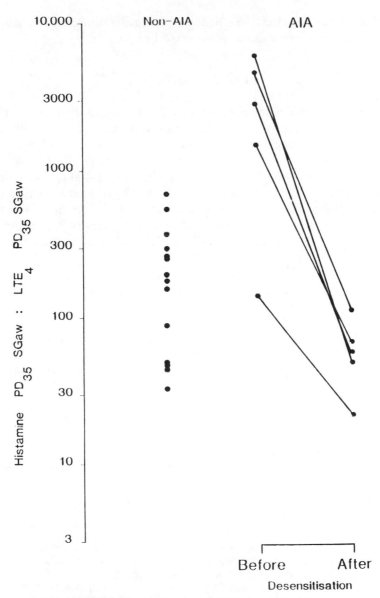

**FIG. 3.** Responsiveness of the airways to LTE₄ relative to histamine in asthmatic subjects tolerant of aspirin (non-AIA), and in subjects with aspirin-induced asthma before and after oral aspirin desensitization (AIA). Relative responsiveness, dose of histamine eliciting a 35% fall in sGaw divided by the dose of LTE₄ eliciting a 35% fall in sGaw. (Reprinted from ref. 93 with permission.)

mechanism of AIA, and that the efficacy of desensitization may relate in part to a downregulation of the airway response to $LTE_4$.

## CONCLUSIONS

$LTC_4$ and $LTD_4$ can be metabolized to $LTE_4$ by human lung, and $LTE_4$ is recovered in BAL fluid of asthmatic subjects. The airways of individuals with asthma demonstrate a relative hyporesponsiveness to $LTC_4$ and $LTD_4$ compared with histamine and methacholine, but are markedly hyperresponsive to inhaled $LTE_4$. Whereas $LTE_4$ is approximately 100-fold less potent than the other cysteinyl leukotrienes in constricting the airways of normal individuals, all three are of similar potency in the more sensitive asthmatic subjects. The airways of individuals with aspirin sensitivity are particularly sensitive to $LTE_4$. $LTE_4$, but not $LTC_4$ and $LTD_4$, enhances the contractile response of guinea pig tracheal smooth muscle to histamine in vitro, an effect that is mediated through the secondary generation of prostanoids. All three cysteinyl leukotrienes enhance the airway responsiveness to histamine of asthmatic individuals

$LTE_4$ therefore has properties distinct from those of $LTC_4$ and $LTD_4$. This may be due to the existence of a separate receptor for $LTD_4$ that is selectively upregulated in the airways of asthmatic subjects. The unique properties of this mediator should be considered in the design and assessment of new leukotriene antagonists for the treatment of bronchial asthma.

## REFERENCES

1. Samuelsson B. *Science* 1983;220:568–75.
2. Weller PF, Lee CW, Foster DW, Corey EJ, Austen KF, Lewis RA. *Proc Natl Acad Sci USA* 1983;80:7626–30.
3. Shaw RJ, Cromwell O, Kay AB. *Clin Exp Immunol* 1984;56:716–22.
4. Borgeat P, de Laclos BF, Rabinovich H, et al. *J Allergy Clin Immunol* 1984;74:310–5.
5. Williams JD, Czop JK, Austen KF. *J Immunol* 1984;132:3034–40.
6. Fels AO, Pawlowski NA, Cramer EB, King TKC, Cohn ZA, Scott WA. *Proc Natl Acad Sci USA* 1982;79:7866–70.
7. Martin TR, Altman LC, Albert RK, Henderson WR. *Am Rev Respir Dis* 1984;129:106–111.
8. Talbot SF, Atkins PC, Goetzl EJ, Zweiman B. *J Clin Invest* 1985;76:650–6.
9. Benyon RC, Lowman MA, Church MK. *J Immunol* 1987;138:861–7.
10. Paterson NAM, Wasserman SI, Said JW, Austen KF. *J Immunol* 1976;117:1356–62.
11. Peters SP, MacGlashan DW, Schulman ES, et al. *J Immunol* 1984;132:1972–9.
12. Leung KBP, Flint KC, Hudspith BN, et al. *Agents Actions* 1987;20:213–5.
13. Edenius C, Heidvall K, Lindgren JA. *Eur J Biochem* 1988;178:81–6.
14. Maclouf JA, Murphy RC. *J Biol Chem* 1988;263:174–81.
15. Feinmark SJ, Cannon PJ. *J Biol Chem* 1986;261:16466–72.
16. Dahinden CA, Clancy RM, Gross M, Chiller JM, Hugli TE. *Proc Natl Acad Sci USA* 1985;82:6632–6.
17. Sirois P, Brousseau Y, Salari H, Borgeat P. *Prostaglandins* 1985;30:21–36.
18. Aharony D, Dobson PT, Krell RD. *Biochem Biophys Res Commun* 1985;131:892–8.
19. Conroy DM, Piper PJ, Samhoun MN, Yacoub M. *Br J Pharmacol* 1989;96:72P.

20. Marom Z, Shelhamer JH, Bach MK, Morton DR, Kaliner M. *Am Rev Respir Dis* 1982; 126:449–51.
21. Coles SJ, Neill KH, Reid LM, et al. *Prostaglandins* 1983;25:155–70.
22. Lewis RA, Drazen JM, Austen KF, Clark DA, Corey EJ. *Biochem Biophys Res Commun* 1980;96:271–7.
23. Drazen JM, Austen KF, Lewis RA, et al. *Proc Natl Acad Sci USA* 1980;77:4354–8.
24. Dahlén S-E, Björk J, Hedqvist P, et al. *Proc Natl Acad Sci USA* 1981;78:3887–91.
25. Soter NA, Lewis RA, Corey EJ, Austen KF. *J Invest Dermatol* 1983;80:115–9.
26. Camp RDR, Coutts AA, Greaves MW, Kay AB, Walport MJ. *Br J Pharmacol* 1983;80: 497–502.
27. Lam S, Chan H, LeRiche JC, Chan-Yeung M, Salari H. *J Allergy Clin Immunol* 1988;81: 711–7.
28. Wardlaw AJ, Hay H, Cromwell O, Collins JV, Kay AB. *J Allergy Clin Immunol* 1989;84: 19–26.
29. Wenzel SE, Larsen GL, Johnston K, Voelkel NF, Westcott JY. *Am Rev Respir Dis* 1990; 142:112–9.
30. Crea AEG, Nakhosteen JA, Lee TH. *Eur Respir J* 1992;5:190–5.
31. Pliss LB, Ingenito EP, Ingram RH, Pichurko B. *Am Rev Respir Dis* 1990;142:73–8.
32. Tagari P, Ethier D, Carry M, et al. *Clin Chem* 1989;35:388–91.
33. Örning L, Kaijser L, Hammarström S. *Biochem Biophys Res Commun* 1985;130:214–20.
34. Maltby NH, Taylor GW, Ritter JM, Moore K, Fuller RW, Dollery CT. *J Allergy Clin Immunol* 1990;85:3–9.
35. Taylor GW, Taylor I, Black P, et al. *Lancet* 1989;1:584–8.
36. Drazen JM, O'Brien J, Sparrow D, et al. *Am Rev Respir Dis* 1992;146:104–8.
37. Smith CM, Christie PE, Hawksworth RJ, Thien F, Lee TH. *Am Rev Respir Dis* 1991;144: 1411–3.
38. Manning PJ, Rokach J, Malo J-L, et al. *J Allergy Clin Immunol* 1990;86:211–20.
39. Kikawa Y, Miyanomae T, Inoue Y, et al. *J Allergy Clin Immunol* 1992;89:1111–9.
40. Dahlén S-E, Hedqvist P, Hammarström S, Samuelsson B. *Nature* 1980;288:484–6.
41. Lee TH, Austen KF, Corey EJ, Drazen JM. *Proc Natl Acad Sci USA* 1984;81:4922–5.
42. Holroyde MC, Altounyan REC, Cole M, Dixon M, Elliott EV. *Lancet* 1981;2:17–8.
43. Weiss JW, Drazen JM, McFadden ER Jr, et al. *JAMA* 1983;249:2814–7.
44. Weiss JW, Drazen JM, Coles N, et al. *Science* 1982;216:196–8.
45. Griffin M, Weiss JW, Leitch AG, et al. *N Engl J Med* 1983;308:436–9.
46. Barnes NC, Piper PJ, Costello JF. *Prostaglandins* 1984;28:629–30.
47. Adelroth E, Morris MM, Hargreave FE, O'Byrne PM. *N Engl J Med* 1986;315:480–4.
48. Smith LJ, Greenberger PA, Patterson R, Krell RD, Bernstein PR. *Am Rev Respir Dis* 1985;131:368–72.
49. Davidson AB, Lee TH, Scanlon PD, et al. *Am Rev Respir Dis* 1987;135:333–7.
50. O'Hickey SP, Arm JP, Rees PJ, Spur BW, Lee TH. *Eur Respir J* 1988;1:913–7.
51. Arm JP, O'Hickey SP, Hawksworth RJ, et al. *Am Rev Respir Dis* 1990;142:1112–8.
52. Drazen JM, Lewis RA, Austen KF, Corey EJ. In: Berti F, Folco G, Velo GP, eds. *Leukotrienes and prostacyclin.* New York: Plenum Press; 1983:125–34.
53. Jacques CA, Spur BW, Johnson M, Lee TH. *Br J Pharmacol* 1991;104:859–66.
54. Snyder DW, Krell RD. *J Pharmacol Exp Ther* 1984;231:616–22.
55. Weichman BM, Tucker SS. *Prostaglandins* 1985;29:547–60.
56. Pong S-S, DeHaven RN. *Proc Natl Acad Sci USA* 1983;80:7415–9.
57. Cheng JB, Townley RG. *Biochem Biophys Res Commun* 1984;118:20–6.
58. Krell RD, Tsai BS, Berdoulay A, Barone M, Giles RE. *Prostaglandins* 1983;25:171–8.
59. Hay DWP, Muccitelli RM, Wilson KA, Wasserman MA, Torphy TJ. *J Pharmacol Exp Ther* 1988;244:71–78.
60. Aharony D, Catanese CA, Falcone RC. *J Pharmacol Exp Ther* 1989;248:581–8.
61. Lewis MA, Mong S, Vessella RL, Crooke ST. *Biochem Pharmacol* 1985;34:4311–7.
62. Buckner CK, Krell RD, Lavaruso RB, Coursin DB, Bernstein PR, Will JA. *J Pharmacol Exp Ther* 1986;237:558–62.
63. Hay DWP, Muccitelli RM, Tucker SS, et al. *J Pharmacol Exp Ther* 1987;243:474–81.
64. Brocklehurst WE. *Prog Allergy* 1962;6:539–58.

65. Kern R, Smith LJ, Patterson R, Krell RD, Bernstein PR. *Am Rev Respir Dis* 1986;133: 1127–32.
66. Kaye MG, Smith LJ. *Am Rev Respir Dis* 1990;141:993–7.
67. Bisgaard H, Groth S. *Clin Sci* 1987;72:585–92.
68. Holgate ST, Beasley CRW, Twentyman OP. *Clin Sci* 1987;73:561–72.
69. Woolcock AJ, Salome CM, Yan K. *Am Rev Respir Dis* 1984;130:71–5.
70. Sterk PJ, Timmers MC, Dijkman JH. *Am Rev Respir Dis* 1986;134:714–8.
71. Bel EH, van der Veen H, Kramps JA, Dijkman JH, Sterk PJ. *Am Rev Respir Dis* 1987; 136:979–84.
72. Bel EH, van der Veen H, Dijkman JH, Sterk PJ. *Am Rev Respir Dis* 1989;139:427–31.
73. Bianco S, Robuschi M, Vaghi A, et al. In: Herzog H, Perruchoud AP, eds. *Progress in respiratory research,* Vol. 19. Basel: Karger; 1985:82–6.
74. Krilis S, Lewis RA, Corey EJ, Austen KF. *J Clin Invest* 1983;71:909–15.
75. Arm JP, Spur BW, Lee TH. *J Allergy Clin Immunol* 1988;82:654–60.
76. O'Hickey SP, Hawksworth RJ, Fong CY, Arm JP, Spur BW, Lee TH. *Am Rev Respir Dis* 1991;144:1053–7.
77. Phillips GD, Holgate ST. *J Appl Physiol* 1989;66:304–12.
78. Samter M, Beers RF. *Ann Intern Med* 1968;68:975–83.
79. Chafee FH, Settipane GA. *J Allergy Clin Immunol* 1974;53:193–9.
80. McDonald JR, Mathison DA, Stevenson DD. *J Allergy Clin Immunol* 1972;50:198–207.
81. Szczeklik A, Gryglewski RJ, Czerniawska-Mysik G. *Br Med J* 1975;1:67–9.
82. Szczeklik A, Gryglewski RJ, Czerniawska-Mysik G. *J Allergy Clin Immunol* 1977;60:276–84.
83. Pleskow WW, Stevenson DD, Mathison DA, Simon RA, Schatz M, Zeiger RS. *J Allergy Clin Immunol* 1982;69:11–9.
84. Toogood JH. *Chest* 1977;72:135–7.
85. VanArsdel PP Jr. *J Allergy Clin Immunol* 1984;73:431–4.
86. Ferreri NR, Howland WC, Stevenson DD, Spiegelberg HL. *Am Rev Respir Dis* 1988;137: 847–54.
87. Ortolani C, Mirone C, Fontana A, et al. *Ann Allergy* 1987;59:106–12.
88. Picado C, Ramis I, Rosellò J, et al. *Am Rev Respir Dis* 1992;145:65–9.
89. Christie PE, Tagari P, Ford-Hutchinson AW, et al. *Am Rev Respir Dis* 1991;143:1025–9.
90. Knapp HR, Sladek K, Fitzgerald GA. *J Lab Clin Med* 1992;119:48–51.
91. Kumlin M, Dahlén B, Björck T, Zetterström O, Granström E, Dahlén S-E. *Am Rev Respir Dis* 1992;146:96–103.
92. Arm JP, O'Hickey SP, Spur BW, Lee TH. *Am Rev Respir Dis* 1989;140:148–53.
93. *Adv Immunol* 1992;51:325–82.

Advances in Prostaglandin, Thromboxane,
and Leukotriene Research, Vol. 22, edited by
S.-E. Dahlén et al. Raven Press, Ltd., New York © 1994

# Eosinophil Eicosanoid Relations in Allergic Inflammation of the Airways

## William W. Busse and Julie B. Sedgwick

*University of Wisconsin Medical School, Allergy Section,
Madison, Wisconsin 53792*

Products of the 5-lipoxygenase pathway of arachidonic acid metabolism $LTB_4$, $LTC_4$, $LTD_4$, and $LTE_4$ can have a profound and potent influence on airway physiology (1,2). These effects include recruitment and activation of inflammatory cells, stimulation of mucous secretion, changes in vascular permeability, and increased airway smooth-muscle tone. The cell sources for these products are multiple and include eosinophils (1,2). This chapter focuses on the evidence that eosinophils generate 5-lipoxygenase products, the specificity of this response, the possibility that eosinophil phenotypes may influence the intensity of this reaction, and factors that regulate and potentially control this metabolic activity.

## GENERATION OF LEUKOTRIENES BY EOSINOPHILS

Over a decade ago, Jörg and colleagues (3) isolated horse eosinophils and incubated them with the calcium ionophore A23187. This resulted in the generation of an SRS-like smooth-muscle–contracting activity. This observation fitted with the observation that eosinophils are important cells in airway inflammation in asthma and could contribute to this process via 5-lipoxygenase products. Furthermore, these investigators (3) found that the generation of SRS activity was fivefold greater from eosinophils than from neutrophils, suggesting that neutrophils do not contribute significantly to the SRS activity generated. Finally, greater than 92% of the eosinophil SRS bioactivity was caused by leukotrienes $C_4$ ($LTC_4$) and $D_4$ ($LTD_4$).

Characterization of leukotriene generation by eosinophils was also observed with human granulocytes by Weller et al. (4). In these experiments, human eosinophils were isolated from five donors with eosinophilia and three normal subjects. A number of significant observations were noted in these early studies. First, $LTC_4$ was the predominant eosinophil leukotriene product generated after activation with ionophore when eosinophilic subjects were the cell source; e.g., $LTC_4$ (69 ± 28 mg/$10^6$ cells) versus $LTB_4$ (1.5

$\pm$ 0.8 mg/$10^6$ cells). Similar findings were also noted by Shaw et al. (5). Second, the major leukotriene product from neutrophils was $LTB_4$. Finally, eosinophil generation of $LTC_4$ was greater when the cell source was patients with eosinophilia. These data indicated not only that the preferential cysteinyl product from eosinophils was $LTC_4$ but the possibility that conditions associated with eosinophilia influenced the intensity by which eosinophils generated leukotrienes. The extension of this differential leukotriene response to the pathogenesis of various allergic inflammatory disease was obvious and has continued to be a source of interest.

Shaw and co-workers (6) extended their observations with human eosinophils and noted that the generation of sulfidopeptides could also occur via activation by physiologic stimuli, i.e., IgG-coated particles, and that a subpopulation of low-density eosinophils had an enhanced capacity to generate leukotrienes. Furthermore, they were able to demonstrate that eosinophil $LTC_4$ generation to IgG-coated beads was significantly enhanced if the cells were first incubated, or primed, with the chemotactic peptide f-Met-Leu-Phe (fMLP). These data were important, and showed that physiologic stimuli could activate eosinophil generation of $LTC_4$ and that the level of this response was likely influenced by the phenotypic characteristics of the eosinophil in study.

Bruynzeel et al. (7) also isolated human eosinophils and evaluated leukotriene generation by opsonized zymosan particles. Opsonized zymosan particles generated $LTC_4$ exclusively in a time- and dose-dependent fashion, with maximal sulfidopeptide formation appearing 60 min after activation. Their studies indicated that C3b and/or IgG receptors on eosinophils were capable of generating significant amounts of $LTC_4$. In contrast, when other activators were evaluated, i.e., fMLP, platelet-activating factor (PAF), $LTB_4$, or phorbol myristate acetate (PMA), eosinophil $LTC_4$ synthesis did not occur. However, fMLP and PAF significantly enhanced the subsequent eosinophil generation of $LTC_4$ to opsonized zymosan particles.

As indicated, a number of physiologic stimuli can induce generation of $LTC_4$ by eosinophils. These have included IgG covalently linked to Sepharose beads (6) and antigen–antibody complexes (8). As a result of these observations, it was proposed that the response of eosinophils to IgG-labeled particles may mimic adherence of these cells to opsonized helminthic larvae and thus may indicate an effector cell action in parasitic disease. To extend these observations with a relevant target, Moqbel and co-workers (9) coated helminthic larvae with IgG and IgE antibodies and then incubated the larvae with eosinophils. Their results provided further insight into factors, both target and effector cell, that influence $LTC_4$ generation. Both live and fixed opsonized schistosomula induced the release of $LTC_4$ from low-density eosinophils (Table 1). However, the amount released was 20% or less than the total amount of $LTC_4$ generated by the calcium ionophore A23187. For example, low-density eosinophils that were adherent to IgG-coated

**TABLE 1.** *Effect of various treatments of FPLC fractions of immune (antischistosome) serum on the levels of specific IgE and IgG antibodies and the elicitation of LTC$_4$ release from and cytotoxicity of human low-density eosinophils*

| | Specific anti–*S. mansoni* | | Eosinophil functional assays | |
|---|---|---|---|---|
| | RAST (% IgE binding) | ELISA (IgG OD units) | LTC$_4$ release (pmol/10$^6$ cells) | Cytotoxicity (% kill) |
| Unfractionated immune serum | 36 | 8–4 | 15 ± 4 | 82 ± 5 |
| IgG-rich fractions | | | | |
| Untreated | 0 | 6–8 | 6.0 ± 0.1 | 40 ± 2 |
| + Protein A | 0 | 0–1 | 0.1 ± 0.1 | 9.4 ± 4 |
| IgE-rich fractions | | | | |
| Untreated | 35 | 7–0 | 7.8 ± 0.4 | 31 ± 1 |
| + Protein A alone | 32 | 0–18 | 5.5 ± 0.4 | 30 ± 1.5 |
| + Protein A and anti-IgE | 0 | 0–2 | 0.2 ± 0.2 | 8 ± 3 |

LTC$_4$ and cytotoxicity data represent the mean ± SEM of three experiments.
OD, optical density.

schistosomulas released $6.0 \pm 0.1$ pmol LTC$_4$/10$^6$ cells; a similar population of eosinophils incubated with an IgE-rich preparation elaborated $7.8 \pm 0.4$ pmol LTC$_4$/10$^6$ cells. In contrast, normal-density eosinophils did not generate detectable levels of LTC$_4$ when incubated with IgE-coated schistosomula; IgG-coated parasites caused 4.6 pmol of LTC$_4$/10$^6$ cells to be released. These data indicate that low-density, presumably primed cells are capable of parasite lysis and generation of LTC$_4$ to both IgE- and IgG-coated schistosomula.

In addition, these investigators compared the effects of PAF, LTB$_4$, and fMLP on the ability of normal- and low-density eosinophils to produce LTC$_4$ in IgE- and IgG-dependent systems. Under these conditions, PAF ($1 \times 10^{-7}$ M) and LTB$_4$ ($1 \times 10^{-7}$ M), but not fMLP, caused normal-density eosinophils to release LTC$_4$ when exposed to IgE-coated parasites. Whether this priming was related to changes in eosinophil density, expression of surface receptors, or other factors was not determined. It was also not determined whether these IgE-dependent activities operated via an IgE-specific receptor or through the stimulation of other receptor ligands. However these and the previously reviewed data indicate that a number of stimuli, both soluble and particulate, can cause eosinophils to generate LTC$_4$ and that this activity is more apparent with "activated" eosinophils, as might be represented by the low-density phenotype.

In addition to stimulus-specific regulation of leukotrienes, the source and species of eosinophils may also influence the amount or type of leukotriene generated. Hirata et al. (10) isolated guinea pig alveolar macrophages and eosinophils. When the alveolar eosinophil suspension was stimulated with both arachidonic acid and the calcium ionophore A23187, LTB$_4$ was produced and LTC$_4$, LTD$_4$ and LTE$_4$ were undetectable in the supernatant fluid. These data suggest that guinea pig alveolar eosinophils contain both cyclooxygenase and 5-lipoxytenase but do not produce peptidoleukotrienes, probably because they lack $LTA_4$ glutathione transferase. These data also raise the question as to the cell source for cysteinyl leukotrienes with lung anaphylaxis.

Tamura et al. (11) also evaluated the effect of PAF on $LTC_4$ generation by human eosinophils. PAF directly stimulated eosinophil generation of $LTC_4$, but the amount generated was about one-tenth that noted with a calcium ionophore. In contrast, other chemotactic stimuli, i.e., eosinophil chemotactic factor of anaphylaxis (ECF-A) or $LTB_4$, had no effect on eosinophil generation of $LTC_4$. Moreover, when the cells were preincubated with PAF and ECF-A, submaximal concentrations of the calcium ionophore markedly enhanced the ability of eosinophils to generate $LTC_4$. Therefore, in addition to functioning as eosinophil attractants, some chemotactic stimuli can also generate $LTC_4$ and prime these cells for subsequent activation.

From these observations, it is apparent that eosinophils are a rich source of the cysteinyl $LTC_4$. Furthermore, a number of factors are capable of stimulating 5-lipoxygenase generation of $LTC_4$. Some of these stimuli, i.e., IgG, C3b, and IgE, have biologic relevance and indicate the possibility that eosinophil generation of $LTC_4$ may also occur in vivo if the activating stimulus is appropriate.

## EOSINOPHIL GENERATION OF $LTC_4$ IN ASTHMA

A number of studies have investigated whether eosinophil phenotypes or eosinophils from different disease states influence the intensity of $LTC_4$ generation. We discussed the findings by Shaw et al. (6), who showed that low-density eosinophils generated more $LTC_4$ when activated with IgG-coated beads. Similar findings have been noted by others. For example, Kajita et al. (12) collected blood samples from patients during a quiescent state of bronchial asthma. Using Percoll gradients, eosinophils of different density were isolated and then activated by the calcium ionophore. A number of significant findings were noted. First, compared with neutrophils, eosinophils generated significantly more $LTC_4$. Moreover, there was a tendency for eosinophils of lower density to generate more $LTC_4$ than cells of normal density. These data raised the possibility that low-density eosinophils were "activated," the end result being a cell with enhanced physiologic response. Because there is an increased concentration of low-density eosinophils in asthma (13,14), this raises the possibility that $LTC_4$ generation from eosinophils is increased in asthma and could thus contribute to a greater airway obstruction when activated.

To extend these observations, Taniguchi et al. (15) isolated normal-density eosinophils from normal subjects and two groups of asthma patients:

allergic and nonallergic. Eosinophils from both groups of asthma patients, allergic and nonallergic, generated more $LTC_4$ than eosinophils from normal subjects. In this population of patients, a number with aspirin sensitivity were found; although eosinophils from these subjects generated more $LTC_4$ than normal, they were not distinct from other asthma subjects.

Schauer and colleagues (16) isolated purified granulocytes from children with asthma. Calcium ionophore A23187 generated significantly more $LTC_4$ from eosinophils when asthma patients were the cell source. The enhanced granulocyte production was associated with increased number of eosinophils and particularly those of low density.

Kauffman and co-workers (17) found somewhat different results. Peripheral blood eosinophils from asthma and allergy subjects were isolated into normal- and low-density fractions. There was significantly less $LTC_4$ generation to the calcium ionophore from low-density cells ($57 \pm 3$ ng/$10^6$ cells) than cells of normal density ($103 \pm 44$ ng/$10^6$ cells). This differential was found with cells from patients with asthma, both quiescent and acute, and allergic disease. In contrast, when these two populations of eosinophils were isolated from four subjects and $LTC_4$ generation was triggered by serum-treated zymosan, low-density eosinophils released more $LTC_4$. However, the suspension of low-density eosinophils was not highly purified. Nevertheless, these observations raise the possibility that cell activators may differ in their ability to stimulate $LTC_4$ secretion, and this factor must be taken into

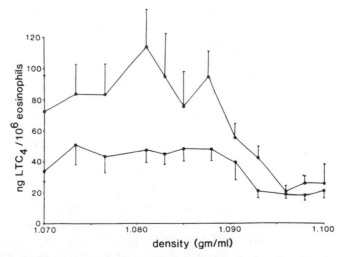

**FIG. 1.** Release of $LTC_4$ by eosinophils from asthmatic (squares) and normal (circles) subjects according to cell density. Cells were stimulated with 1µg/ml A23187 for 15 min. Each point represents the mean nanograms of $LTC_4$ released per $10^6$ eosinophils ($\pm$SEM) for fractions of equivalent density obtained from eight normal and eight asthmatic subjects. $LTC_4$ released was quantitated by RIA. The difference between $LTC_4$ release by eosinophils from asthmatic and normal subjects with a density of 1.093 g/ml or less was significant ($p < 0.05$). (From ref. 18 with permission.)

consideration in evaluating leukotriene synthesis and the effects of disease on this eosinophil response.

Hodges and colleagues (18) have reached conclusions similar to those of Kauffman et al. (17). In their study, peripheral blood eosinophils were fractionated on suspensions of different densities, and cells were obtained from normal and asthmatic subjects. Although there was a shift to eosinophils of lower density in asthma, the $LTC_4$ response to ionophore was not dictated by the presence of asthma (Fig. 1). There was, however, a greater amount of $LTC_4$ generation from lower-density eosinophils, but low-density eosinophils from normals, not asthmatics, secreted more $LTC_4$. These observations indicate that $LTC_4$ generation to the calcium ionophore is influenced by cell density but that this particular response, at least to the ionophore, does not distinguish asthmatics from normal subjects.

## THE INFLUENCE OF LEUKOTRIENES ON EOSINOPHIL FUNCTION

Recruitment of eosinophils in the airway is an essential step for their involvement in allergic inflammation. Although a number of important and potent eosinophil attractants have been identified, the role of leukotrienes in asthma and allergic airway diseases has not been fully established. Woodward et al. (19) evaluated the effect of $LTD_4$ on eosinophil migration into guinea pig conjunctiva. $LTD_4$ and $LTE_4$ caused eosinophil migration to guinea pig conjunctiva. In contrast, $LTB_4$ and $LTC_4$ had little to no effect. When similar analyses were attempted in the skin, $LTC_4$, $LTD_4$, and $LTE_4$ had no effect on eosinophil movement. These data indicate that some leukotrienes can stimulate eosinophil migration but that, at least with $LTD_4$ and $LTE_4$, this response may be species- and organ-specific.

$LTB_4$ has been shown to be an important attractant for neutrophils and also an activator of their oxidative burst. Based on the observation that $LTB_4$ is chemotactic for eosinophils, an $LTB_4$ receptor has also been suggested to be present on these cells. Ng and co-workers (20) used isolated guinea pig eosinophils to evaluate this possibility. They found that $LTB_4$ is an effective attractant for guinea pig eosinophils. Furthermore, $LTB_4$ is capable of activating the respiratory burst of these eosinophils; however, in comparison to other stimuli, i.e., the ionophore and PMA, this response, as measured by chemiluminescence, is small and transient. Finally, these investigators were able to identify a single high-affinity $LTB_4$-receptor population on the guinea pig eosinophil. Therefore, in guinea pigs, eosinophils respond to $LTB_4$ with cell migration or possess a receptor for this factor on their cell surface.

Almost two decades ago, a mast cell-derived chemotactic factor for eosinophils was identified. In recent studies, Shemi and co-workers in London (21) set out to more specifically identify the nature of this factor. In their studies, the release of ECF-A from challenged presensitized guinea pig lung fragments closely paralleled the release of immunoreactive $LTB_4$ and histamine. With the use of HPLC and specific RIA, greater than 60% of the derived ECF-A was attributable to $LTB_4$. Furthermore, PAF and histamine had negligible chemotactic activity for guinea pig eosinophils. Similar studies have not been conducted with human cells to determine whether lung-derived ECF-A activity is found with $LTB_4$.

## REGULATION OF AIRWAY CYSTEINYL GENERATION

Challenge of sensitized airway tissue with antigen has proven an informative model for the study of allergic inflammation. When nasal tissue is challenged with antigen, there is immediate release of histamine and tryptase. Furthermore, there is also release of cysteinyl leukotrienes (22). Although the cell source of these mediators is not specifically established, the kinetics of these activities suggest the nasal mast cell.

We have begun to use a segmental bronchoprovocation with antigen to evaluate the lower airway response to antigen (23). With this technique, segments of the pulmonary tree are identified and challenged with either saline (control) or antigen. The segments are lavaged immediately after antigen challenge and 48 hr later. Lavage from the immediate sample contains high concentrations of histamine and tryptase, suggesting mast cell activation; $LTC_4$ was detected, but in elevated concentration only from the segments given a high concentration of antigen. In contrast, the lavage fluid obtained 48 hr after segmental antigen challenge exhibited a marked increase in cells, particularly eosinophils, and large concentrations of $LTC_4$. The cell source for $LTC_4$ could not be determined, but $LTC_4$ was strongly corrected with eosinophil recruitment to the airways (Fig. 2).

A number of factors have been shown to modify the eosinophil's capacity to generate $LTC_4$. Siberstein et al. (24) have shown that culture with granulocyte/macrophage colony-stimulating factor (GM-CSF) markedly enhances eosinophil generation of $LTC_4$ by the ionophore. Similar promotion was noted by Fabian et al. (25). In contrast, Debbaghi et al. (26) found that incubation of guinea pig eosinophil with IL-1$\beta$ for 30 to 180 min, inhibits the release of arachidonic acid by suppressing phospholipase $A_2$ activity. Therefore, the influence of cytokines on eosinophil function may relate to the function tested as well as to cytokine specificity.

In addition, eosinophil release of $LTC_4$ can be influenced by agents of potential importance for control of allergic inflammation. For example, Cromwell et al. (27) showed that inhibitors of the 5-lypoxygenase pathway (9BW755C and U60257) were capable of inhibiting $LTC_4$ generation when A23187 was the activating stimulus; inhibition was maximal at $1 \times 10^{-5}\,M$ of these antagonists. Furthermore, we were able to inhibit human eosinophil

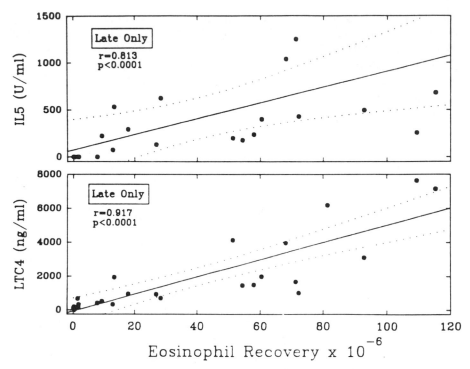

**FIG. 2.** Correlation of eosinophil counts with IL-5 and $LTC_4$ levels in the late (48-hr) BAL samples. The regression line (solid line) and 95% confidence levels (dotted lines) are shown. (From ref. 23 with permission.)

generation of $LTC_4$ to ionophore with nedocromil sodium when concentrations of 1 and 10 m$M$ were used (28). Therefore, the therapeutic potential exists for regulation of eosinophil generation of $LTC_4$ by medications that are either currently in use or that have potential importance for the treatment of asthma.

## SUMMARY

Eosinophils are prominent features of allergic inflammation and can contribute to this process through release of inflammatory enzymes, granule-associated proteins, and leukotriene products. There is considerable interest in the fact that selected cytokines enhance eosinophil generation of leukotrienes. Therefore, future directions must include efforts to identify factors that regulate eosinophil synthesis of leukotrienes and therapeutic agents that might control these specific inflammatory responses.

## REFERENCES

1. Holtzman MJ. *Am Rev Respir Dis* 1991;143:188–203.
2. Drazen JM, Austen KF. *Am Rev Respir Dis* 1987;136:985–9.

3. Jörg A, Henderson WR, Murphy RC, Klebanoff SJ. *J Exp Med* 1982;155:390–402.
4. Weller PF, Lee CW, Foster DW, Corey EJ, Austen KF, Lewis RA. *Proc Natl Acad Sci USA* 1983;80:7626–30.
5. Shaw RJ, Cromwell O, Kay AB. *Clin Exp Immunol* 1984;56:716–22.
6. Shaw RJ, Walsh GM, Cromwell O, Moqbel R, Spry CJF, Kay AB. *Nature* 1985;316:150–2.
7. Bruynzeel PLB, Kok PTM, Hamelink ML, Kijne AM, Verhagen J. *FEBS Lett* 1985;189: 350–4.
8. Cromwell O, Moqbel R, Fitzharris P, et al. *J Allergy Clin Immunol* 1988;82:535–44.
9. Moqbel R, MacDonald AJ, Cromwell O, Kay AB. *Immunology* 1990;69:435–42.
10. Hirata K, Maghni K, Borgeat P, Sirois P. *J Immunol* 1990;144:1880–5.
11. Tamura N, Agrawal DK, Townely RG. *J Immunol* 1988;141:4291–7.
12. Kajita T, Yui Y, Mita H, Taniguchi N, Saito H, Mishima T. *Int Arch Allergy Appl Immunol* 1985;78:406–10.
13. Fukuda T, Dunnette SL, Reed CE, et al. *Am Rev Respir Dis* 1985;132:981–5.
14. Shult PA, Lega M, Jadidi S, et al. *J Allergy Clin Immunol* 1988;81:429–37.
15. Taniguchi N, Mita H, Saito H, Yui Y, Kajita T, Shida T. *Allergy* 1985;40:571–3.
16. Schauer U, Eckhart A, Müller R, Gemsa D, Rieger CHL. *Int Arch Allergy Appl Immunol* 1989;90:201–6.
17. Kauffman H, van der Belt B, deMonchy JGR, Boelens H, Köeter GH, deVries K. *J Allergy Clin Immunol* 1987;79:611–9.
18. Hodges MK, Weller PK, Gerard NP, Ackerman SJ, Drazen JM. *Am Rev Respir Dis* 1988;138:799–804.
19. Woodward DF, Krauss AH-P, Nieves AL, Spada CS. *Drugs Exp Clin Res* 1991;XVII: 543–8.
20. Ng CI, Sun FF, Taylor BM, Wolin MS, Wong PY-K. *J Immunol* 1991;147:3096–3103.
21. Shemi R, Cromwell O, Taylor GW, Kay AB. *J Immunol* 1991;147:2276–83.
22. Creticos PS, Peters SP, Atkinson NF Jr, et al. *N Engl J Med* 1984;310:1626–30.
23. Sedgwick JB, Calhoun WJ, Gleich GJ, et al. *Am Rev Respir Dis* 1991;144:1274–81.
24. Silberstein DS, Owen WF, Gasson JL, et al. *J Immunol* 1986;166:129–41.
25. Fabian I, Kletter Y, Mor S, et al. *Br J Haematol* 1992;80:137–43.
26. Debbaghi A, Hidi R, Vargrafts BB, Touqui L. *J Immunol* 1992;149:1374–80.
27. Cromwell O, Shaw RJ, Walsh GM, Mallet AI, Kay AB. *Int J Immunopharmacol* 1985;7: 775–81.
28. Sedgwick JB, Bjornsdottir U, Geiger K, Busse WW. *J Allergy Clin Immunol* 1992;90:202–9.

Advances in Prostaglandin, Thromboxane,
and Leukotriene Research, Vol. 22, edited by
S.-E. Dahlén et al. Raven Press, Ltd., New York © 1994

# Role of Cysteinyl Leukotrienes in Spontaneous Asthmatic Responses

J. M. Drazen, C. M. Lilly, *R. Sperling, †P. Rubin, and
E. Israel

*Combined Program in Pulmonary and Critical Care Medicine, Departments of
Medicine, Beth Israel Hospital and Brigham and Women's Hospital, and Harvard
Medical School, Ina Sue Perlmutter Laboratory, Children's Hospital, and
Respiratory Biology Program, Harvard School of Public Health, Boston,
Massachusetts 02215; *Department of Rheumatology and Immunology, Brigham
and Women's Hospital, and Harvard Medical School, Boston, Massachusetts
02115; and †Abbott Research Laboratories, Abbott Park, Illinois 60064*

Clinical trials examining the effects of antagonists at the $LTD_4/LTE_4$ receptor or inhibitors of 5-lipoxygenase function in the amelioration of induced or spontaneous human asthma have provided the first "proof of principle" for the importance of leukotrienes in asthma. Although the conclusion of most of these studies is that leukotrienes have a role to play in asthma, by considering the studies in the aggregate it is possible to draw conclusions beyond those that derive from the individual studies. Three types of such studies have been conducted: studies of induced asthma attacks; studies of the short-term (0- to 6-hr) airway effects of administration of $LTD_4/LTE_4$-receptor antagonists or 5-lipoxygenase inhibitors; and studies of such agents on airway function and symptoms in chronic spontaneous asthma. We review here the implications of a number of these studies when considered in the aggregate.

## AGENTS ACTIVE ON THE 5-LIPOXYGENASE PATHWAY USED IN CLINICAL ASTHMA TRIALS

### Antagonists at the $LTD_4/LTE_4$ Receptor

Many agents capable of antagonizing the pharmacologic effects of $LTD_4$ or $LTE_4$ at their receptors in the airway have been described (1–15). However, only a few have been used in clinical trials in patients with asthma. Of the agents studied, a number have been found clinically ineffective or minimally effective (16–19), and one agent has not been studied by more than one investigative group (20). These agents will not be considered further. Three antagonists have been employed in multiple clinical trials, i.e., LY171883 (21), MK-571 (22), and ICI204219 (23) (Table 1). These agents are

**TABLE 1.** *Potency of leukotriene $D_4$-receptor antagonists used in asthma trials*

| Antagonist | Route of administration (dose) | Shift in $LTD_4$ dose–response curve (ref.) |
|---|---|---|
| LY171,883 | Oral (400 mg) | 3–4-fold (21) |
| MK-571 | IV/Oral (28 mg i.v.) | 44-fold (22) |
| ICI204,219 | Oral/Inhaled (40 mg p.o.) | ≈100-fold (23) |

Potency of the antagonists at the $LTD_4/LTE_4$ receptor that has been studied in human asthma. The potency may vary depending on the dose given or route used. The data cited reflect the amounts used in clinical trials.

each capable of inhibiting the bronchospasm that results from inhalation of aerosols generated from solutions of $LTD_4$. Comparisons among the three agents are particularly useful because they vary in potency by approximately 30-fold. Therefore, if the effectiveness of an agent is limited by its potency, then one would expect effectiveness in asthma models to vary in concert with potency.

### Inhibitors of 5-Lipoxygenase

Although three chemically distinct inhibitors of 5-lipoxygenase have been studied in clinical asthma (24–26), only one, zileuton (A64077), has been

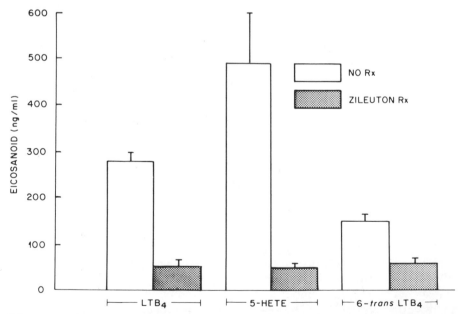

**FIG. 1.** A23187-induced 5-lipoxygenase product formation, in whole blood ex vivo isolated from asthma patients before and after treatment with 800 mg of zileuton. The treatment was associated with a decrease in the amount of $LTB_4$, 6-*trans*-$LTB_4$, and 5-HETE recovered.

shown to have the capacity to inhibit the formation of leukotrienes ex vivo (26) or in vivo. When given as a single dose, 800 mg of this agent resulted in a 74% decrease in the ionophore-stimulated production of $LTB_4$ ex vivo (27,28). Furthermore, RP-HPLC resolution of the products resulting from ionophore stimulation of whole blood removed from subjects 3 hr after ingestion of zileuton, when compared to the products recovered from ion-ophore-stimulated blood from the same subjects before zileuton treatment, demonstrated not only that the amount of $LTB_4$ was decreased but that the amounts of 5-HETE and 6-*trans*-$LTB_4$ produced were also decreased (Fig. 1), consistent with action as a 5-lipoxygenase inhibitor rather than a stimu-lator of $LTB_4$ metabolism.

## EFFECTS OF AGENTS ACTIVE ON THE 5-LIPOXYGENASE PATHWAY IN INDUCED ASTHMA

### Antigen-Induced Asthma

The effects of a single 400-mg dose of LY171883 or placebo given orally on the airway effects of inhaled antigen was examined by Fuller and co-workers (29) in six subjects with both early asthmatic reactions (EAR) and late asth-matic reactions (LAR). The investigators used the maximal expiratory flow rate measured at 40% of vital capacity above residual volume from a partial flow–volume curve ($\dot{V}$) as an index of airway narrowing. Antigen inhalation on the day when placebo was taken resulted in a 54.7% decrease in the $\dot{V}$, whereas after administration of LY171883 the same inhalation challenge was associated with a significantly diminished 35.8% decrease in the $\dot{V}$. To dis-tinguish effects on the EAR from those on the LAR, the area under the $\dot{V}$ time curve (AUC) from 0 to 60 min was compared to that achieved from 4 to 6 hr. Antigen inhalation resulted in a decrease in the AUC 0 to 60 min after inhalation of 3,539 and 2,142 units after placebo or LY171883, respectively; this improvement was statistically significant ($p < 0.05$). In contrast, the AUC measured from 4 to 6 hr after antigen was not improved by adminis-tration of LY171883: $-2,438$ units after placebo and $-4,028$ units after LY171883 ($p$ = NS).

MK-571 (37.5 mg administered as an intravenous infusion for 8 hr) inhib-ited both the EAR and the LAR, measured as the area under the $FEV_1$ time curve, by 47% and 31%, respectively ($p$ = 0.09 for both) (30). When 450 mg of MK-571 was given by intravenous infusion over 8 hr, the EAR and LAR were inhibited by 88% and 63%, respectively ($p$ = 0.01). Over this dose range, the effects of MK-571 on the $LTD_4$ dose–response curve are directly related to the dose of the drug given (22). Therefore, there is a direct rela-tionship between the ability of MK-571 to shift the dose–response curve to $LTD_4$ and its ability to inhibit antigen-induced asthma.

There are two archivally published studies of the effects of ICI-204219 on antigen-induced airway narrowing. Taylor and co-workers (31) studied the effects of a single 40-mg oral dose of ICI204219 on the airway response and alterations in airway responsiveness to histamine induced by inhalation of antigen. Compared to placebo, 2 hr after treatment with ICI204219 there was a significant decrease in both the EAR and LAR. The AUC for $\Delta FEV_1$ versus time for the first 2 hr after antigen exposure decreased from 2,480 to $-49$ ($p < 0.005$). During the period from 2 to 6 hr after antigen inhalation (i.e., the LAR), the AUC decreased from 4,047 after placebo treatment to 510 after ICI204219 ($p < 0.03$). The decrease in the magnitude of the EAR and LAR was associated with a decrease in the airway hyperresponsiveness to histamine resulting from exposure to antigen by approximately one doubling dilution; the $PC_{20}$ decreased 2.38 doubling dilutions after placebo and 1.35 doubling dilutions after ICI204219 ($p < 0.01$). Findlay and colleagues (32) examined the effects of ICI204219 on the amount of cat dander, administered by aerosol, required to decrease the $FEV_1$ by 20%. ICI204219 treatment resulted in a mean increase in the amount of cat dander required for this effect of 15.2-fold, with 8 of the 12 subjects requiring between three- and 30-fold greater amounts of dander. The magnitude of the bronchospastic response, assessed as the AUC for $FEV_1$ versus time for 0 to 5 hr after inhalation, after antigen exposure was decreased by 86% after ICI204219 treatment. Airway responsiveness to histamine was not tested. The effects of LY171883, MK-571 and ICI204219 on antigen-induced airway narrowing are compared in Fig. 2. Note that as agents with the capacity to induce a greater shift in the $LTD_4$ dose–response curve are used, the magnitude of the inhibition of the antigen response is increased.

Further evidence for the involvement of leukotrienes in the asthmatic

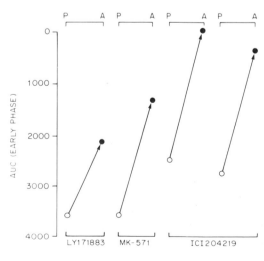

FIG. 2. Comparison of the magnitude of inhibition of the antigen-induced asthma response by $LTD_4/LTE_4$-receptor antagonists. The ordinate is the area under the curve during the early asthmatic response. Data are summarized from the studies as indicated: LY171883 (29), MK-571 (30), and ICI204219 (31,50). Note that as more potent receptor antagonists were used, a greater inhibition of response was achieved. P, placebo; A, active drug.

response to inhaled antigen has been the enhanced recovery of $LTE_4$ from the urine of subjects with asthma after antigen challenge. A number of investigative groups have demonstrated recovery of $LTE_4$ from the urine after antigen inhalation (16,33–37). In some of these studies the investigators were able to show that the amount of $LTE_4$ recovered in the urine was proportional to the degree of bronchospasm. Taylor et al. (31) demonstrated that a bronchospastic response was not required for the amount of $LTE_4$ in the urine to increase. They showed that antigen inhalation was associated with a similar magnitude of increase in urinary $LTE_4$ when the bronchospastic response occurred or when it was blocked by inhalation of salmeterol.

Hui and co-workers (38) examined the effects of zileuton, an inhibitor of 5-lipoxygenase, on the response to inhaled antigen. They found that a single oral dose of 800 mg of zileuton decreased the amount of $LTE_4$ recovered from the urine by 48%. However, the timing of the doses of zileuton and antigen was such that the bronchospastic response to antigen, although decreased, was not decreased significantly. After antigen inhalation, the $FEV_1$ decreased by 1.08 L during the placebo treatment period and by 0.83 L during the zileuton treatment period ($p = 0.08$).

Taken together, these data demonstrate a pivotal and predominant role for the cysteinyl leukotrienes in the airway response to inhaled antigen. Importantly, the close relationships between the recovery of $LTE_4$ from the urine and the magnitude of induced EARs, as well as the relationship between the magnitude of inhibition achieved by the various agents active on the 5-lipoxygenase pathway and all components of the antigen airway response, strongly suggest that the cysteinyl leukotrienes are critical to the antigen response.

### Cold Air/Exercise-Induced Asthma

The same agents active on the 5-lipoxygenase pathway that have been studied in antigen-induced asthma have been studied in asthma induced by cold air exposure or exercise. The results, although qualitatively similar, have been quantitatively different. LY171883 given as 600 mg twice a day for 2 weeks inhibited the bronchospastic response to cold air hyperventilation compared to placebo (39). A cold air hyperventilation challenge that resulted in a 35% decrease in the $FEV_1$ when placebo was administered resulted in a 24% decrease in the $FEV_1$ when LY171883 was administered. Although the effects of this dosing schedule on the $LTD_4$ response were not tested in this study, there is reason to believe that the dose–response curve to inhaled $LTD_4$ would have been shifted by approximately three- to sixfold (21). MK-571, in a dose that would probably shift the $LTD_4$ dose–response curve by about 75-fold, was compared to placebo, using a double-blind crossover trial design, by Manning and colleagues (40). They found an average 69.5% inhibition of the bronchospastic response to exercise. When the subgroup of five subjects who responded to the exercise stimulus with a 30% or greater fall in the $FEV_1$ are considered separately, the average fall in the $FEV_1$ was 37% during the placebo period and 16% during the active treatment period. This selection of subjects allows more uniform comparison among different leukotriene receptor antagonists, as can be appreciated in Fig. 3. ICI204219 also significantly ($p < 0.01$) inhibited the bronchospastic response to exercise (41). In this study, during the placebo treatment period the exercise stimulus resulted in a 36% drop in the $FEV_1$; during treatment with ICI204219 the same exercise stimulus resulted in a 21.6% decrease in the $FEV_1$. Zileuton, a 5-lipoxygenase inhibitor, at a dose that inhibited the ex vivo production of $LTB_4$ by 80% (27) was associated with a 50% increase in the amount of cold dry air ventilation required to achieve a given physiologic effect.

As summarized in Fig. 3, the effects of agents that vary in potency as antagonists at the $LTD_4/E_4$ receptor by over 30-fold have very similar effects on airway narrowing induced by cold air and/or exercise. In particular, it appears that once an agent with the capacity to shift the $LTD_4$ dose–response curve by eight- to tenfold is administered, increasing potency is not associated with increasing effect. Furthermore, the effects of the approximately 80% inhibition of 5-lipoxygenase achieved by zileuton are similar in magnitude to those resulting from MK-571 and ICI204219. Therefore, the alteration of the bronchoconstrictor response to exercise/cold air appears to be relatively independent of the degree of inhibition of the 5-lipoxygenase pathway, once an adequate level of inhibition is reached. Based on the data available, this level appears to be equivalent to an eight- to tenfold shift of the $LTD_4$ dose–response curve or an 80% to 90% inhibition of $LTB_4$ production ex vivo. Importantly, only 35% to 50% of the bronchospastic re-

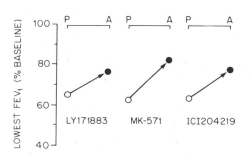

**FIG. 3.** Comparison of the magnitude of the inhibition of the exercise/cold air-induced asthmatic response by $LTD_4/LTE_4$-receptor antagonists. The ordinate is the maximal percent change in the $FEV_1$ after stimulus exposure during placebo (P) or active (A) agent treatment. Data are summarized from studies as indicated: LY171883 (2), MK-571 (40), and ICI204219 (41). The data shown for MK-571 were selected to allow comparison of equivalent asthmatic responses. Note that similar effects on the bronchospastic response were achieved despite a 30-fold difference in potency of antagonists studied.

sponse to exercise appears to be mediated by production of the cysteinyl leukotrienes.

## EFFECTS OF AGENTS ACTIVE ON THE 5-LIPOXYGENASE PATHWAY ON SPONTANEOUS AIRWAY TONE

In the studies noted above, antagonists at the $LTD_4/LTE_4$ receptor or 5-lipoxygenase inhibitors were administered before the initiation of the challenge. This enabled the investigators to follow airway function for an appropriate period of time before application of the bronchoconstrictor stimulus. In each case there was no effect on baseline airway function resulting from the intervention (27,29–32,38–41). In contrast, Hui and Barnes (42) found that oral administration of 40 mg ICI204219 resulted in a significant ($p <$ 0.0005) 8.5% increase in the $FEV_1$ noted 3.5 hr after administration of the drug. These investigators also demonstrated that salbutamol, administered by aerosol after the ICI204219, was associated with an additional increase in the $FEV_1$ of approximately 20%. Although the studies, as noted above, in which the effects of $LTD_4/LTE_4$ antagonists or 5-lipoxygenase inhibitors on the $FEV_1$ before induced asthma (27,29–32,38–41) appear to be in conflict with the results of Hui and Barnes (42), the conflict is at best a superficial one and probably results from the more severely deranged baseline function of the subjects studied by latter investigators (42). The findings of Hui and Barnes (42) have been confirmed in studies by others (43,44). We monitored airway function after administration of zileuton in patients with chronic, stable asthma and demonstrated a 13% increase in $FEV_1$ over the next 2 hr. Therefore, not only are $LTD_4/LTE_4$ receptors occupied in patients with asthmatic airway narrowing but the synthesis of bronchoactive leukotrienes is a continuous ongoing process.

## EVIDENCE FOR THE PRODUCTION OF LEUKOTRIENES DURING SPONTANEOUS ASTHMATIC EPISODES

Taylor and co-workers (45) demonstrated among subjects who required emergency care for asthma that some, but not all, had large amounts of $LTE_4$ in their urine. The investigators found no relationship between the amount of $LTE_4$ recovered from the urine and the degree of airway narrowing. A possible interpretation of these data is that only a subset of individuals with asthma have airway obstruction mediated by leukotrienes.

We reasoned that we could identify a subset of individuals with acute spontaneous airway narrowing due to muscle constriction on the basis of their response to inhalation of bronchodilators. We further reasoned that because the cysteinyl leukotrienes are potent contractile agonists for airway smooth muscle, individuals with muscle airway narrowing would have evidence of hyperproduction of the leukotrienes. To test this hypothesis, the bronchodilator responsiveness of 89 patients presenting to the emergency service for treatment of an acute spontaneous asthmatic episode was examined (46). Individuals who enrolled in the trial gave written informed consent to provide a urine sample and to receive during their first hour in the emergency service only three treatments with inhaled albuterol at 20-min intervals. In addition, a recording of peak flow was made at the time of entry into the study, before initiation of any treatment of asthma, and 10 min after the third treatment with inhaled albuterol.

Of the 89 subjects originally enrolled in the study, one subject's urine contained inadequate creatinine to be considered an adequate sample, and 12 others were not considered in the data analysis because they had only minimal airflow obstruction (i.e., a peak flow on enrollment in the study of 250 L/m or greater). The changes in peak flow rate in response to three treatments with inhaled albuterol at 20-min intervals in the 76 remaining patients are shown in Fig. 4. The responses were widely distributed, with the single greatest response in a patient whose peak flow increased from 130 to 470 L/min, or 362%. Seven subjects had a decrease in peak flow rate over the first hour of treatment, with the least responsive subject having an initial peak flow of 155 L/min, which decreased to 105 L/min over the first hour of treatment. The mean (± SD) response of the peak flow rate as a percentage of the original response was 178.3 ± 66.9%; the median response was 160%

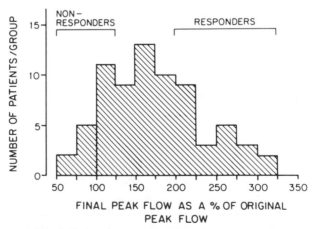

**FIG. 4.** Histogram of peak flow responses to three consecutive treatments with inhaled albuterol within the first hour of emergency treatment for asthma. The vertical solid line separates subjects with a bronchodilator response from those without a bronchodilator response. The responder group was defined as those subjects with a peak flow rate after treatment with inhaled albuterol that was greater than 200% of pretreatment value. The nonresponder group was those subjects whose peak flow after treatment with inhaled albuterol was less than 125% of pretreatment value. (From ref. 46 with permission.)

of the original peak flow. Approximately one-quarter of the patients, termed "responders," had more than a doubling of their peak flow rate with this treatment regimen. Another quarter of the patients, termed "nonresponders," had a less than 25% improvement in peak flow over the 1-hr period of observation in the emergency service. The remainder of the patients had responses to inhaled albuterol between these two extremes. Most subjects in both patient groups were using $\beta$-agonist inhalers and theophylline. There were a few subjects in each group using systemic and inhaled corticosteroids; there was no significant difference between the groups in the proportion of subjects using corticosteroids.

Because the diagnosis of asthma could be questioned in individuals who failed to manifest bronchodilatation when treated with inhaled albuterol, follow-up peak flow recordings were obtained from hospital records or home peak flow readings to ensure that the patients studied did not have fixed airway obstruction. The follow-up peak flow readings were all recorded within 2 months of the readings obtained on the emergency unit. Follow-up data were available from nine of the 12 acute nonresponders in whom urinary $LTE_4$ values were available. In these subjects the mean peak flow, after completion of the third treatment with inhaled albuterol in the emergency service, was 42.1 ± 6.0% of that predicted. Over the follow-up period there was an average increase in peak flow of 46.4 ± 8.4%. The highest peak flow recorded in these subjects during follow-up was significantly ($p < 0.005$) greater, 88.7 ± 7.3% of that predicted, than the flow rate after the third treatment with inhaled albuterol.

The amount of $LTE_4$ in the urine was determined in a number of the responder and nonresponder patients and compared to the amount of $LTE_4$ recovered from the urine of nonatopic, nonasthmatic healthy volunteers. Urinary $LTE_4$ was determined by concentration on a $C_{18}$ solid-state support, followed by elution onto analytical RP-HPLC. The fractions obtained from RP-HPLC were assayed using a solid-phase ELISA for $LTE_4$. As described in detail elsewhere (46), $LTE_4$ values were corrected for recovery of an internal standard and normalized by the amount of creatinine in the urine. The $LTE_4$ excretion rate in the normal group was significantly ($p < 0.0001$) less than in the responder group but not significantly less than that of the nonresponder group ($p = 0.071$, Wilcoxon two-sample test). Urinary $LTE_4$ excretion rates varied about 1,000-fold. We subdivided the subjects into those with low (i.e., less than 10 pg $LTE_4$/mg creatinine), medium (i.e., 10 to 99.9 pg $LTE_4$/mg creatinine) and high (i.e., greater than 100 pg $LTE_4$/mg creatinine) excretion rates. Of the normal subjects, 53.8%, 46.2%, and 0.0% had low, medium, or high urinary $LTE_4$ excretion rates, respectively. The proportion of responder subjects with low, medium, or high urinary $LTE_4$ excretion was 0.0%, 18.8%, and 81.2%, respectively. The proportion of nonresponder subjects with high, medium, or low urinary $LTE_4$ excretion was 33.3%, 33.3%, and 33.3% respectively. There was no significant correlation between age, initial peak flow, or degree of reversibility and the rate of urinary $LTE_4$ excretion among all subjects. The mean urinary $LTE_4$ excretion was not significantly different between the subjects using oral steroids and those not using oral steroids in the nonresponder and responder subject groups. These data clearly demonstrate that subjects with acute, spontaneous, reversible airway narrowing excrete large amounts of $LTE_4$.

These data support the hypothesis that subjects with spontaneous, acute, reversible airway narrowing produce large quantities of the cysteinyl leukotrienes. Among the subjects with asthma whose airway narrowing was equally severe, but not reversible, some had evidence for hyperexcretion of leukotrienes, whereas in others the amount of $LTE_4$ recovered from the urine was within the normal range. There are a number of possible, but not necessarily mutually exclusive, explanations for this finding. First, if the irreversible nature of the airway obstruction in all the nonresponders was due to nonmuscular factors (i.e., to edema and airway secretions), then the high urinary $LTE_4$ levels observed in these subjects may reflect the release of leukotrienes at a time when the airway obstruction due to nonmuscular factors was so severe as to preclude further narrowing in response to any spasmogen. Whether cysteinyl leukotrienes were released in the lungs of these subjects before their arrival in the emergency service and whether the actions of leukotrienes could account for the proposed presence of edema and cell infiltration is not known. However, the beneficial effect observed with the more potent leukotriene receptor antagonists on the LAR (31,32), as well as the beneficial effects of leukotriene receptor antagonists or 5-lipoxygenase inhibitors that occur over weeks of treatment with these agents (47,48), suggests that the cysteinyl leukotrienes have potent proinflammatory properties and could account for some of the nonmuscular changes in the airway. Second, $LTE_4$ is not the only product of leukotriene metabolism. It is possible that $LTE_4$ was produced endogenously but that metabolites other than $LTE_4$ could have been recovered from the urine of the subjects who had airway narrowing and a low urinary $LTE_4$. Finally, the slowly reversible airway narrowing in the subjects with low urinary $LTE_4$ levels reflects the actions of nonleukotriene spasmogens.

## SPECULATIVE CONCLUSIONS ON THE ROLE OF LEUKOTRIENES IN SPONTANEOUS REVERSIBLE AIRWAY NARROWING IN ASTHMA

The data available to date, as reviewed above, clearly demonstrate that there is endogenous production of the cysteinyl leukotrienes in a majority of patients with asthma. The observation that patients with spontaneous reversible airway narrowing uniformly had high levels of $LTE_4$ in their urine, coupled with the knowledge that the $LTD_4/LTE_4$ receptor antagonists or 5-lipoxygenase inhibitors have the capacity to reverse spontaneous airway narrowing, strongly implicates the leukotrienes as important mediators of this obstruction. Furthermore, the studies using exercise/cold air- or antigen-induced airway narrowing as asthma models clearly suggest that there is stimulus-related heterogeneity in the endogenous mediators that are released in bronchospastic responses. In the antigen model, leukotrienes are probably the major mediator of acute bronchospasm, whereas in the exercise model leukotrienes play an important contributory role but there are clearly other mechanisms leading to the observed obstructive response. It seems reasonable to speculate that in spontaneously occurring asthma both types or even mixed stimuli are likely to be encountered. If the models of induced bronchospasm reflect natural exposure, then there is strong reason to believe that the cysteinyl leukotrienes are pivotal molecules in the acute obstructive response.

## REFERENCES

1. Weichman BM, Wasserman MA, Gleason JG. *J Pharmacol Exp Ther* 1984;228:128–132.
2. Fleisch JH, Rinkema LE, Haisch KD, et al. *J Pharmacol Exp Ther* 1985;233:148–157.
3. Jones TR, Young R, Champion E, et al. *Can J Physiol Pharmacol* 1986;64:1068–75.
4. Krell RD, Giles RE, Yee YK, Snyder DW, Keith RA. *J Pharmacol Exp Ther* 1987;243: 548–56, 557–64.
5. Hay DW, Muccitelli RM, Tucker SS, et al. *J Pharmacol Exp Ther* 1987;243:474–81.
6. Krell RD, Giles RE, Yee, Snyder DW. *J Pharmacol Exp Ther* 1987;243:557–64.
7. Jones TR, Zamboni R, Belley M, et al. *Can J Physiol Pharmacol* 1989;67:17–28.
8. Hand JM, Aucn MAMZHC, Englebach IM. *Int Arch Allergy Appl Immunol* 1989;89:78–82.
9. Dillard RD, Hahn RA, Mccullough D, et al. *J Med Chem* 1991;34:2768–78.
10. Wahedna I, Wisniewski AS, Tattersfield AE. *Br J Clin Pharmacol* 1991;32:512–5.
11. Odonnell M, Crowley HJ, Yaremko B, O'Neill N, Welton AF. *J Pharmacol Exp Ther* 1991;259:751–9.
12. Jones TR, Zamboni R, Belley M, et al. *Can J Physiol Pharmacol* 1991;69:1847–54.
13. Salmon JA, Garland LG. *Prog Drug Res* 1991;37:9–90.
14. Brown FJ, Cronk LA, Aharony D, Snyder DW. *J Med Chem* 1992;35:2419–39.
15. Salmon JA, Garland LG. *Prog Drug Res* 1991;37:9–90.
16. Britton JR, Hanley SP, Tattersfield AE. *J Allergy Clin Immunol* 1987;79:811–6.
17. Barnes N, Piper PJ, Costello J. *J Allergy Clin Immunol* 1987;79:816–21.
18. Bel EH, Timmers MC, Dijkman JH, Stahl EG, Sterk PJ. *J Allergy Clin Immunol* 1990;85: 1067–75.
19. Rasmussen JB, Eriksson LO, Andersson KE. *Allergy* 1991;46:266–73.
20. Robuschi M, Riva E, Fuccella LM, et al. *Am Rev Respir Dis* 1992;145:1285–8.
21. Phillips GD, Rafferty P, Robinson C, Holgate ST. *J Pharmacol Exp Ther* 1988;246:732–8.
22. Kips JC, Joos GF, Delepeleire I, et al. *Am Rev Respir Dis* 1991;144:617–21.
23. Smith LJ, Geller S, Ebright L, Glass M, Thyrum PT. *Am Rev Respir Dis* 1990;141:988–92.
24. Mann JS, Robinson C, Sheridan AQ, Clement P, Bach MK, Holgate ST. *Thorax* 1986;41: 746–52.
25. Fuller RW, Maltby N, Richmond R, et al. *Br J Clin Pharmacol* 1987;23:677–81.
26. Rubin P, Dube L, Braeckman R, et al. *Prog Inflam Res Ther* 1991;35:103–16.
27. Israel E, Dermarkarian R, Rosenberg M, et al. *N Engl J Med* 1990;323:1740–4.
28. Knapp HR. *N Engl J Med* 1990;323:1745–8.
29. Fuller RW, Black PN, Dollery CT. *J Allergy Clin Immunol* 1989;83:939–44.
30. Rasmussen JB, Margolskee DJ, Eriksson LO, Williams VC, Andersson KE. *Ann NY Acad Sci* 1991;629:436.
31. Taylor IK, O'Shaughnessy KM, Fuller RW, Dollery CT. *Lancet* 1991;337:690–4.
32. Findlay SR, Barden JM, Easley CB, Glass M. *J Allergy Clin Immunol* 1992;89:1040–5.

33. Sladek K, Dworski R, Fitzgerald GA, et al. *Am Rev Respir Dis* 1990;141:1441–5.
34. Manning PJ, Rokach J, Malo JL, et al. *J Allergy Clin Immunol* 1990;86:2311–20.
35. Westcott JY, Smith HR, Wenzel SE, et al. *Am Rev Respir Dis* 1991;143:1322–8.
36. Smith CM, Christie PE, Hawksworth RJ, Thien F, Lee TH. *Am Rev Respir Dis* 1991;144:1411–3.
37. Hartnell A, Kay AB, Wardlaw AJ. *J Immunol* 1992;148:1471–8.
38. Hui KP, Taylor IK, Taylor GW, et al. *Thorax* 1991;46:184–9.
39. Israel E, Juniper EF, Callaghan JT, et al. *Am Rev Respir Dis* 1989;140:1348–53.
40. Manning PJ, Watson RM, Margolskee DJ, Williams VC, Schwartz JI, O'Byrne PM. *N Engl J Med* 1990;323:1736–9.
41. Finnerty JP, Wood-Baker R, Thomson H, Holgate ST. *Am Rev Respir Dis* 1992;145:746–9.
42. Hui KP, Barnes NC. *Lancet* 1991;337:1062–3.
43. Busse W. *Am Rev Respir Dis* [in press].
44. Kips JC, Joos GF, Pauwels RA. *Lancet* 1991;337:1618.
45. Taylor GW, Taylor I, Black P, et al. *Lancet* 1989;1:584–8.
46. Drazen JM, O'Brien J, Sparrow D, et al. *Am Rev Respir Dis* 1992;146:104–8.
47. Cloud ML, Enas GC, Kemp J, et al. *Am Rev Respir Dis* 1989;140:1336–9.
48. Israel E. *Am Rev Respir Dis* 1992;145:A16(Abstract).
49. Sala A, Voelkel N, Maclouf J, Murphy RC. *J Biol Chem* 1990;265:21771–8.
50. Smith HR, Larsen GL, Cherniack RM. *J Allergy Clin Immunol* 1992;89:1076–84.

*Advances in Prostaglandin, Thromboxane, and Leukotriene Research*, Vol. 22, edited by
S.-E. Dahlén et al. Raven Press, Ltd., New York © 1994

# Summary: The Pharmacology of Leukotrienes in Asthma

John Costello, *Susan Meltzer, and *Eugene R. Bleecker

*King's College School of Medicine and Dentistry, London SE5 9PJ, England; and
*University of Maryland School of Medicine, Baltimore, Maryland 21201*

Although the treatment of clinical asthma has not changed significantly in the past 30 years, our understanding of underlying mechanisms in asthma has increased exponentially during the same period. This has occurred because of the development of new clinical and research approaches and of advances in cellular and molecular biology.

The concept of asthma as a condition in which acute and chronic inflammatory change in the airways plays a fundamental role is now well-established; moreover, the role of formation and release of leukotrienes as a crucial element of these inflammatory processes is now supported by abundant laboratory and clinical evidence (Fig. 1). The function of effector cells, eosinophils, lymphocytes, macrophages, and neutrophils, and the role of individual cysteinyl leukotrienes, are considered here, with emphasis on the contribution of leukotriene antagonists to our understanding of the pathogenesis of asthma and of their potential for clinical benefit of patients.

Leukotrienes appear to be of central importance in the events that occur in the inflamed airways of asthmatics. These substances are metabolites of the arachidonic acid pathway, which are formed in the membranes of inflammatory cells and in the bronchial epithelium. They were identified by Jorg et al. (1) in horse eosinophils, when their ability was demonstrated to contract smooth muscle, and they were known for some years as a slow-reacting substance of anaphylaxis (SRS-A). This group of substances includes $LTA_4$, $LTB_4$, $LTC_4$, $LTD_4$, and $LTE_4$. $LTB_4$ has the neutrophil as its primary target, whereas the products of the glutathione 5-transferase pathway, $LTC_4$, $LTD_4$, and $LTE_4$, known as the cysteinyl leukotrienes, primarily affect contractile cells, including bronchial smooth-muscle cells. In addition, $LTC_4$ and $LTD_4$ increase mucous production in cultured human lung tissue. The cysteinyl leukotrienes are believed to be primary effectors of the asthmatic responses, and the evidence for their role in asthma is the result of many studies that have been published during the last decade.

The in vitro evidence for the involvement of leukotrienes in asthma has

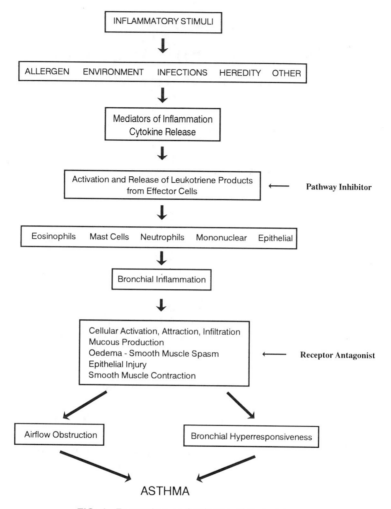

**FIG. 1.** Formation and release of leukotrienes.

been reviewed by Arm and Lee (*this volume*). They emphasize that much of our existing information has been developed with animal models and that relatively few in vitro human data are available. Unfortunately, much of that comes from experiments on tissue samples from nonasthmatics. The measurement of urinary leukotrienes after various pharmacologic manipulations has produced data regarding the possible action of leukotrienes in the respiratory system. More recently, the measurement of leukotrienes in broncho-alveolar lavage fluid has produced more direct information about the role of these mediators in airway disease. Arm and Lee emphasize the greater relative bronchoconstrictor potency of $LTE_4$ in asthmatic airways and suggest that this may be due to upregulation of a separate $LTE_4$ receptor.

Eosinophilia in asthma is well established, but the relationship between eosinophils and leukotrienes in asthmatic responses is still not clearly defined. Busse and Sedgwick (*this volume*) have reviewed this topic and have presented evidence confirming that a causative relationship has not been established, although Taniguchi et al. (2) and Schauer et al. (3) both found that eosinophils of subjects with asthma secrete more leukotrienes than those of normal controls. Similar studies by Kauffmann et al. (4) and by Hodges and co-workers (5) have produced conflicting results.

Eosinophils are an important source of $LTC_4$ and are susceptible to a number of biologically relevant stimuli for $LTC_4$ production. The ability of eosinophils to synthesize $LTC_4$ does not appear to differ between cells obtained from asthmatics and those from normals, but the $LTC_4$ generation is influenced by cell density, with low-density eosinophils demonstrating a greater capacity for $LTC_4$ production. The effect of leukotrienes in the migration of the eosinophil itself is probably species- and organ-specific, with $LTB_4$ and the cysteinyl leukotrienes varying in their roles. There is no clear pattern of action of leukotrienes on eosinophil function in asthmatic airways. The *production* of leukotrienes by eosinophils is regulated by cytokine action and can be influenced by therapy; this may therefore be a novel approach to new therapeutic possibilities.

Dahlén et al. (6) elicited bronchial contractions in atopic asthmatics in vitro, extracting leukotrienes in amounts that correlated with the severity of the reaction. They also challenged human lung tissue from asthmatics with leukotrienes, producing long-lasting contraction of smooth airway muscle. Bronchoconstriction produced by leukotrienes has a longer duration than that produced by histamine. Inhaled $LTD_4$ is a potent bronchoconstrictor in normal subjects as well as in patients with rhinitis and asthma (7), is 1,000 times more potent than histamine in normal subjects (8), but is only several times more potent in asthmatics (9). O'Byrne et al. (*this volume*) propose that tachyphylaxis is responsible for the relative hyporesponsiveness of asthmatics to leukotrienes. Activation of the cyclooxygenase pathway and secretion of inhibitory prostaglandins ameliorate eicosanoid-induced bronchoconstriction. Cyclooxygenase inhibition with indomethacin decreases the refractoriness of exercise-induced bronchoconstriction in sensitive asthmatics (10), and inhaled $PGE_2$ inhibits hyperresponsiveness and both the early and late responses to antigen (11). The inhibition of exercise-induced bronchospasm by leukotriene antagonism but not by $H_1$-blockers suggests a fundamental role for leukotrienes in exercise-induced asthma. The role of the cyclooxygenase pathway in asthma remains elusive, but the concept of inhibitory prostaglandins is intriguing.

The use of leukotriene antagonists in aspirin-sensitive asthmatics illustrates the interaction between the cyclooxygenase and lipoxygenase pathways. Baseline urinary $LTE_4$ has been shown to be elevated in aspirin-sensitive asthmatics compared with other asthmatics, and increases further in susceptible individuals after challenge with lysine–aspirin inhalation (12). The leukotriene receptor antagonist MK-0679, given before aspirin provocation, still resulted in increased urinary $LTE_4$, but increased the $PD_{20}$ $FEV_1$ to aspirin challenge, thus decreasing bronchoconstriction (Dahlén et al., *this volume*). The interdependence of the cyclooxygenase and 5-lipoxygenase pathways is illustrated by these results.

Drazen's study of emergency room patients with acute airflow obstruction provides further evidence for leukotriene involvement in asthma (13; and *this volume*). Patients who responded to β-agonist therapy with significant improvement in peak expiratory flow measurements had significantly higher urinary leukotriene levels than the nonresponders. The reason for the nonresponders' lack of response is not clear, although a number of the subjects had a slower but significant improvement in asthma parameters on followup. The roles of other inflammatory mediators, nonreversible airflow obstruction (COPD), or pathophysiologic mechanisms such as edema or cell infiltration rather than smooth-muscle contraction, are proposed as alternate explanations.

$LTC_4$ has been found in bronchoalveolar lavage fluid in asymptomatic and symptomatic asthmatics but not in normal subjects (14,15), implying that "leukotriene tone" may account for chronic airflow obstruction in asthma, and may be reduced by treatment with leukotriene pathway inhibitors or receptor antagonists. The specific mediators and mechanisms of the early and late asthmatic responses have yet to be definitively clarified, but elevated levels of leukotrienes have been measured in bronchoalveolar fluid in both phases of the allergic reaction (16).

Many of the current studies of leukotriene antagonists are difficult to compare owing to the lack of standardization in procedures. Despite these criticisms, there is substantial evidence that leukotrienes are an integral component of the asthmatic response. The most convincing data are from recent studies in human subjects demonstrating attenuation of symptoms, improvement in airflow obstruction, reductions in inflammatory cells, and reduction in mediators by leukotriene antagonism (Barnes and Kuitert, *this volume*).

Controversy persists regarding the utility, safety, and role of β-agonists as primary therapy in asthma. Evidence for their contribution to the increasing mortality rate in asthma has yet to be definitively refuted. Various studies have shown both tachyphylaxis and increased bronchial hyperresponsiveness with repetitive and chronic use, although it is difficult to separate the effect of the drug from that of the disease process itself. Anti-inflammatory agents, corticosteroids and, to a lesser extent, cromolyn, are now considered to represent primary therapy for mild to moderate asthma. The search therefore continues for more selective targeted therapy, pharmacologically and possibly in relation to specific types of asthmatic response.

The development of leukotriene antagonists appears to represent the first promising new therapy for asthma in the past 40 years, specifically targeting the inflammatory mechanism(s) responsible for the pathophysiologic abnormalities in asthma. The ultimate goal is to develop better alternatives to inhaled and oral corticosteroids as anti-inflammatory interventions for asthma therapy. Two main classes of leukotriene inhibitors are presently being developed. 5-Lipoxygenase inhibitors inhibit the formation of $LTA_4$ from arachidonic acid, thus affecting the formation of leukotrienes ($LTB_4$, $LTC_4$, $LTD_4$, $LTE_4$). The second class of agents, receptor antagonists, inhibit specific mediators. The results of early clinical trials were disappointing owing to erratic absorption, short half-lives, and low potency. More recent work with receptor antagonists has shown more promising control of asthmatic and allergic symptoms. At present, a variety of agents are in various stages of clinical development.

Bronchial hyperresponsiveness to $LTD_4$ and antigen is significantly attenuated in both asthmatics and normal subjects by leukotriene antagonists (17–20). Leukotriene-induced bronchoconstriction is usually resolved within 1 to 2 hr and, unlike antigen-induced bronchoconstriction, is not associated with a late response. However, leukotriene antagonists have been shown to decrease both the early and late asthmatic responses after antigen (21), and there is a correlation between the ability of these antagonists to inhibit $LTD_4$-induced hyperresponsiveness and the antigen response (22–23). Therefore, the leukotrienes appear to play a causative role in both the early and the late asthmatic response, either directly, as a mediator causing bronchoconstriction, or secondarily, via airway narrowing caused by edema and other cell responses. Inhibition of exercise-induced bronchoconstriction by leukotriene antagonists (24–26) has identified a causal role of these mediators and has partially clarified the responsible mechanism for this response, and leukotriene antagonists attenuate the asthmatic response to cold air (27). When zileuton, a 5-lipoxygenase inhibitor, was given before allergen provocation, urinary $LTE_4$ was significantly decreased compared to placebo and the early response was attenuated (28). The late asthmatic response and metacholine responsiveness have been shown to be variably affected. These results suggest that inhibition was not complete and that other mediators are involved. In a study by Israel and colleagues (29), a modest improvement in pulmonary function was noted in 139 asthmatics after 4 weeks of zileuton; symptoms improved and β-agonist use decreased concurrently. These results illustrate the effectiveness of inhibition but further reinforce the concept that other mediators are involved. A leukotriene receptor antagonist, ICI204,219, was shown to improve baseline pulmonary function in mild asthmatics after a single 40-mg dose (30).

In summary, the role of leukotrienes in asthma is well-established. The development of specific antagonists has clarified certain aspects of the disease that were previously not well-understood. The clinical role of these agents is presently under active study. There may well be a role for them in the treatment of obstructive airway disease, attenuating the effects of chronic inflammation. Further studies will clarify their specific utility. The most promising areas appear to involve exercise-susceptible individuals and moderate asthmatics with chronic airflow obstruction.

## REFERENCES

1. Jorg A, Henderson WR, Murphy RC, Klebanoff SJ. *J Exp Med* 1982;155:390–420.
2. Taniguchi N, Mita H, Saito H, Yui Y, Kajita T, Shida T. *Allergy* 1985;40:571–3.
3. Schauer U, Echhart A, Miller R, Gemsa D, Riger CHL. *Int Arch Allergy Appl Immunol* 1989;90:201–6.
4. Kauffman H, van der Belt B, de Monchy JGR, Boelens H, Koeter GH, de Vries K. *J Allergy Clin Immunol* 1987;79:611–9.
5. Hodges MK, Weller PK, Gerard NP, Acherman SJ, Drazen JM. *Am Rev Respir Dis* 1988;138:799–804.
6. Dahlén S-E, Hansson G, Hedqvist P, Bjorck T, Granstrom E, Dahlén B. *Proc Natl Acad Sci USA* 1983;80:1712–6.
7. Smith LJ, Greenberger PA, Patterson R, Krell RD, Bernstein PR. *Am Rev Respir Dis* 1985;131:368–72.
8. Dahlen SE, Hedquist P, Hammarstrom S, Samuelsson B. *Nature* 1980;288:484–6.
9. Griffin M, Woodrow W, Leitch AG, et al. *N Engl J Med* 1983;308:436–9.
10. O'Byrne PM, Jones GL. *Am Rev Respir Dis* 1986;134:69–72.
11. Yamaguchi T, Kohrogi H, Honda I, et al. *Am Rev Respir Dis* 1992;146:923–9.
12. Kumlin M, Dahlen B, Bjorck T, Zetterstrom D, Granstrom E, Dahlen SE. *Am Rev Respir Dis* 1992;146:96–103.
13. Drazen JM, O'Brien J, Sparrow D, et al. *Am Rev Respir Dis* 1992;146:104–8.
14. Lam S, Chan H, LeRiche JC, Chan-Yeung M, Salari H. *J Allergy Clin Immunol* 1988;81:711–7.
15. Wardlaw AJ, Hay H, Cromwell O, Collins JV, Kay AB. *J Allergy Clin Immunol* 1989;84:19–26.
16. Wenzel SE, Westcott JY, Larsen GL. *J Allergy Clin Immunol* 1991;87:540–8.
17. Kips JC, Joos G-F, Lepeleire ID, et al. *Am Rev Respir Dis* 1991;144:617–21.
18. Holroyde MC, Altounyan REC, Cole M, Dixon M, Elliott EV. *Lancet* 1981;2:17–8.
19. Barnes N, Piper PJ, Costello J. *J Allergy Clin Immunol* 1987;79:816–21.
20. Smith LJ, Geller S, Ebright L, Glass M, Thyrum PT. *Am Rev Respir Dis* 1990;141:988–92.
21. Rasmussen JB, Eriksson L-O, Margolskee DJ, Tagari P, Williams VC, Andersson K-E. *J Allergy Clin Immunol* 1992;90:193–201.
22. Findlay SR, Barden JM, Easley CB, Blass M. *J Allergy Clin Immunol* 1992;89:1040–5.
23. Fuller RW, Black PN, Dollery CT. *J Allergy Clin Immunol* 1989;83:939–44.
24. Israel E, Dermarkarian R, Rosenberg M, et al. *N Engl J Med* 1990;323:1740–4.
25. Finnerty JP, Wood-Baker R, Thomson H, Holgate ST. *Am Rev Respir Dis* 1992;145:746–9.
26. Manning PJ, Watson RM, Margolskee DJ, Williams VC, Schwartz JI, O'Byrne PM. *N Engl J Med* 1990;323:1736–9.
27. Israel E, Juniper EF, Callaghan JT, et al. *Am Rev Respir Dis* 1989;140:1348–53.
28. Hui KP, Taylor IK, Taylor GW, et al. *Thorax* 1991;46:184–9.
29. Israel E, Rubin P, Kemp JP, et al. (Submitted.)
30. Hui KP, Barnes NC. *Lancet* 1991;337:1062–3.

# 5. Mediators and Mechanisms in Nasal and Rheumatic Inflammation

Advances in Prostaglandin, Thromboxane,
and Leukotriene Research, Vol. 22, edited by
S.-E. Dahlén et al. Raven Press, Ltd., New York © 1994

# The Mediators of the Early and Late Phases of Allergic Rhinitis

## Michael A. Kaliner

*Institute for Asthma and Allergy, Washington Hospital Center,
Washington, D.C. 20010*

Allergic rhinitis is the most common immunologic disease and the most common chronic disease experienced by humans. About 10% to 20% of the American population experiences allergic rhinitis. More than 1 billion dollars is spent yearly on over-the-counter and prescription allergy preparations. In addition, allergic rhinitis accounts for 2.5% of all physician visits for all diseases, and another 0.5% of all visits are for the purpose of receiving allergy immunotherapy (1). To understand the pathophysiology of allergic rhinitis, it is first necessary to be knowledgeable about nasal anatomy.

### ANATOMY OF THE NASAL MUCOSA

The nasal mucosa is lined with a pseudostratified columnar epithelium resting on a basement membrane that separates it from the deeper submucosal structures. On the epithelial surface is the bilayered epithelial lining fluid layer. The outer layer consists of a sticky mucous blanket which serves to trap foreign particles including bacteria, viruses, and allergens, as well as to hold and concentrate certain glandular and vascular proteins. This outer mucous or gel layer is constantly being swallowed and replaced about every 15 min by glandular secretions. The lower layer of the epithelial lining fluid is an aqueous periciliary layer. It is this periciliary layer in which the cilia beat, transporting the mucous layer only by the tips of the cilia during the propulsive portion of the stroke. The periciliary layer is where the aqueous proteins secreted by the serous cells of the submucosal glands are concentrated. This layer provides most of the antimicrobial functions of secretions, whereas the outer gel layer acts to trap and transport foreign particles through mucociliary clearance (2).

Four types of cells contribute to the epithelium: ciliated columnar epithelial cells, nonciliated columnar epithelial cells, goblet cells, and basal cells. The goblet cells constitute the glandular portion of the epithelium. These cells, as well as the deeper submucosal glands, secrete mucous glycoproteins and other proteins onto the epithelial surface. All of the columnar epithelial cells contain microvilli, nonmobile projections that increase cell surface area and contribute to hydration. In addition, most of the columnar cells contain cilia, which beat in a wavelike pattern through the sol layer of the mucous blanket to propel the sticky upper mucous layer. This process represents the first line of defense against respiratory pathogens, and failure of this system leads to sinusitis, as in Kartagener's syndrome.

Deep to the epithelial basement membrane is a submucosa rich in glands. Three types of glands can be found: mucous, seromucous, and serous glands. In seromucous glands, the mucous cells from the central portion of the gland, and serous cells form a crescent over the mucous cells. Mucous glycoproteins localize immunohistochemically to the mucous cells, and lysozyme, lactoferrin, neutral endopeptidase, secretory leucoprotease inhibitor, and secretory IgA localize to the serous cells (2). The interstitial cells of the nasal mucosa are composed primarily of lymphocytes, with interspersed fibroblasts and mast cells. In normal subjects there are about 150 lymphocytes/mm of basement membrane in the nasal mucosa (3). Two-thirds of these cells are $CD_4$-positive and the remainder are $CD_8$-positive (3). The relative proportions and total population of $CD_4$- and $CD_8$-positive cells do not change during the allergy season (4). There are about 10 mast cells/mm basement membrane, most of which are of the $MC_{TC}$ subtype (4,5). The mast cells are located in close proximity to the nerves and blood vessels and are occasionally seen between epithelial cells. Most nasal mast cells are found in the superficial 200 μm of mucosa, usually clustered beneath the basement membrane and in the epithelium. In normal subjects there are about 7,000 mast cells/mm$^3$ in the tissue and only 50/mm$^3$ in the epithelium. The epithelial mast cell is of the $MC_T$ subtype (5), and the number of these epithelial mast cells is reported to increase during the allergy season (6). The total number of mast cells and lymphocytes does not increase during the allergy season (4). Interestingly, the only cells bearing IgE in the human nasal mucosa are mast cells (5).

The nose is one of the most vascular organs of the body, with total blood flow per cubic centimeter of tissue in excess of that in muscle, brain, and liver (7). The blood flow in the superficial mucosa has been found to be 42 ml/100 g tissue/min, which is also exceptionally high (8). Blood vessels feeding the epithelium and glands contain fenestrations in their basement membranes similar to those of the renal glomeruli. This anatomic arrangement facilitates rapid extravasation of fluid through the vascular walls, presumably to assist in the hydration of inspired air. Although the typical flow of blood from arteries to capillaries and into veins occurs in the nose, there are also many arteriovenous anastomoses in the nasal mucosa. In addition, cavernous sinusoids occur between the capillaries and venules. These vessels, which are found most densely in the inferior and middle turbinates, contain smooth-muscle cells that are under sympathetic control (9). Normally, the cavernous sinuses are contracted, but under conditions of reduced sympathetic tone or cholinergic stimulation, this erectile tissue becomes engorged, resulting in considerable nasal obstruction.

## NASAL NEUROPEPTIDES

Although the veins and venules in the nasal mucosa are predominantly innervated by sympathetic nerves, the arterial vessels that supply the glands, as well as the glands themselves, are innervated by both cholinergic and sympathetic fibers (10). Cholinergic stimulation causes arteriolar dilatation, in theory enhancing passive diffusion of plasma protein into the glands. In addition, the same cholinergic stimulation simultaneously induces active secretion from serous and mucous cells (11). Most of the cholinergic receptors on nasal glands and blood vessels are of the M3 type (12,13). In addition to containing the classical neurotransmitters, the three types of nerve fibers innervating the nose (the sensory, cholinergic, and sympathetic nerves) also contain neuropeptides. Sensory fibers from the trigeminal nerve are capable of responding to noxious stimuli such as mechanical or thermal injury, mediators such as bradykinin or histamine, and acute injury (14). These nerves form the afferent limb of several central reflexes and also participate in local vascular responses that are similar to the cutaneous wheal and flare response. Several neurotransmitters, including CGRP, the tachykinins SP and NKA, and GRP, have been found in sensory nerves (14). Parasympathetic neurons contain acetylcholine as well as VIP and a related neuropeptide called peptide histidine methionine (PHM). Sympathetic neurons contain norepinephrine and NPY, a peptide that causes many of the same effects as norepinephrine, including very long-lasting vasoconstriction.

The exact role of these neuropeptides in allergic diseases is still being evaluated. Immunohistochemical studies have demonstrated weak staining for CGRP, SP, and NKA fibers in the nasal mucosal epithelium. The submucosal glands, arterioles, and venous sinusoids are innervated by fibers staining for GRP, CGRP, SP, NKA, and VIP. Assuming that these neuropeptides can affect only structures that contain specific receptors, the distribution of neuropeptide binding sites has also been studied. The only neuropeptide for which both fibers and receptors were localized to the epithelium was SP (15). Submucosal glands were rich in both receptors and fibers for GRP > VIP > SP (15–17). The venous sinusoids, however, contained only a few neuropeptide receptors for CGRP, SP, and VIP. In contrast, arterioles contained receptors for all of the neuropeptides studied except for GRP; however, most of the receptors were for CGRP, which causes vasodilatation (18), or for NPY, which induces vasoconstriction (19). To assess the effect of these neuropeptides on glandular secretion, nasal turbinate explants were incubated ex vivo with control fluids or with various neuropeptides, and the secretion of glycoconjugates from mucous cells and of lactoferrin from serous cells was measured. GRP and VIP were both potent secretagogues for serous cells > mucous cells. SP and NKA were weak mucous cell secretagogues, and the latter was also a weak serous cell secretagogue (11).

Analysis of nasal secretions for the presence of neuropeptides after allergen challenge has recently led to the appreciation that there is a close relationship between antigen activation of mediators and the generation of neuropeptides into secretions. Specifically, SP, CGRP, and VIP are all increased significantly within 3 min of positive allergen challenge (20). The mechanism for this neuropeptide secretion is unknown, except that histamine is capable of causing VIP but not SP or CGRP release. We assume that the histamine-induced VIP secretion reflects the cholinergic stimulation that results from histamine release, and that VIP is released along with acetylcholine in this process. The mediators responsible for eliciting SP and CGRP release are unknown at this time. These data indicate that neuropeptides are secreted during allergic reactions and that they might play some role in causing symptoms.

## MEDIATORS OF ALLERGIC RHINITIS

To assess which mediators are important in inducing the symptoms of allergic rhinitis, it is important to know which mediators are released during an allergic reaction. Mast-cell activation after antigen challenge is well-described. In electron micrographic studies of resting mast cells, the ubiquitous, densely stained secretory granules are roughly spherical, and most are 0.2 to 0.5 μm in diameter. Most granules comprise a dense, amorphous matrix with embedded or interspersed crystalline constituents in the form of scrolls, gratings, or lattices. Scrolls are found most commonly in cells undergoing degranulation. It should be noted that even in experimentally unstimulated nasal tissue, variable numbers of degranulating mast cells are present. In unstimulated nasal epithelium, one-third of mast cells may be degranulated, and the percentage progressively increases from the lamina propria to the mucosal surface. Early events after IgE-mediated stimulation of human lung mast cells include granule swelling with loss of stainable matrix, an increase in the proportion of granules demonstrating a scroll pattern, and the appearance of electron-dense clumps in the granules. Granules progressively become more ropelike, with eventual solubilization of granule contents. In nasal and lung mast cells, extruded granules are never observed intact in the external environment of the degranulated nasal mast cell. Over the course of a few minutes, the degranulating mast cell may discharge the solubilized contents from 1,000 secretory granules into the surrounding interstitial fluid.

Within minutes after allergen exposure, the mast-cell products histamine,

$LTC_4$, and $PGD_2$ can be measured in nasal washings (21). Mast cells are found near superficial postcapillary venules (which respond with increased vascular permeability), sensory nerves (which respond by initiating the sensation of itch and elicit the sneeze reflex), and glands that respond by secretion. Many of the effects associated with acute allergic rhinitis can be reproduced by a histamine challenge (22), and antihistamines prevent many of the symptoms of acute allergic rhinitis (23). Histamine challenge to the nose leads to pruritus, sneezing, nasal congestion induced by vasodilatation, increased vascular permeability, and reflex cholinergic stimulation of glandular secretion on both the ipsilateral and contralateral nares. Activation of mast cells also leads to the generation of the 5-lipoxygenase products $LTC_4$, $LTD_4$, and $LTE_4$, which can induce vascular permeability, vasodilatation and mucous secretion. Concomitant with the increase in mast-cell mediators, an increase in the neuropeptides CGRP, SP, and VIP in secretions can also be observed (24), as well as an increase in bradykinin (25). In addition, mast-cell activation in vitro leads to the transcription and/or translation and release of a number of cytokines including TNF-$\alpha$, interleukins 1, 3, 4, 5, and 6, and GM-CSF (26–29).

The nasal mucosa also contains many inflammatory cells that might contribute cytokines to the allergic response. Lymphocytes comprise the majority of cells in the nasal submucosa. Lymphocytes in the mucosa of allergic individuals transcribe message for the TH-2 products IL-4 and IL-5, as well as GM-CSF (30) and IL-3, after allergen challenge. There are only scant data on cytokines recovered in lavages after antigen challenge; however, interleukins 1, 2, 3, 4, 5 and GM-CSF have been recovered (31–35), the former two cytokines during the first 30 min and all of them during the ensuing 10 hr.

## SYMPTOMS OF ALLERGIC RHINITIS AND RESPONSIBLE MEDIATORS

The cardinal symptoms of allergic rhinitis include pruritus, sneezing, rhinorrhea, and nasal congestion. Pruritus and sneezing are induced by sensory nerve stimulation, and congestion results from vasodilatation with resultant engorgement of cavernous sinusoids. Rhinorrhea can be induced by increased vascular permeability as well as direct glandular secretion. During the first 30 min after antigen challenge, concomitant with an increase in mediators, one can measure an enormous increase in the plasma proteins albumin and IgG as well as a smaller increase in the glandular proteins lysozyme, lactoferrin, and secretory IgA in nasal lavage fluids (36). In the nares contralateral to antigen challenge, rhinorrhea also occurs and consists entirely of glandular proteins. This contralateral rhinorrhea can be inhibited by pretreatment with atropine, suggesting that it is cholinergically mediated.

Therefore, antigen-induced rhinorrhea involves mostly vascular permeability on the ipsilateral side only and reflex mediated glandular secretion on both the ipsilateral and contralateral sides (11). This pattern is identical to that of histamine-induced rhinorrhea. In addition, antigen challenge leads to a late inflammatory response that is associated with prolonged congestion (37) and increased responsiveness to both antigen and histamine challenge (38).

Each of the symptoms of acute allergic rhinitis, as well as the secretion of plasma and glandular proteins, can largely be inhibited by pretreatment with an $H_1$ antagonist. Sneezing and pruritus are caused exclusively by stimulation of histamine $H_1$ receptors on sensory nerve endings. Histamine-induced vasodilatation and increased vascular permeability are also directly mediated via $H_1$ receptors on blood vessels. In contrast, histamine-induced glandular secretion is not mediated directly but rather by stimulation of a cholinergic reflex. Therefore, histamine is capable of inducing all of the features of acute allergic rhinitis except for the late-phase reaction (Table 1).

Although it is clear that histamine is a major mediator in acute allergic rhinitis, other mediators are also important in causing congestion (vasodilatation) and rhinorrhea (vascular permeability and glandular secretion). In addition to histamine, newly generated leukotrienes and bradykinin can induce both vasodilatation and increased vascular permeability, and leukotrienes can also induce glandular secretion. Both parasympathetic and sensory neurons are stimulated during allergic reactions, and several of the

**TABLE 1.** *Symptoms and pathologic features of allergic rhinitis and proposed mediators*

| Symptom | Pathologic feature | Proposed mediator |
|---------|-------------------|-------------------|
| Pruritus | Sensory nerve stimulation | Histamine ($H_1$) Prostaglandins |
| Nasal obstruction | Mucosal edema and vasodilatation | Histamine ($H_1$) Kinins Leukotrienes $C_4$, $D_4$, and $E_4$ TNF-$\alpha$ CGRP, SP |
| Sneezing | Sensory nerve stimulation | Histamine ($H_1$) Leukotrienes $C_4$, $D_4$, and $E_4$ |
| Rhinorrhea (see also edema above) | Increased mucous secretion | Histamine (via muscarinic reflex) Leukotrienes $C_4$, $D_4$, and $E_4$ Bradykinin |
| Hyperirritability and prolonged congestion | Late-phase reaction | SP, VIP Inflammatory factors Eicosanoids, PAF Chemotactic factors IL-1, IL-5, IL-6, IL-8, TNF-$\alpha$ |

neuropeptides localized to these neurons have been shown to rise in nasal secretions after antigen challenge. The neuropeptides SP and VIP are capable of inducing glandular secretion, and CGRP, which is co-localized with SP to sensory fibers, is capable of inducing vasodilatation and contributing to congestion. Mast cell-derived chemotactic factors, as well as PAF, IL-5, and IL-8, are probably instrumental in attracting inflammatory cells into the late-phase reaction. IL-1, IL-6, and TNF-α probably also play a role in inducing inflammation through up-regulation of adhesion molecule expression (39). IL-2 might be important in activating lymphocytes after allergen challenge, thus providing the message for additional cytokine production. Finally, interleukins 3, 4, 6, and possibly 10 play a role in promoting mast-cell growth and differentiation and in enhancing IgE synthesis.

In summary, histamine is the major mediator of the immediate allergic reaction, although other inflammatory mediators as well as neuropeptides also may play a role in producing rhinorrhea and congestion. Therefore, the use of antihistamines alone is insufficient to prevent all of the symptoms of allergic rhinitis. The late-phase reaction is triggered by the release from mast cells of chemotactic factors and by generation and release of inflammatory and chemotactic cytokines. Because the combination of antihistamines and topical corticosteroids is capable of inhibiting the generation, release, and activity of most if not all of the mediators potentially involved in the allergic response, this combination therapy represents a logical and effective approach to the treatment of allergic rhinitis.

## REFERENCES

1. Kaliner MA, Lemanske R. *JAMA* 1992;268:2807–29.
2. Kaliner MA. *Am Rev Respir Dis* 1991;144:S52–66.
3. Igarashi Y, Scott TA, Hausfeld JH, Kaliner MA, White MV. *J Allergy Clin Immunol* 1992;89:204.
4. Bentley AM, Jacobson MR, Cumberworth V, et al. *J Allergy Clin Immunol* 1992;89:877–83.
5. Igarashi Y, White M, Hausfeld J, Irani A, Schwartz L, Kaliner M. *FASEB J* 1992;6: A2005(abst).
6. Lozewizc S, Gomez E, Clague J, Gatland D, Davies RJ. *J Allergy Clin Immunol* 1990;85: 125–31.
7. Drettner B, Aust R. *Acta Otolaryngol* 1974;78:259–65.
8. Druce HM, Bonner RF, Patow C, Choo P, Kaliner MA. *J Appl Physiol* 1984;57:1276–83.
9. Atkinson TP, Kaliner MA. In: Busse W, Holgate S, eds. *Asthma and rhinitis*. Cambridge, MA: Blackwell Scientific [in press].
10. Raphael GD, Meredith SD, Baraniuk JN, Kaliner MA. *Am J Rhinol* 1988;2:109–16.
11. Raphael GD, Baraniuk JN, Kaliner MA. *J Allergy Clin Immunol* 1991;87:457–67.
12. Okayama M, Mullol J, Baraniuk JN, et al. *Am J Respir Cell Mol Biol* 1993;8:176–87.
13. Baraniuk JN, Kaliner MA, Barnes PJ. *Am J Rhinol* 1992;6:H5–8.
14. Baraniuk JN, Kaliner MA. In: Busse W, Holgate S, eds. *Asthma and rhinitis*. Cambridge, MA: Blackwell Scientific [in press].
15. Baraniuk JN, Lundgren JD, Okayama M, et al. *Am J Respir Cell Mol Biol* 1991;4:228–36.
16. Baraniuk JN, Lundgren JD, Goff J, et al. *J Clin Invest* 1990;85:998–1005.
17. Baraniuk JN, Lundgren JD, Okayama M, et al. *J Clin Invest* 1990;86:825–31.
18. Baraniuk JN, Lundgren JD, Goff J, et al. *J Appl Physiol* 1990;258:81–8.

19. Baraniuk JN, Castellino S, Lundgren JD, et al. *Am J Respir Cell Mol Biol* 1990;3:165–74.
20. Mosimann B, White M, Kaulbach H, Goldrich M, Kaliner M. *Am Rev Respir Dis* 1002;145:A47(Abstract).
21. Naclerio RM, Meier HL, Kagey-Sobotka A, et al. *Am Rev Respir Dis* 1983;128:597–602.
22. Raphael GD, Meredith SD, Baraniuk JN, Druce HM, Banks SM, Kaliner MA. *Am Rev Respir Dis* 1989;139:791–800.
23. Simmons, E. *J Allergy Clin Immunol* 1992;90:705–15.
24. Mosimann B, White MV, Kaulbach HK, Goldrich M, Kaliner MA. *J Allergy Clin Immunol* 1992;89:210.
25. Proud D, Baumgarten CR, Naclerio RM, Ward PE. *J Immunol* 1987;138:428–34.
26. Burd PR, Rogers HW, Gordon JR, et al. *J Exp Med* 1989;170:245–57.
27. Gordon JR, Galli SJ. *Nature* 1990;346:274–6.
28. Plaut M, Pierce JII, Watson CJ, Hanley-Hyde J, Nordan RP, Paul WE. *Nature* 1989;339:64–7.
29. Gurish MF, Ghildyal N, Arm J, et al. *J Immunol* 1991;146:1527–33.
30. Durham SR, Ying S, Varney VAS, et al. *J Immunol* 1992;148:2390–4.
31. Moss RB, Ohkubo K, Paciotti G, et al. *J Allergy Clin Immunol* 1992;89:179.
32. Bochner BS, Charlesworth EN, Lichtenstein LM, et al. *J Allergy Clin Immunol* 1990;86:830–9.
33. Sim TC, Alam R, Hilsmeier KA, Grant JA. *J Allergy Clin Immunol* 1992;89:216.
34. Steinberg DG, Rosenwasser LJ. *J Allergy Clin Immunol* 1992;89:217.
35. Sur S, Hunt LW, Weiler DA, Ohnishi T, Gleich GJ. *J Allergy Clin Immunol* 1992;89:215(abst).
36. Raphael GD, Igarashi Y, White MV, Kaliner MA. *J Allergy Clin Immunol* 1991;88:33–42.
37. Naclerio RM, Proud D, Togias AG, et al. *N Engl J Med* 1985;313:65–70.
38. White M, Goldrich M, Daniel A, Kaliner M. *J Allergy Clin Immunol* 1992;89:206.
39. Gundel RH, Wegner CD, Torcellini CA, et al. *J Clin Invest* 1991;88:1407–11.

Advances in Prostaglandin, Thromboxane,
and Leukotriene Research, Vol. 22, edited by
S.-E. Dahlén et al. Raven Press, Ltd., New York © 1994

# Leukotrienes as Mediators of Nasal Inflammation

Howard R. Knapp and *John J. Murray

*Division of Clinical Pharmacology, University of Iowa, Iowa City, Iowa
52242-1081; and *Allergy Division, Vanderbilt University,
Nashville, Tennessee 37232*

Leukotrienes are produced by a variety of cell types involved in allergic and inflammatory processes (1), but their role as the primary mediators of particular pathologic processes in humans has been difficult to establish with certainty (2). In nasal inflammation, one must differentiate between several etiologies that are characterized by different degrees of specific symptoms, such as that resulting from viral infection versus allergic rhinitis. There have been few studies of leukotriene involvement in the nasal inflammatory response to infection, for example, but it would not be surprising to find that with different cell populations and different types of symptoms, various mediators might be involved to a very different extent than in allergic rhinitis. Because leukotrienes were first described as substances originating from allergic responses, it is logical that most of the studies of nasal leukotrienes have involved allergic rhinitis. The studies described below deal primarily with our efforts to associate changes in leukotriene synthesis with changes in symptoms in a nasal allergen challenge model.

## LEUKOTRIENES IN NASAL ALLERGY

The nasal allergen challenge model has been utilized to study both the early and late phases of human allergic rhinitis (3,4). Differences have been noted between the types and proportions of mediators recovered in nasal lavage fluids, and inferences have been made regarding the types of cells that are most likely to be responsible for these processes. The accurate quantitation of labile compounds in low concentrations remains technically challenging, however, and the many possible transformation products of the mediators known to be present can rarely be assessed. As a result, it may not be possible to determine the primary cell populations involved in particular aspects of nasal inflammation by noting the types of mediators measurable in lavage fluids, just as it will be more convincing to establish a specific compound as responsible for a particular symptom complex when effective receptor antagonists are available.

It has been noted that $PGD_2$ and leukotrienes are both present in the early phase of the nasal allergic response and that only leukotrienes, but not $PGD_2$, are present in the late response (5). On this basis, it has been suggested that mast cells are mainly involved in the early phase and that basophils, which have not been shown to make $PGD_2$, are involved in the late phase. Recent histologic evidence has also been presented to further support this idea (6). It is known, however, that $PGD_2$ is rapidly isomerized to other products in the presence of albumin or enzymes likely to be present in inflammatory infiltrates (7), so it is also possible that $PGD_2$ is being produced in increased amounts but is undetectable in the late-phase samples because of rapid metabolism. Leukotrienes are less stable chemically than $PGD_2$ and are also rapidly transformed both by specific and nonspecific enzymes, as well as by reactive oxygen species associated with inflammation. As a result, their absence or increase must be assessed with caution unless some information is available about the extent of their alteration. With the many possible sources of variation in leukotriene production, transport, and metabolism, it is not surprising that some disagreements have appeared over their possible role in nasal allergy (8). These could arise from differences in nasal challenge or lavaging procedures, as well as in the analytical methods used to measure the mediators involved.

Despite the many methodologic challenges, there have emerged a number of reports agreeing that acute nasal allergen challenge is associated with the release of leukotrienes, prostaglandins, histamine, kinins, and other inflammatory cell mediators (8). The primary products of the 5-lipoxygenase pathway include 5-HETE, cysteinyl leukotrienes, and $LTB_4$, and nonenzymatic products of $LTA_4$ hydrolysis, the *trans*-$LTB_4$ isomers (2). All of these products can be converted by a number of pathways into other products under the right in vivo conditions, and it has been found that the degree of inflammation has a marked influence on the rapidity of such metabolism. Studies on the oxidation of $LTB_4$, for example, have shown that isolated neutrophils metabolize it rapidly to more polar products, primarily via ω-oxidation (9). The neutrophils induced by chemical injection to form a dense pleural infiltrate metabolize $LTB_4$ more slowly (10), however, and in stimulated whole blood little metabolism of $LTB_4$ takes place (11). It is possible that different stages of nasal inflammation may have widely different metabolic "density," and have much different tendencies to demonstrate metabolism of $LTB_4$. It has also been noted that the proportion of cysteinyl leukotrienes recovered as $LTE_4$ is increased in late versus early-phase nasal lavage fluids (12), and that there is a high degree of interindividual variability in both the total leukotriene generation as well as in the proportion of $LTC_4$, $LTD_4$, and $LTE_4$ recovered. We have also found that there can be marked intraindividual differences in the amount of $LTB_4$ recovered after repetitive nasal chal-

nasal challenge and that, as with levels of histamine (13), there is no correlation between the degree of nasal symptoms and the absolute amount of mediator in the fluid (14).

As a result of this extreme variability, it is necessary to conduct comparative studies under conditions that are as closely matched as possible. Examining atopic individuals before or during the allergy season, for example, could understandably produce different patterns of mediator release. The basis for such differences may be difficult to understand if only a few primary mediators can be measured, since the differing degrees of metabolism for the different eicosanoids will not be able to be assessed. As a result, it is essential that individuals be studied with the same extent of baseline nasal inflammation if their results are to be compared. It has been shown that repeated allergen challenge causes a "priming" effect with regard to symptoms and the release of some mediators, but it is not known to what extent the metabolism of different eicosanoid pathways is influenced by this phenomenon (15,16). Interestingly, we have found that repeated challenge of the same subject over a period too brief to allow a late-phase response to develop resulted in the recovery of steadily increasing amounts of histamine, whereas stimulated $LTB_4$ concentrations continuously declined. Clearly, complex allergen–cell reactions can lead to great differences in mediator removal even if the rates of synthesis are the same, which they probably are not because the number and types of cells present in the nasal mucosa are changing during such prolonged challenges (17), in a similar way to what actually occurs during the allergy season.

## LEUKOTRIENE EFFECTS IN THE NOSE

Because it is established that the nasal allergic response results in markedly increased synthesis of leukotrienes, the next question is whether leukotrienes can actually produce any part or all of the nasal allergic symptom complex. Nasal instillation of histamine causes congestion, sneezing, itching, and rhinorrhea, but it has been known for many years that $H_1$-receptor antagonists block itching and sneezing and decrease rhinorrhea but provide little relief from the congestion that accompanies nasal allergic reactions (18). This suggests that other mediators must be involved, so it was of interest that nasal challenge with $LTD_4$ produced an increase in nasal blood flow (19) and nasal congestion (20) without itching or sneezing. $LTD_4$ was used in these studies because of the rapidity and variability of metabolism of $LTC_4$ in the nose, and it would be expected that this factor alone could lead to marked interindividual responses in a challenge test.

Because leukotrienes are produced in response to nasal allergic reactions and provoke specific allergic symptoms when administered nasally, it is likely that they play a role in the development of allergic symptoms in vivo.

Proof of this, however, requires the additional observation that blocking the synthesis of leukotrienes or their action on specific cell receptors markedly reduces the nasal allergic response. A first step in this is the development of a drug that has demonstrable ability to perform one of these effects in human subjects. The drug must then be tested in a suitable human model of nasal allergy and, finally, to understand the role of leukotrienes in chronic hay fever symptoms, the drug must be tested "in the field" in actual free-living patients. We describe below how some of the initial steps in this direction have been accomplished.

## LEUKOTRIENE INHIBITION IN NASAL ALLERGY

With many potential applications in clinical allergy and inflammatory diseases, there has been a great effort to develop effective 5-lipoxygenase inhibitors and antagonists of leukotriene receptors (21). From a pharmacologic standpoint, eicosanoids are usually produced in vast excess in response to potent in vivo stimuli, and it is difficult to achieve adequate concentrations of receptor antagonists at pathologically important sites throughout an achievable dosing interval. The antagonists that have been available thus far have not been especially potent, and this could explain the lack of effect in a nasal challenge model (22). More potent agents are under development, and some may have a sufficiently long half-life that a clinically detectable degree of nasal receptor antagonism can be achieved.

A number of compounds have been synthesized that exhibit inhibitory activity against 5-lipoxygenase in vitro but have yielded negative results in clinical testing. If a drug is able to achieve inhibition of 5-lipoxygenase in tissues, it should be expected that it would also exhibit inhibition of the enzyme in blood, and stimulated leukotriene synthesis in whole blood has been developed as an index of such potential (23). Naturally, a compound may inhibit neutrophils in blood undergoing a capacity-related leukotriene stimulus, such as with the calcium ionophore A-23187, but may fail to achieve adequate tissue levels for a sufficient portion of the dosing interval to exhibit a clinically detectable effect. On the other hand, it would be surprising for a drug to inhibit the 5-lipoxygenase in tissues and not in stimulated blood, yet some unsuccessful compounds have entered clinical testing without this information. The high potency of A-64077 in inhibiting neutrophil $LTB_4$ synthesis in vitro held out the promise that, even with a half-life of less than 3 hr, peak levels could be reached that would allow a high degree of enzyme inhibition in blood (24) and, potentially, in tissues as well. This led to our adapting the nasal allergen challenge model specifically to test whether A-64077 could significantly inhibit 5-lipoxygenase activity in human tissues during in vivo stimulation of leukotriene synthesis (14).

From the reported half-life of A-64077 (24), we estimated that nasal aller-

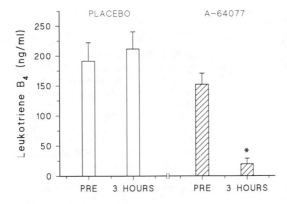

**FIG. 1.** Effect of A-64077 on the release of LTB$_4$ from whole blood ex vivo. Bars show means and SEM for LTB$_4$ present in blood from the eight subjects after addition of ionophore A-23187. The blood was drawn before (PRE) or 3 hr after (3 HOURS) dosing with 800 mg A-64077 or an identical placebo. *Significant inhibition at $p < 0.01$ by a two-tailed comparison using the Wilcoxon signed-rank test.

gen challenge should be performed at about 3 hr after oral dosing in order to occur at peak plasma levels of the drug. At this time point we also drew blood for measurement of drug levels and assessment of drug specificity by noting the effects on the activities of 5-lipoxygenase, cyclooxygenase, and 12-lipoxygenase. The latter two points were approached by measurement of thromboxane B$_2$ and 12-HETE generation during serum formation for 1 hr at 37°C. The timing of this incubation is important, because although thromboxane generation during blood clotting is essentially complete after 45 min (25), elaboration of 12-HETE by the platelets continues in a linear fashion for some hours (26). Figure 1 shows the marked degree of 5-lipoxygenase inhibition achieved in the subjects' blood at 3 hr after dosing, and Fig. 2 shows the lack of effect of A-64077 on 12-HETE formation by platelets. It is interesting that both thromboxane B$_2$ (not shown) and 12-HETE generation showed slight increases during the nasal challenge study performed after placebo administration. This is reminiscent of reports of in vivo platelet activation during allergic bronchospasm (27), and perhaps relates to in vivo "priming" of platelets with epinephrine released by the stress of untreated nasal allergic symptoms. When active drug was given, however, there was a diminished severity of nasal congestion response (Fig. 3) and a lack of

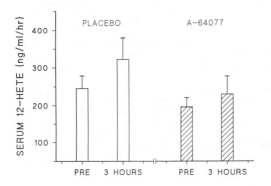

**FIG. 2.** Effect of A-64077 on the generation of 12-HETE in serum. Bars show means and SEM for 12-HETE (ng/ml/hr) in the serum of eight subjects whose blood was sampled before (PRE) or 3 hr after (3 HOURS) oral dosing with 800 mg A-64077 or identical placebo.

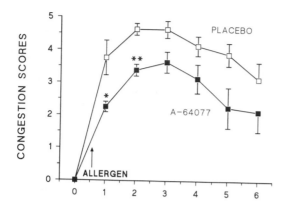

**FIG. 3.** Time course of nasal congestion symptoms during allergen challenge after administration of A-64077 or placebo. Values are means ± SEM (bars) for the eight subjects, obtained at the end of each 12-min assessment period. Significant effect of A-64077 at *$p < 0.05$ and **$p < 0.02$, respectively, using a two-tailed comparison by the Wilcoxon signed-rank test. (From ref. 14 with permission.)

increase in ex vivo generation of 12-HETE (Fig. 2) and thromboxane $B_2$ (not shown) by platelets.

The reduction in nasal congestion was correctly noted to occur with active drug in this double-blind study by seven of the eight participants. Administration of A-64077 was remarkably free of cardiovascular or any other side effects that could have indicated the order of dosing to the subjects; the one subject who had similar responses on both placebo and active drug was found to have had much lower drug levels than any of the other seven subjects and to have achieved only a 34% inhibition of stimulated $LTB_4$ release in blood ex vivo in comparison to the mean of 92% reached by the others (Table 1).

In addition to selective inhibition of the 5-lipoxygenase pathway in blood ex vivo, A-64077 was found to reduce the concentrations of both $LTB_4$ and 5-HETE in nasal rinse fluid obtained after antigen instillation. Together, these two compounds provide a reflection of concomitant inhibition of two portions of the 5-lipoxygenase pathway, and no significant effect on the nasal release of prostaglandin $D_2$ was observed (Fig. 4). Overall, the findings

**TABLE 1.** *Congestion scores and subject assessment of dosing order*

| | Subject | | | | | | | |
|---|---|---|---|---|---|---|---|---|
| | 1 | 2 | 3 | 4 | 5 | 6 | 7 | 8 |
| A-64077[a] | 9 | 25 | 23 | 17 | 16 | 18 | 9 | 18 |
| Placebo[a] | 30 | 30 | 27 | 19 | 25 | 16 | 22 | 24 |
| Subject assessment correct? | + | + | + | + | + | ? | + | + |
| Inhibition of W-B $LTB_4$ at T = 3 hr | 82% | 95% | 97% | 100% | 99% | 34% | 87% | 91% |

[a] Total congestion scores for each subject during the challenge test 3 hr after receiving A-64077 (800 mg) or an identical placebo. After both challenge tests, performed at least 2 weeks apart, the subjects were asked to identify the occasion when they had received active drug. The inhibition of $LTB_4$ release stimulated by ionophore A-23187 in whole-blood ex vivo (W-B $LTB_4$) at 3 hr after dosing is expressed as a percent of that obtained before dosing on that occasion.

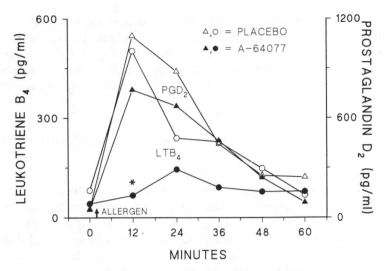

**FIG. 4.** Time course of nasal $LTB_4$ and prostaglandin $D_2$ release during allergen challenge after administration of placebo (open symbols) or A64077 (solid symbols). Median values for the eight subjects, obtained at the end of each 12-min assessment period, are shown. Stimulation of $LTB_4$ was blunted in seven of the eight subjects ($p < 0.010$) and total $LTB_4$ released during the study was significantly reduced ($p = 0.05$). In contrast, the release of prostaglandin $D_2$ was reduced after administration of A-64077 in only three of the eight subjects at any point. *Significant difference ($p < 0.02$) by the Wilcoxon signed-rank test. (From ref. 14 with permission.)

in this study provided the first direct demonstration of in vivo 5-lipoxygenase inhibition in human subjects, as well as a strong suggestion that leukotrienes play a significant role in the development of nasal congestion after allergen challenge. Further work will be needed to extend these observations from our nasal allergen challenge model to clinical hay fever, however, as our initial chronic study in the ragweed season yielded a positive but statistically nonsignificant trend toward symptom improvement. Analysis of urinary $LTE_4$ excretion during that study may provide a clue as to how to improve on this effort, as the dosing regimen selected yielded only a 50% to 60% inhibition over the 24-hr period. It may well be that a higher degree of 5-lipoxygenase inhibition than this will have to be achieved throughout the dosing interval to produce clinically significant symptomatic improvement for hay fever sufferers.

We have also tested another putative 5-lipoxygenase inhibitor, SC-45662, in our nasal challenge model. This drug is believed to inhibit 5-lipoxygenase by acting as a intramolecular antioxidant, and it offered promise because of its long biologic half-life (28). Unfortunately, the high degree of drug binding to plasma proteins caused it to provide only a 25% inhibition of stimulated $LTB_4$ in blood, which was less than that found in the sole subject in the study of A-64077 who had no symptomatic improvement with the drug. Although there was some tendency toward improvement in each of the individual symptoms assessed (nasal and conjunctival) and the investigators' global assessment score showed significant improvement ($p < 0.05$), none of the symptoms or mediators alone exhibited a statistically significant reduction in response to active drug administration, but all shared the same degree of nonsignificant tendency toward improvement.

## THE 5-LIPOXYGENASE PATHWAY AND DIETARY MODIFICATION

An alternative approach to inhibition of leukotriene effects has been proposed to be via dietary enrichment with long-chain $\omega$-3 polyunsaturated fatty acids (2). These marine oil components include eicosapentaenoic acid, which has been described as a good substrate for 5-lipoxygenase. When tested on normal (not EPA-supplemented) neutrophils, the EPA-derived $LTB_5$ had much less chemotactic activity than did arachidonate-derived $LTB_4$ (29). The activity of EPA-derived $LTC_5$, however, has not been found to be any less than that of $LTC_4$ (30). A further observation on marine oil supplementation is that it results in a reduction of total 5-lipoxygenase product release, based on observations with A-23187 stimulation of isolated neutrophils (31). This is a maximal, capacity-related stimulus, however, and when we assessed the effect of even very high-dose fish oil supplementation on neutrophil function and leukotriene release in response to receptor-mediated stimuli, we did not find any reduction in total $LTB_4$ release at all (32). In fact, ex vivo $LTB_4$ release was not reduced by fish oil ingestion, and total $LTB_4$ + $LTB_5$ was increased. To test the hypothesis that such dietary modification would modify leukotriene release and symptom development in response to allergen challenge in vivo, we performed nasal allergen challenges in six subjects who were participating in our studies on fish oil supplementation (providing 9 g EPA/day). A substantial amount of $LTB_5$ was synthesized from the EPA during this in vivo allergen challenge, but no decrease, and in fact an increase, in the release of $LTB_4$ was seen (33). In accordance with the idea that nasal leukotrienes are involved in nasal congestion responses after allergen challenge, no reduction in allergic symptoms was found in these subjects while they were taking the fish oil.

## SUMMARY AND CONCLUSIONS

The three sets of studies that we have described support the notion that leukotrienes play a role in the nasal inflammatory response to allergen challenge. Strong inhibition of both leukotrienes and symptoms by A-64077, a trend toward inhibition of both leukotrienes and symptoms by SC-45662, and a lack of effect on either leukotrienes or symptoms by dietary eicosapentaenoic acid provide a consistent association between alterations of leukotrienes and nasal symptoms. A great deal of evidence has now accumulated that leukotrienes are important mediators of inflammation in vivo, but we also know that the chronic stimulus of hay fever produces a much more complex picture than seen in an acute challenge model and that many other mediators such as kinins, other peptides, histamine, and eicosanoids produced outside the 5-lipoxygenase pathway are involved (34,35). Further clinical research will be needed to develop optimal dosing regimens and delivery systems to achieve high concentrations of potent and safe 5-lipoxygenase inhibitors at sites that are critical for producing clinically useful results by modulation of the 5-lipoxygenase pathway.

## ACKNOWLEDGMENT

These studies were supported by NIH grants HL-35380, GM-15431, and HL-48877 to Dr. Knapp, as well as by grants from Abbott Laboratories and G. D. Searle and Company. Dr. Knapp is an Established Investigator of the American Heart Association.

## REFERENCES

1. Samuelsson B. *Science* 1983;220:568–75.
2. Lewis RA, Austen KF, Soberman RJ. *N Engl J Med* 1990;323:645–55.
3. Creticos PS, Peters SP, Adkinson NF, et al. *N Engl J Med* 1984;310:1626–30.
4. Shaw RJ, Fitzharris P, Cromwell O, Wardlaw AJ, Kay AB. *Allergy* 1985;40:1–6.
5. Naclerio RM, Proud D, Togias AG, et al. *N Engl J Med* 1985;313:65–70.
6. Bascom R, Wachs M, Naclerio RM, et al. *J Allergy Clin Immunol* 1988;81:580–9.
7. Ito S, Narumiya S, Hayaishi O. *Prostaglandins Leukot Essent Fatty Acids* 1989;37:219–34.
8. Naclerio RM, Baroody FM, Togias AG. *Am Rev Respir Dis* 1991;143:S91–5.
9. Shack S, Goldstein IM. *J Biol Chem* 1984;259:10181–7.
10. Taylor W, Sun F. *Biochem Pharmacol* 1985;34:3495–3502.
11. Reilly IA, Knapp HR, FitzGerald GA. *J Clin Pathol* 1988;41:1163–7.
12. Pipkorn U, Proud D, Lichtenstein LM, et al. *J Clin Invest* 1987;80:957–61.
13. Mygind N, Secher C, Kirkegaard J. *Eur J Respir Dis* 1983;128(suppl):16–20.
14. Knapp HR. *N Engl J Med* 1990;323:1745–8.
15. Connell JT. *J Allergy* 1969;43:33–44.
16. Wachs M, Proud D, Lichtenstein LM, Kagey-Sobotka A, Norman PS, Naclerio RM. *J Allergy Clin Immunol* 1989;84:492–501.
17. Bascom R, Pipkorn U, Lichtenstein LM, Naclerio RM. *Am Rev Respir Dis* 1988;138:406–12.
18. Laduron PM, Janssen PF, Gommeren W, Leysen JE. *Mol Pharmacol* 1981;21:294–300.
19. Bisgaard H, Olsson P, Bende M. *Clin Allergy* 1986;16:289–97.
20. Okuda M, Watase T, Mazawa A, Jiu C-M. *Ann Allergy* 1988;60:537–40.
21. Busse WW, Gaddy JN. *Am Rev Respir Dis* 1991;143:S103–7.
22. Flowers BK, Proud D, Kagey-Sobotka A, Lichtenstein LM, Naclerio RM. *Otolaryngol Head Neck Surg* 1990;102:219–24.
23. Sweeney FJ, Eskra JD, Carty TJ. *Prostaglandins Leukot Med* 1987;28:73–93.
24. Rubin PD, Kesterson J, Swanson L, et al. *Clin Pharmacol Ther* 1989;45:187[Abstract].
25. Patrono C. *Circulation* 1990;81(suppl I):I-12–5.
26. Hwang DH. *Lipids* 1982;17:845–52.
27. Woolcock AJ. *Am Rev Respir Dis* 1988;138:730–44.
28. Alexander J, Keane B, Metcalf LE, et al. *J Allergy Clin Immunol* 1992;89:208 [Abstract].

29. Goldman DW, Pickett WC, Goetzel EJ. *Biochem Biophys Res Commun* 1983;117:282–338.
30. Leitch AG, Lee TH, Ringel EW, et al. *J Immunol* 1984;132:2559–65.
31. Lee TH, Hoover RL, Williams JD, et al. *N Engl J Med* 1985;312:1217–24.
32. Knapp HR. *Clin Res* 1986;34:390A.
33. Knapp HR. *Clin Res* 1991;39:319A.
34. Miadonna A, Tedeschi A, Leggieri E, et al. *Am Rev Respir Dis* 1987;136:357–62.
35. Freeland HS, Pipkorn U, Schleimer RP, et al. *J Allergy Clin Immunol* 1989;83:634–42.

*Advances in Prostaglandin, Thromboxane,*
*and Leukotriene Research,* Vol. 22, edited by
S.-E. Dahlén et al. Raven Press, Ltd., New York © 1994

# Basic Mechanisms in Rheumatoid Arthritis: The Role of T Lymphocytes in Rheumatoid Synovitis

Saifeddin Alsalameh, Gerd R. Burmester, and
Joachim R. Kalden

*Institute of Clinical Immunology and Rheumatology, Department of Medicine III,*
*University of Erlangen–Nürnberg, 91054 Erlangen, Germany*

Rheumatoid arthritis (RA) is a chronic systemic inflammatory disease of unknown etiology that develops in genetically susceptible hosts, as demonstrated by the association with certain HLA class II (DR 4) antigens. RA is not a homogeneous disease entity, as there are different clinical manifestations in individual patients, variable outcomes, the presence or absence of serum rheumatoid factors, and different genetic backgrounds (1). RA has a worldwide distribution and involves most racial and ethnic groups, with a prevalence ranging between 1% and 2%. Although the etiology of RA remains elusive, data on the pathogenesis of tissue destruction, including mechanisms of cellular activation and cytokine release, are accumulating rapidly (2). There is no doubt that the immune system plays an integral role in the pathogenesis of RA. This article presents a short summary of pathogenic mechanisms in RA, with special emphasis on the role of T cells.

## PATHOGENIC MECHANISMS IN RHEUMATOID ARTHRITIS

According to current knowledge, the development of rheumatoid synovitis is a cell-mediated process involving various cellular elements, including T cells, macrophages, antigen-presenting cells (APC), synoviocytes, chondrocytes, and plasma cells, producing rheumatoid factors with the subsequent formation of immune complex. Additional factors, such as cytokines, their inhibitors, and growth factors are also involved. Within the different cell populations and soluble factors, T cells and macrophages are the most prominent partners playing a central role in the processes that lead to synovitis and the destruction of cartilage and bone.

On the basis of available clinical and experimental data, the hypothesis can be put forward that T lymphocytes become activated by a thus far unknown rheumatoid antigen (self-peptides or peptides from microbial agents) via HLA class II molecules with specific motifs on APC. Subsequently, activated T cells undergoing clonal proliferation in an autocrine or paracrine manner stimulate other cells such as T cells, monocytes/macrophages, B cells, synovial lining cells, and chondrocytes to release cytokines, growth factors, rheumatoid factors, arachidonic acid products, and proteolytic enzymes. These factors then play a major part in causing synovitis with pannus formation, resulting in cartilage and bone destruction. Associated with this hypothesis is the requirement for persistent antigens to maintain chronicity.

The central role of T lymphocytes in the development of rheumatoid inflammation is underlined by the following observations. First, chronic arthritis can be induced in healthy animals by the transfer of small numbers of specific T-cell lines or clones from arthritic animals. These T lymphocytes injected into the animals in the absence of additional antigens initiate inflammatory events that ultimately result in cartilage destruction (3). Second, T-cell–directed therapy has been shown to exhibit beneficial effects in RA patients and animal models (4–8). Third, rheumatoid synovial T cells can, however, be stimulated under appropriate conditions, particularly with antigens, suggesting that RA synovial T cells belong to a selection of antigen-reactive T cells with characteristics of memory T cells. Finally rheumatoid synovial T cells show an activated phenotype as indicated by the presence of MHC class II antigens, CD29, CD69, CDw60, and other activation markers. This is paralleled by a higher precursor frequency of cells responsive to IL-2. This in vivo activated phenotype is strikingly different from T cells activated in vitro. The phenotypical hallmark of many cell systems present in the inflamed synovium is the intense expression of HLA class II antigens both on cells that constitutively express these cell surface molecules, including macrophages, and on other mesenchymal cells that normally do not express these antigens, such as activated fibroblasts and even chondrocytes (9,10). The expression of MHC class II antigens is the prerequisite for foreign and autologous antigens that are presented to T cells. On the basis of these observations, many investigators have focused their interest on the characterization of T cells both in blood and the synovial sites in RA and on the identification of antigens and autoantigens responsible for the T-cell activation. Although no autoantigen has been clearly defined until now, possible candidates for autoantigens are collagen type II, proteoglycans and, more recently, chondrocyte membrane components (11,12). Even though both cellular and humoral immune responses are demonstrated against these components, it is not clear whether these antigens actually initiate the inflammatory processes or whether they merely represent attempts by immune cells to discard damaged cartilage tissues.

## PHENOTYPICAL AND FUNCTIONAL PROPERTIES OF INTRA-ARTICULAR T LYMPHOCYTES

Many findings indicate that RA intra-articular T lymphocytes have been activated in vivo. These observations include the presence of HLA class II (Ia) antigens, which are absent from resting T cells, the expression of the CD2R antigens, and other markers such as the very late antigen (VLA) family (13–15). HLA class II antigens are preferentially expressed on the T-cell subset with the suppressor/cytotoxic (CD8 +) phenotype (13). In contrast, analysis of the expression of the interleukin-2 receptor (IL-2R) revealed that this receptor is present only on a minority of blood or intra-articular T cells (usually 5% to 10%, as detected by anti-Tac antibodies), which are primarily of the helper/inducer (CD4 +) phenotype (16,17). The lack of IL-2R suggests that either the majority of RA synovial tissue T cells have become frozen in a late postactivation stage, i.e., the so-called "incomplete" or "frustrated" activation, or have been activated via T-cell receptor (TCR)-independent pathways (18). These cells are responsive to IL-2 in vitro and can effectively be cloned from intra-articular sites (19). The phenotypical data suggest that two in principle mutually exclusive activated T-cell populations exist in RA, i.e., the HLA class II +/CD8 + T cells and the IL-2R +/CD4 + T-cell population (Fig. 1). In contrast to the latter cells, however, T cells activated in vitro are IL-2R–positive to a large extent.

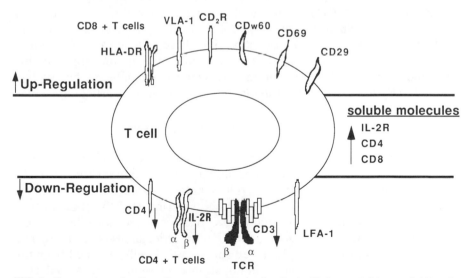

**FIG. 1.** Expression of cell surface molecules on "activated" rheumatoid synovial T cells. The scheme shows the up- and downregulation of cell surface molecules and soluble receptors, such as IL-2R, CD4, CD8, and transferin receptor (TfR) detected in synovial fluid of RA patients.

Another major difference between in vivo activated RA T cells and in vitro mitogen- or antigen-activated T cells is the low staining intensity and the small nonblastoid appearance of the rheumatoid T cells in contrast to the T-cell blasts in vitro, which are of larger size and express higher amounts of activation antigens per cell (16). Moreover, the analysis of T-cell derived cytokines at the mRNA and protein levels, with rather low levels of IL-2, IL-4, and interferon-$\gamma$ (20), which in general implies that rheumatoid T cells, particularly at the intra-articular sites, have been activated to some extent, implies either that the activation process has not been carried out completely or that activated cells have rapidly reverted to resting state. Studies of the T-cell subset distribution have shown consistent data, with elevated CD4/CD8 ratios in blood primarily in active patients and decreased CD4/CD8 ratios in the synovial fluid in the majority of RA patients (13,21). In the synovial tissue there is a differential distribution of the T-cell subsets, with the CD4+ T cells primarily present in the lymphoid aggregates and the CD8+ T cells located in the diffuse lymphocyte infiltration (22). Analysis of the CD3/TCR–complex revealed downregulation of the CD3 antigen on synovial T cells, with an antigen expression per synovial T cell reduced by roughly one-third (17). Moreover, the CD4 antigen appears to be more moderately downregulated as well (23). These findings (Fig. 1) support the hypothesis that synovial T cells have been activated in vivo, presumably by antigen contact resulting in downregulation of molecules involved in antigen recognition. Analysis of RA synovial T cells has been extended to the expression of the CD29/CD45 antigens, showing that most of the intra-articular T cells with the helper/inducer CD4+ phenotype bear the CD29 as well as the CD45RO antigen (24,25) suggesting that these cells are of the memory type. With regard to expression of the CD29 molecule, its receptor function for tissue matrix components is of interest, which might indicate the involvement of CD29 in invasion and homing mechanisms of intra-articular T cells.

## Preferential Use of T-Cell Receptor Gene

The TCR recognizes a particular antigen in the context of an MHC allele. Most human T cells express $\alpha/\beta$ TCR, and a minority express the $\gamma/\delta$ TCR. Several groups have investigated the role of antigen-specific T cells in RA by searching for a restricted clonality by the assessment of the $\beta$-chain use. These studies, carried out by many investigators, have not convincingly demonstrated clonality or oligoclonality of intra-articular T cells. The results obtained were controversial. Repeated analyses of T cells obtained from the same joint at various time points did not show consistently rearranged TCR gene patterns, which suggested that the TCRs used by RA synovial T cells are heterogeneous (26). Recently, oligoclonality was found in a sample of synovial T cells with an overpresentation of the V$\beta$14 TCR gene, which was absent from peripheral blood T cells (27). This observation led to the hypothesis that, because Vβ14 is used in the immune response to bacterial superantigens, RA might be mediated/driven by such a mechanism (27). Another preliminary report indicted that freshly isolated T cells from inflamed joints primarily used the Vβ14 and Vδ1 families (28). The same group demonstrated that the T cells expressing the Vδ1 gene segment in the synovium were derived from a polyclonal expression (29). Pluschke et al. (30) and Bucht et al. (31) reported that T-cell subsets expressing certain Vα families are expanded in the inflamed synovium. Other investigators (32) showed a clonal dominance in RA and osteoathritic (OA) synovial membrane T cells but not in the peripheral blood cells. More recently, analysis of the total TCR-repertoire examined by generating "representative" T-cell clone panels which were subsequently tested for clonality by restriction mapping of the TCRβ gene locus did not reveal clonality in rather large TC clone panels generated from three patients with RA. In contrast, using in vivo preactivated, IL-2-responsive T cells, clonality of the T cell repertoire was found in two of four RA patients (33). In this study, analysis of clonal TCR of one RA patient showed that the TCRβ chain was composed of a Vβ5 family region, a novel D region, and Jβ1.2. The reason for this polyclonal overexpansion of T-cell subsets is unclear. One explanation could be the stimulation of T cells with certain HLA class II alleles plus antigen or stimulation with an (unidentified?) superantigen (34,35). Differences in study populations, probe selection, and techniques of cell handling before examination (e.g., expansion of cells with different stimuli, such as IL-2, anti-CD3, or mitogens) might account for the discrepancies in the above-mentioned data.

Despite the presence of an activated phenotype, a strikingly decreased responsiveness of intra-articular T cells in RA has been shown in global functional assays. Diminished mitogenic responsiveness, reduced production of IL-2 and interferon-γ on mitogen stimulation, and a decreased response in the mixed leukocyte reaction have been consistently observed (36,37). The report of a significantly reduced proliferative response of synovial T cells on stimulation with anti-CD3 monoclonal antibodies is in agreement with the decreased expression of the CD3 antigen in intra-articular T lymphocytes (17). Many experimental studies aiming at restoration of T-cell function have failed, including the addition of cytokines such as IL-1 or IL-2, the depletion of the CD8+ T-cell subset, or the co-incubation of synovial T cells with peripheral blood monocytes (17). Despite the reduced T-cell responsiveness of intraarticular T cells, co-cultivation of synovial T cells with peripheral T cells enhanced the response of the latter cell population (17). In addition, a helper augmentation effect of synovial T cells has been demonstrated, resulting in enhanced frequency of immunoglobulin-producing peripheral blood B cells (38).

## WHAT TRIGGERS T CELLS?

The hallmark of many inflammatory and degenerative joint diseases is the destruction of cartilage. Normally, cartilage is an immunologically privileged, sequestered tissue that has been shown to possess tissue-specific matrix and cell surface antigens (39). In RA the cartilage is invaded by aggressive tissue elements, ultimately leading to the complete destruction of joint structures. The reasons for the infiltration by the pannus tissue have not been elucidated. However, the presence of large numbers of activated T lymphocytes and macrophages in the surrounding synovial membrane (13, 23,40,41) strongly suggests an (auto?)antigen-driven process. Attempts to define the (auto?)antigen responsible for the induction of RA have initially focused on the investigation of collagen type II, which is almost exclusively expressed in cartilage, and the response to mycobacterial antigens, which have been proposed to initiate the autoantigenic immune response by a molecular mimicry-like mechanism. The latter idea has been supported by reports on T-cell lines and clones (e.g., A2b clone) reactive to *M. tuberculosis* that were strongly arthritogenic in a rat model of adjuvant arthritis (42). Cartilage proteoglycan was suggested to be the self-antigen responsible for this effect. By testing the A2b clone on antigens that could possibly serve as a target structure within the joints, it was found that in addition to mycobacteria, crude cartilage extracts, and proteoglycan proteins in particular, were also capable of stimulating the A2b clone (43). When a series of recombinant proteins or protein fragments of mycobacteria was used to further characterize the fine specificity of the arthritogenic rat T-cell clones, a response to a 65 kDa protein expressed in many microbacterial species was observed (4). This protein belongs to the 60 kDa family of heat shock proteins (HSP). In previous studies it had been shown that this 65 kDa protein comprises dominant epitopes recognized by a significant number of T cells, both in animals and in humans with antimycobacterial immune response (43). There was, however, no evidence that the clone A2b was arthritogenic due to the recognition of the rat HSP 65 itself (44). In patients with bacterial infections, antibodies against HSP 65 may easily dominate (45). Even in healthy human subjects, T-cell reactivity to HSP 65 can be found against epitopes shared between human and bacterial HSP 65 (46,47).

The immunodominant region recognized by generated synovial fluid T-cell clones (pulsed with fragments of the 65 kDa HSP) appears to be the amino terminus of the peptide fragments of the 65 kDa HSP (48). Additional observations appeared to indicate that the human T-cell response to the 65 kDa mycobacterial protein was related to inflammatory joint diseases. Responsiveness of synovial T cells to this antigen had been found in one-third of RA patients and in the majority of patients with other chronic inflammatory arthritis (49).

Investigations performed in our laboratory applying a panel of mycobacterial antigens, including particulate antigens of several mycobacterial species, purified protein derivative (PPD), and the recombinant 65 kDa protein, along with the nonmycobacterial protein antigen tetanus toxoid (TT), demonstrated a reduced proliferative response toward all antigens in blood T cells from RA patients compared to the non-RA group and to healthy donors. However, because of wide variations in the stimulation values, these differences did not reach statistical significance, with the exception of a lower response to *M. tuberculosis* in RA patients compared to the non-RA group. There was no peripheral blood T-cell reactivity to the 65 kDa protein in all patients with RA and in non-RA controls. However, there was a discrepancy between the cell responses obtained in blood and synovial T cells. In both patient groups, synovial T cells usually responded far more strongly to the antigens used compared to their counterparts from peripheral blood. Likewise, the 65 kDa protein induced marked responses in synovial T cells from four of eight RA patients and in three of four patients with non-RA diseases. Markedly elevated responses to TT were found in synovial T cells in half of the patients investigated (50).

The lower stimulation indices observed in our experiments in comparison with the initial studies by Res et al. (49) may be explained by the highly purified 65-kDa protein used in our study. In addition, the response of the synovial T cells of the most of the RA patients to several crude mycobacterial preparations, including the 65-kDa protein, the nonmycobacterial antigen TT and, more recently, spirochetal antigens and lipopolysaccharide (LPS), indicates an accumulation of T cells of the CD29/CD45RO memory type. This phenotyping analysis of synovial T cells responsive to mycobacterial antigens and tetanus toxoid was shown for the CD4 + /CD29 + phenotype and the remainder of a population of 5% expressing the CD45RA antigen, in contrast to only 60% CD29 + versus 45% CD45RA + in peripheral blood. The accumulation of T cells in the rheumatoid joints, with a predominance of CD4 + /CD29 + antigens, may be mediated by adhesion molecules present on the TC subsets and/or on the endothelial cells in the inflammatory lesions (15,23,52). In summary, our study and an additional study by Res et al. (51) following up their initial observations do not provide evidence that the 65 kDa protein or other mycobacterial antigens can stimulate T cells in RA or non-RA joint diseases with any preference. Therefore, the role of mycobacterial antigens as potential triggering elements in human chronic arthritis remains elusive.

Based on findings in other autoimmune diseases, such as thyroiditis and juvenile diabetes (53,54), chondrocytes, representing the cellular elements in cartilage tissue, have been proposed to be especially involved in autoimmune processes. This hypothesis is supported by the presence of HLA class II (Ia) antigens on chondrocytes, either ex vivo in RA (9) or induced by interferon-γ on normal human cartilage cells (17), as well as by the antigen-presenting capacity of rabbit or human chondrocytes (55,56). In mixed chondrocyte/leukocyte reactions, however, the antigenicity of autologous or allogeneic chondrocytes, either HLA class II antigen-negative or interferon-γ-treated HLA class II-positive chondrocytes, was rather weak (12,56). Therefore, in our own experiments, we studied the T-cell activation toward isolated chondrocyte membranes. Membrane vesicles were thought to be better targets as autoantigens after being processed by "professional" antigen-presenting cells in the inflamed synovium. The data obtained revealed that there was a striking TC reactivity toward chondrocyte membrane components in patients with RA, both in blood (Fig. 2) and in synovial tissue (Table 1), which was strongly dependent on the presence of monocytes (Table 2) and had all the characteristics of an antigen-driven response (11) The observed T-cell response toward chondrocyte membranes far exceeded the T-cell stimulation induced by membranes from other sources, such as fibroblasts or epithelial cells, as well as by other cartilage components, including collagen type II (11). Clonal analysis demonstrated a high precursor frequency of blood T cells reactive to chondrocyte membranes in patients with RA.

Figure 2 shows that there was a significantly increased stimulatory response to chondrocyte membranes in approximately 50% of RA patients, where there was no or only marginal reactivity toward membranes from other sources. Normal donor cells usually were not stimulated by either membrane preparation. The difference in reactivity toward chondrocyte membrane preparations between patients and normal donors was significant at the level of $p < 0.02$ (Fig. 2). The highest T-cell proliferation was measured with human adult chondrocyte membranes, whereas human infant and fetal chondrocyte membranes were less effective in enhancing T-cell proliferation (Table 1). Xenogenic membranes from chicken chondrocytes strongly stimulated T-cell proliferation. The data obtained indicate that the pattern of reactivity differs from individual to individual; some patients showed similar responses to all preparations, and others reacted preferentially to membranes obtained from human and chicken sources (11,12).

Additional evidence for the hypothesis that chondrocytes might be involved in immunologic reactions within the joint has recently been provided by the demonstration of autoantibodies against chondrocyte surface membrane antigens in patients with destructive joint diseases (12,57). Patients with RA and OA had significant titers of antichondrocyte membrane antibodies as measured by ELISA. The autoantibodies recognized a number of antigens that could be visualized by electrophoretic separation and subsequent blotting of sucrose density-gradient–enriched membrane proteins (Fig. 3). Table 3 lists polypeptides frequently recognized by RA sera. These reactions were absent when membranes prepared from human fibroblasts or from epithelial tumor cells were applied, whereas antibody response was highly crossreactive against cartilage cell membranes derived from other species. The initial immunologic and biochemical analysis of the RA 65 kDa polypeptide (CH65) isolated from chondrocyte membranes, which is the

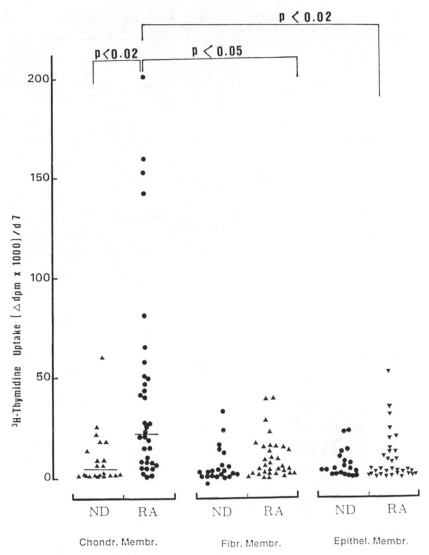

**FIG. 2.** Response of peripheral blood mononuclear cells toward isolated membranes from various cell types as determined by [³H]thymidine uptake after 7 to 9 days of culture. There was a significantly higher T cell proliferation toward chondrocyte membranes ($p < 0.02$) in patients with RA compared to normal donors (ND). In addition, chondrocyte membranes induced a significantly higher stimulatory response than fibroblast ($p < 0.05$) or epithelial ($p < 0.02$) cell material.

**TABLE 1.** *Effect of monocytes on the response of T cells from peripheral blood of RA patients toward chondrocyte membrane preparations[a]*

| Experiment | Subject | T cells | Mono-cytes | T cells + chondrocyte membranes | T cells + mono-cytes | T cells + monocytes + chondrocyte membranes |
|---|---|---|---|---|---|---|
| 1 | Normal donor | 1,889 | ND | 3,918 | 4,917 | 6,444 |
| 2 | RA | 5,979 | 989 | 7,333 | 8,889 | 28,091 |
| 3 | RA | 3,875 | 2,103 | 6,298 | 8,219 | 70,121 |

[a] Values are the difference in [$^3$H]thymidine uptake ($\Delta$dpm) in samples containing antigen minus that in controls. T cells were used at a concentration of $1 \times 10^5$/well, monocytes at $5 \times 10^3$/well. Chondrocyte membranes were used at a final concentration of 14 $\mu$g/ml. ND, not done.

**TABLE 2.** *Reactivity of T cells from rheumatoid synovial tissue toward various cell membrane constituents*

| Patient | Cell source | PaTull | HFF | SFB | Human cell membranes Adult ch. | Fetal ch. | Infant ch. |
|---|---|---|---|---|---|---|---|
| RA 1 | ST | 4.340[a] | 6.445 | 15.053 | 39.703 | 8.749 | 15.280 |
| RA 2 | ST | 0.844 | 1.315 | 8.999 | 35.165 | 5.784 | 6.053 |
| RA 3 | ST | 3.205 | 8.639 | ND | 13.914 | ND | ND |

[a] [$^3$H]thymidine incorporation ($\Delta$dpm).
ch, chondrocytes; HFF, foreskin fibroblasts; SFB, synovial fibroblasts; PaTull, epithelial pancreatic tumor cell line; ST, rheumatoid synovial tissue; ND, not done.

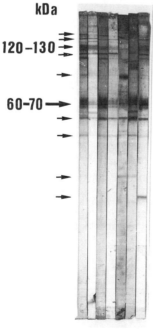

kDa

120–130

60–70

RA  1 2 3 4 5 6 7

**FIG. 3.** SDS-PAGE (10% gel) analysis of chondrocyte membranes with a subsequent immunoblotting procedure using sera obtained from typical RA patients (1 to 7). The RA sera preferentially recognized the 60–70 kDa protein. The high molecular weight areas, probably represent cell surface-attached polypeptides from the extracellular matrix (see Table 3).

**TABLE 3.** *Polypeptides from chondrocyte membrane preparations (source chicken) recognized by RA sera in immunoblotting[a]*

| Molecular weight (kDa) | RA sera ($n = 10$) | ND sera ($n = 10$) |
|:---:|:---:|:---:|
| 150 | + | − |
| 135 | + | (+) |
| 120 | + | − |
| 115 | + | − |
| 95 | + | − |
| 76 | + | − |
| 60–70 | + | − |
| 50 | + | − |
| 45 | + | − |
| 30 | + | − |

[a] Dilution of sera 1:100; the bands in the high molecular weight range probably represent cell surface-attached polypeptides from the extracellular matrix, such as collagens. ND, normal donor; RA, rheumatoid arthritis.

most commonly recognized antigen by immunoblotting with RA sera, excluded an identity between heat shock protein 60–65 from *M. tuberculosis* or *M. butyricum* and CH65. Sera from patients with RA exhibited a differential reaction pattern to HSP 60–65 and CH65, which suggested a significant immunologic and probably a structural difference between the two polypeptides (12). The amino acid composition and structure of CH65 should clarify these differences. In any case, these finding indicate that there is a strong cellular and humoral reactivity toward chondrocyte membrane components in RA that may significantly contribute to the pathogenic processes that lead to cartilage destruction. Moreover, chondrocytes not only may be targets of the immune response, but may also act as antigen-presenting cells for possible cell surface antigens (55,56).

Cartilage proteoglycans are found within the extracellular matrix in the form of multimolecular aggregates associated with a network of collagen fibrils. It has been suggested that autoimmunity to cartilage proteoglycan components plays a role in the etiology of arthritis, particularly in animal models. Intraperitoneal injection of human fetal cartilage proteoglycans (depleted of chondroitin sulfate) in Freund's complete or incomplete adjuvant induced a chronic erosive polyarthritis and spondylitis in all female BALB/C mice (58). This occurrence was strain-specific but not haplotype-specific and was sex-related. Development of arthritis was associated with the presence of cellular immunity to the immunizing antigen and to chondroitinase ABC-related mouse cartilage proteoglycans (59). Interestingly, associated with the arthritis was the development of cytotoxicity to human and mouse chondrocytes in the presence of complement. In arthritis rabbits, a preferentially humoral immune reactivity was observed in the majority of sera against hyaluronic acid and/or chondroitin sulfate bound to the core protein (60).

Spleen cells from arthritic rabbits responded to both native and degraded proteoglycans. These in vitro blastogenic responses were completely dependent on the presence of T lymphocytes in the cultures. Some rabbits injected with homologous human proteoglycans developed both cellular and humoral immunity to the immunizing proteoglycans but failed to mount a cellular immunity to rabbit. The induction of immunity to proteoglycans was not accompanied by any demonstrable synovitis in these rabbits. A strongly arthritogenic T-cell clone (A2b) specific for *M. tuberculosis* antigens in adjuvant arthritis in rats also recognized antigens present in proteoglycans purified from cartilage, human synovial fluid, and the medium from chondrocyte cultures, as mentioned above, indicating that target epitopes for the TC clone may be present in proteoglycan components of cartilage. The development of this arthritis was accompanied by the expression of cell-mediated and humoral immunity to the immunizing antigen. Intravenous injections of proteoglycans synergized with CFA in the induction of adjuvant arthritis in rats and induced both humoral and cellular reactivity to proteoglycan, whereas immunity induced by proteoglycan alone was not sufficient for the induction of arthritis. Rats immunized with proteoglycan had high titers of anti-proteoglycan and a strong delayed-type hypersensitivity to proteoglycans, which was also enhanced by pretreatment with PGs intravenously, although none of these animals developed arthritis (61).

In human patients with RA or OA, peripheral blood lymphocytes did not exhibit a significant proliferative response to homologous cartilage proteoglycan (62). Furthermore, both the autologous and the heterologous peripheral blood lymphocyte proliferation in patients with RA, OA, and ankylosing spondylitis were unaltered by the addition of cartilage fragments and purified bovine articular proteoglycans (63). Analysis of arthritic articular cartilage proteoglycans failed to demonstrate the presence of antigen(s) stimulating peripheral blood lymphocytes. With regard to the minimal response, it has been suggested that serum antibodies to the proteoglycan link protein may be more common in patients with rheumatic diseases than in healthy controls. However, antibodies against highly purified cartilage link protein were found in the sera of only approximately 25% of patients with RA. There were no significant differences between the nonarthritic control population and the RA patient group with regard to either prevalence or the mean titer of anti-link protein antibodies (64). In contrast to chondroitinase-digested proteoglycans, it is likely that the putative arthritogenic protein epitopes on PGs are sterically masked or are expressed as new determinants after modification of the tertiary structure of the core protein by the removal of the negatively charged chondroitin sulfate side chains. In human subjects proteoglycans have not been shown conclusively to induce a marked humoral or cellular immunity.

## CYTOKINES IN RHEUMATOID SYNOVITIS PRODUCED BY T LYMPHOCYTES

Cytokines are soluble hormone-like factors that act as local and systemic signals. They are produced primarily by immune cells, enabling intercellular communication between cells and modulation of the local environment. In RA, cytokines and growth factors have been implicated in a variety of events including activation and proliferation of synoviocytes, recruitment of cells into the joint cavity, such as lymphocytes and monocytes, and the degradation of the cartilage and bone matrices. The cytokines produced exclusively by T lymphocytes are IL-2, IL-3, IL-4, IL-5, IL-6, interferon-$\gamma$ and GM-CSF, IL-10 and other peptides. By using sensitive and specific immunoassays to identify cytokines in RA synovial fluids, IL-2 and interferon-$\gamma$ could be detected at low levels (65). In contrast, factors secreted by articular fibroblasts, chondrocytes, and macrophages, such as IL-1, IL-6, GM-CSF, and TNF-$\alpha$, transforming growth factor-$\beta$ (TGF-$\beta$) and basic fibroblast growth factor (bFGF) were abundant in synovial fluids (2,66–69). Specific detection of cytokines is difficult, and caution must be used in interpreting immunoassays of synovial fluids because of false-positive results due to rheumatoid factors (unpublished observation). In such situations it is useful to combine protein and mRNA studies.

In the case of IL-2, in contrast to early studies indicating IL-2 activity in synovial fluids, previous reports (70) have indicated the presence of IL-2 mRNA without detectable secreted protein. IL-4 mRNA and protein could not be detected in synovial fluids, synovium supernatants, or the synovium itself, even by PCR (71). Interferon-$\gamma$ is another T-cell cytokine that was detected at low levels in the rheumatoid joints (2). It downregulates the stimulatory effects of other cytokines. For example, interferon-$\gamma$ blocks IL-1$\beta$-induced synoviocyte proliferation, prostaglandin E$_2$ production, and collagenase synthesis (72). Moreover, interferon-$\gamma$ blocked TNF-$\alpha$-mediated proliferation, collagenase production, and GM-CSF synthesis, whereas TNF-$\alpha$ inhibited the induction of HLA-DR expression mediated by interferon-$\gamma$ (73). The detectable low levels of T-cell cytokines may be explained by specific regulatory functions in low concentrations. Interferon-$\gamma$ strongly increases the production of proinflammatory cytokines such as IL-1, TNF-$\alpha$, and IL-6 by monocytes/macrophages, which could be inhibited by IL-4 and IL-10. Interferon-$\gamma$ induced the expression of HLA class II antigens (HLA-DR, $-$DP, and partially $-$DQ) on macrophages and mesenchymal cells, including synovial fibroblast-like cells and chondrocytes (73,74). It is not clear whether the expression of such molecules is important for the local immune reactions by improving the antigen-presenting capacity of such cells or in the control of mesenchymal tissue metabolism under inflammatory conditions. Interleukin-6, a 23- to 28-kDa protein, induces the synthesis of acute-phase proteins in hepatocytes (76). In addition, IL-6 stimulates immunoglobulin production by B lymphocytes. IL-1, TNF-$\alpha$, and lipopolysaccharide (endotoxin) induce the synthesis of IL-6 by monocytes and fibroblasts (77). However, IL-6 was not able to induce prostaglandin E$_2$ release and collagenase production in chondrocytes and synovial fibroblasts (78; and our unpublished data). In vitro, IL-6 inhibited IL-1–induced prostaglandin E$_2$ secretion (79). The exact role of IL-6 in the inflamed joint is unknown. It is possible that IL-6 modulates and reduces the biologic effects of the proinflammatory cytokines IL-1 and TNF-α. Furthermore, it might be involved in the induction of acute-phase protein synthesis and the local production of rheumatoid factors. GM-CSF is a predominant growth factor produced by various cell types, including activated T lymphocytes. GM-CSF potentiated the HLA-DR expression by synovial macrophages and fibroblasts, stimulated IL-1 production and activated neutrophilic granulocytes and monocytes (80–84). GM-CSF and monocyte-CSF (M-CSF) stimulated in vitro the resorption of bone (85). This effect might be mediated via the generation of osteoclasts, as it is known that growth factors stimulate the growth of osteoclast-like cells in culture (85).

The imbalance in the equilibrium of the cytokine network represents the combination of increased destruction and reduced repair activity in RA synovium. The excessive production of proinflammatory cytokines induced by abnormal control of T cells, associated with an inadequate inhibition of their actions, results in the breakdown of cartilage. Control of the cytokine network in rheumatoid joints is rather complex, as cytokine inhibitors and neutralizing antibodies against abundantly produced inflammatory cytokines and soluble receptors are also present in intra-articular sites.

## SUMMARY AND CONCLUSION

Undoubtedly, synovitis is a cell-mediated process involving various cell types, such as T cells, B cells, APC, monocytes/macrophages, synoviocytes, chondrocytes, and cytokines. Therefore, it is difficult to clarify the cell type that plays the central role in the inflammatory process. Despite this difficulty, there is strong evidence that T cells mediate the disease in collaboration with APC that bear specific antigenic peptides. The mediators released could perpetuate an ongoing inflammatory process in the joints irrespective of the nature of the initiating agents. Therefore, many approaches to a more specific immunotherapy for RA have been developed, directed toward the modulation of T cell function. Thus far, various forms of chemical and biologic treatment have been used, such as cyclosporin A and monoclonal antibodies directed against T-cell epitopes and IL-2 receptor, with some beneficial effects on the course of RA. The development of a more specific immunotherapy using reagents directed against the T-cell receptor and vaccination with specific T cells await further studies, since we still do not know the inciting antigen(s) in RA. Nevertheless, we are hopeful that the ongoing search for the still unknown antigen(s) will be successful, thus providing new and better treatment regimens for a still uncurable disease.

## ACKNOWLEDGMENT

This work was supported by the Deutsche Forschungsgemeinschaft, Sonderforschungsbereich SFB 263.

# REFERENCES

1. Zvaifler NJ. In: Schumacher R, Klippel JH, Robinson DR, eds. *Primer on the rheumatic diseases*. Atlanta: Arthritis Foundation;1988:83–7.
2. Firestein GS. In: McCarty DJ, ed. *Current opinion in rheumatology*. Philadelphia: Current Science;1991:398–406.
3. Holoshitz J, Naparstek Y, Ben-Nun A, Cohen IR. *Science* 1983;219:56–8.
4. Waalen K, Førre Ø, Linker-Israeli M, Thoen J. *Scand J Immunol* 1987;25:367–73.
5. Holoshitz J, Matitiau A, Cohen IR. *J Clin Invest* 1984;73:211–5.
6. Tugwell P, Bombardier C, Gent M, et al. *Lancet* 1990;335:1051–5.
7. Ranges GE, Sriram S, Cooper SM. *J Exp Med* 1985;162:1105–10.
8. Horneff G, Burmester GR, Emmrich F, Kalden JR. *Arthritis Rheum* 1991;34:129–40.
9. Burmester GR, Bona AD, Waters SJ, Winchester RJ. *Scand J Immunol* 1983;17:69–82.
10. Burmester GR, Menche D, Merryman P, Klein M, Winchester RJ. *Arthritis Rheum* 1983; 26:1187–95.
11. Alsalameh S, Mollenhauer J, Hain N, Kalden JR, Burmester GR. *Arthritis Rheum* 1990; 33:1477–86.
12. Burmester GR, Alsalameh S, Mollenhauer J. In: Smolen JS, Kalden JR, Maini RN, eds. *Rheumatoid arthritis: recent research advances*. Berlin: Springer-Verlag; 1992:91–111.
13. Burmester GR, Yu DTY, Irani AM, Kunkel HG, Winchester RJ. *Arthritis Rheum* 1981; 24:1370–6.
14. Potocnik AJ, Menninger H, Yang SY, et al. *Scand J Immunol* 1991;34:351–8.
15. Hemler ME, Glass D, Coblyn JS, Jacobson JG. *J Clin Invest* 1986;78:696–704.
16. Burmester GR, Jahn B, Gramatzki M, Zacher J, Kalden JR. *J Immunol* 1984;133:1230–4.
17. Jahn B, Burmester GR, Gramatzki M, Stock P, Kalden JR. *Scand J Immunol* 1987;26:745–54.
18. Pitzalis C, Kingsley GH, Lauchbury JSS, Murphy J, Panayi GS. *J Rheumatol* 1987;14:662–6.
19. Hain N, Alsalameh S, Bertling WM, Kalden JR, Burmester GR. *Rheumatol Int* 1991;10:203–10.
20. Firestein GS, Xu WD, Townsend K, et al. *J Exp Med* 1988;168:1573–86.
21. Duclos M, Zeidler H, Liman W, Peter HH. *Rheumatol Int* 1982;2:75–82.
22. Kurosaka M, Ziff M. *J Exp Med* 1983;158:1191–1200.
23. Cush JJ, Lipsky PE. *Arthritis Rheum* 1988;31:1230–8.
24. Kingsley G, Pitzalis C, Kyriazis N, Panayi GS. *Scand J Immunol* 1988;225–32.
25. Lasky HP, Bauer K, Pope RM. *Arthritis Rheum* 1988;31:52–9.
26. Cush JJ, Duby AD, Lightfoot E, Lipsky PE. *Arthritis Rheum* 1990;33:S37.
27. Paliard X, West SG, Lafferty JA, et al. *Science* 1991;253:325–9.
28. Sioud M, Kjeldsen-Kragh J, Quayle A, et al. *Scand J Immunol* 1990;31:415–20.
29. Sioud M, Førre Ø, Natvig JB. *Eur J Immunol* 1991;21:239–41.
30. Pluschke G, Ricken G, Taube H, et al. *Eur J Immunol* 1991;21:2749–54.
31. Bucht A, Oksenberg JR, Lindblad S, Gronberg A, Steinman L, Klareskog L. *Scand J Immunol* 1992;35:159–65.
32. Stamenkovic I, Stegagno M, Wright KA, et al. *Proc Natl Acad Sci USA* 1988;85:1179–83.
33. Broker BM, Korthäuer U, Heppt P, et al. *Arthritis Rheum* 1993;36:1234–43.
34. Kronenberg M. *Cell* 1989;65:357–42.
35. Friedmann SM, Posnett DN, Tumang JR, Cole BC, Crow MK. *Arthritis Rheum* 1991;34:468–80.
36. Burmester GR, Kalden JR, Peter HH, Schedel I, Beck P, Wittenborg A. *Scand J Immunol* 1978;7:405–17.
37. Seitz M, Napiersky J, Augustin R, Hunstein W, Kirchner H. *Scand J Immunol* 1987;16:262–75.
38. Romain PL, Burmester GR, Enlow RW, Winchester RJ. *Rheumatol Int* 1982;2:121–7.
39. Glant T, Mikecz K. *Cell Tissue Res* 1986;244:359–69.
40. Burmester GR, Dimitru-Bona A, Waters SJ, Winchester RJ. *Scand J Immunol* 1983:17:69–82.
41. Janossy G, Panayi G, Duke O, Bofill M, Poulter LW, Goldstein G. *Lancet* 1981;2:839–42.
42. van Eden W, Thole JER, van der Zee, et al. *Nature* 1988;331:171–3.
43. van Eden W, Holoshitz J, Nevo Z, Frenkel A, Klajman A, Cohen IR. *Proc Natl Acad Sci USA* 1985;82:5064–7.

44. van Eden W, Boog CJP, Hogervorst EJM, Wauben MHM, van der Zee R, van Embden JDA. In: Smolen JS, Kalden JR, Maini RN, eds. *Rheumatoid arthritis: recent research advances.* Berlin: Springer-Verlag; 1992:167–79.
45. Kaufmann SHE. *Immunol Today* 1990;11:129–36.
46. Munk ME, Schoel B, Modrow S, Karr RW, Young RA, Kaufmann SHE. *J Immunol* 1989;143:2844–9.
47. Lamb JR, Bal V, Mendez-Samperio P, et al. *Int Immunol* 1989;1:191–6.
48. Gatson JSH, Life PF, Jenner PJ, Colston MJ, Bacon PA. *J Exp Med* 1990;171:831–41.
49. Res PC, Scharr CG, Breedveld FC, et al. *Lancet* 1988;1:478–80.
50. Burmester GR, Altstidl U, Kalden JR, Emmrich F. *J Rheumatol* 1991;18:171–6.
51. Res PC, Telgt D, van Laar JM, Ouderk Pool M, Breedveld FC, de Vries RRP. *Lancet* 1990;336:1406–8.
52. Hale LP, Martin ME, McCollum DE, et al. *Arthritis Rheum* 1989;32:22–30.
53. Hanafusa T, Pujol-Borell R, Chiovato L, Russel RGG, Doinach D, Bottazzo GF. *Lancet* 1983;2:1111–5.
54. Bottazzo GF, Path MRF, Dean BM, et al. *N Engl J Med* 1985;313:353–60.
55. Tiku ML, Lui S, Weaver CW, Teodorescu M, Shosey IL. *J Immunol* 1985;135:2923–8.
56. Alsalameh S, Jahn B, Krause A, Kalden JR, Burmester GR. *J Rheumatol* 1991;18:414–21.
57. Mollenhauer J, von der Mark K, Burmester GF, Glückert K, Lütjen-Drecoll E, Brune K. *J Rheumatol* 1988;15:1811–7.
58. Mikecz K, Glant TT, Poole AR. *Arthritis Rheum* 1987;30:306–18.
59. Glant TT, Mikecz K, Arzoumanian A, Poole AR. *Arthritis Rheum* 1987;30:201–12.
60. Poole AR, Reiner A, Roughley PJ, Champion B. *J Biol Chem* 1985;260:6020–5.
61. Van Vollenhofen RF, Soriano A, MacCarthy PE, et al. *J Immunol* 1988;141:1168–73.
62. Golds EE, Stephan IB, Esdaile JM, Strawczynski H, Poole AR. *Cell Immunol* 1983;82:196–209.
63. Schurman DJ, Palathumpat MW, DeSilva A, Kajiyama G, Smith RL. *J Orthop Res* 1986;4:255–62.
64. Austin AK, Hobbs RN, Anderson JC, Butler RC, Ashton BA. *Ann Rheum Dis* 1988;47:886–92.
65. Miossec P, Naviliat M, Dupuy D'Angeac A, Sany J, Banchereau J. *Arthritis Rheum* 1990;145:2514–9.
66. Alsalameh S, Firestein GS, Oez S, Kurrle R, Kalden JR, Burmester GR. *J Rheumatol* 1994;21:993–1002.
67. Miossec P. In: Emery P, ed. *Bailliere's clinical rheumatology. International practice and research,* Vol. 6. London: Baillire Tindall; 1992:373–92.
68. Fava R, Olsen N, Keski-Oja J, Moses H, Pincas T. *J Exp Med* 1989;169:291–6.
69. Alsalameh S, Kalden JR, Burmester GR. *Z Rheumatol* 1991;50:347–59.
70. Brennan FM, Field M, Chu CQ, Feldman M, Maini RN. *Br J Rheumatol* 1991;30:76–80.
71. Miossec P, Naviliat M, Dupuy d'Angeac A, Sany J, Banchereau J. *Arthritis Rheum* 1990;33:1180–7.
72. Nakajima H, Hiyama Y, Tsukada W, Warabi H, Uchida S, Hirose S. *Ann Rheum Dis* 1990;49:312–6.
73. Alvaro-Gracia JM, Zvaifler NJ, Firestein GS. *J Clin Invest* 1990;86:1790–8.
74. Amento EP, Bhan AK, McCullough KG, Krane SM. *J Clin Invest* 1985;76:837–48.
75. Jahn B, Burmester GR, Schmid H, Weseloh G, Rohwer P, Kalden JR. *Arthritis Rheum* 1987;30:64–74.
76. Gauldie J, Richards C, Hamish D, Baumann J. *J Leukocyte Biol* 1987;42:554–60.
77. Kohase M, Henriksen-DeStefano P, May LT, Vilcek J, Sehgal PB. *Cell* 1986;45:659–66.
78. Guerne P-A, Zuraw BL, Vaughan JH, Carson DA, Lotz M. *J Clin Invest* 1989;83:585–92.
79. Arend WP, Dayer J-M. *Arthritis Rheum* 1990;33:305–15.
80. Weisbart SC, Golde DW, Clark SC, Wong GG, Gasson JC. *Nature* 1985;314:361–3.
81. Gasson JC, Weisbart RH, Kaufman SE, et al. *Science* 1984;226:1339–42.
82. Wang M, Friedman H, Djeu JY. *J Immunol* 1989;143:671–5.
83. Wang JM, Colella S, Ailavena P, Mantoviani A. *Immunology* 1987;60:469–75.
84. Fischer H-G, Frosch S, Reske K, Reske-Kunz AB. *J Immunol* 1988;141:3882–7.
85. MacDonald BR, Mundy GR, Clark S, et al. *J Bone Miner Res* 1986;1:227–38.

Advances in Prostaglandin, Thromboxane,
and Leukotriene Research, Vol. 22, edited by
S.-E. Dahlén et al. Raven Press, Ltd., New York © 1994

# Summary: Allergic Rhinitis and Rheumatoid Arthritis

Marc E. Goldyne and *Dwight R. Robinson

Medicine and Dermatology Department, University of California, Veterans Affairs
Medical Center, San Francisco, California 94121; and *Arthritis Unit,
Massachusetts General Hospital, Boston, Massachusetts 02114

This section focused on two immunologic diseases: allergic rhinitis and rheumatoid arthritis. Allergic rhinitis involves a relatively localized immediate hypersensitivity reaction primarily mediated by the mast cell. Rheumatoid arthritis presents with chronic synovial inflammation accompanied by a variable degree of systemic manifestations and is mediated primarily by lymphocytes and monocytes.

In the context of leukotrienes and their potential for producing some of the symptoms associated with immunologic diseases, Drs. Kaliner and Knapp provided compelling evidence for the contribution of leukotrienes to the symptoms of allergic rhinitis. The mast cell, which is believed to be essential to the pathogenesis of allergic rhinitis, is a documented source of sulfidopeptide leukotrienes. While recognizing the plurality of mediators that can be recovered after the initiation of allergic rhinitis, Dr. Kaliner reviewed data that cast mast-cell–derived histamine as the central agonist. This mediator directly or indirectly can produce the acute symptoms of itching, sneezing, and increased nasal secretions (rhinorrhea) that are the hallmark of this disease. Furthermore, these symptoms can be largely reversed by therapy with $H_1$ antagonists.

However, as Dr. Knapp noted, the late-phase congestion that characterizes allergic rhinitis is not as responsive to $H_1$ antagonists as are the acute symptoms, and it is the late-phase reaction that seems to be generated by nonhistamine mediators released by the mast cell. In nasal allergy, leukotrienes are present during the late phase of the allergic response, and leukotriene $D_4$ derived from mast cells is capable of inducing congestion without the itching or sneezing characteristic of histamine challenge. Dr. Knapp's investigations demonstrate that inhibiting leukotriene synthesis alleviates the symptoms of allergic rhinitis.

Evidence for the involvement of leukotrienes in other chronic inflammatory diseases, including inflammatory bowel disease and rheumatoid arthritis, is at present inconclusive. In rheumatoid arthritis, measurements of the levels of leukotrienes in synovial tissues are unconvincing, and the effects of leukotriene inhibitors on the course of this disease have not been reported in detail. Drs. Alsalameh, Burmester, and Kalden reviewed current concepts of the pathogenesis of rheumatoid arthritis and conclude, as do many investigators, that the T cell plays a central role. Synovial tissue histology resembles that of a delayed hypersensitivity reaction, with infiltration of large numbers of both CD4 and CD8 types of T cells. In addition, large numbers of B cells and plasma cells, which produce immunoglobulins including the autoantibody rheumatoid factor, are present. Hyperplasia of the synovial lining cells, prominent infiltration of monocyte/macrophages, neovascularization and fibroblast proliferation, and mast cells are prominent features. Neutrophils are characteristically absent from the synovial tissue, although these cells are the dominant cell type in the surrounding synovial fluid. Therefore, several cell types that are potential sources of leukotrienes and other eicosanoids are present in rheumatoid joints.

Dr. Alsalameh et al. discuss the important topic of the pathogenesis of this synovial pathology. Although the pathology resembles an intense delayed hypersensitivity reaction, the antigen(s) toward which this reaction is directed remains elusive. The T-cell phenotype suggests that these cells have previously undergone activation, and T-cell–generated lymphokines are not prominent. On the other hand, macrophage activation appears prominent, and macrophage-generated cytokines, including IL-1, TNF-$\alpha$, and IL-6, are present in synovial tissues. The strong association of rheumatoid arthritis with major histocompatibility complex class II alleles, such as DR4 epitopes, implies that antigen-driven reactions of T4 cells are important, and the prominence of CD4-positive T cells in rheumatoid synovial tissue supports this concept. Yet the antigens responsible for this T-cell–mediated response have not been identified. Evidence for oligoclonality of the synovial T cells exists, but the results of other studies are conflicting. Although many investigators have postulated that the rheumatoid lesion is a response to an infectious etiologic agent, exhaustive searches for such agents have been negative. Alsalameh et al. noted that in established rheumatoid arthritis the initiating agent may be replaced by previously hidden epitopes on joint tissues, such as type II collagen, articular cartilage proteoglycans, or heat shock proteins. In any event, the postulated importance of the $T_4$ lymphocyte in rheumatoid synovial pathology has directed therapeutic efforts toward suppressing or eliminating these cells in rheumatoid patients. Yet inhibition of inflammatory mediators of the effector limb of the immune response, such as the eicosanoids, may be useful, as typified by the nonsteroidal anti-inflammatory drugs.

The chapters in this section provide support for leukotrienes as pivotal mediators, along with histamine, in allergic rhinitis, and although their role in rheumatoid arthritis is less well defined, the leukotrienes also are likely to contribute to the expression of this disease. Further studies of the therapeutic effects of leukotriene inhibitors in both allergic rhinitis and rheumatoid arthritis are eagerly anticipated.

# 6. Lipoxygenase Products and Cytokine Regulation

Advances in Prostaglandin, Thromboxane,
and Leukotriene Research, Vol. 22, edited by
S.-E. Dahlén et al. Raven Press, Ltd., New York © 1994

# Human 15-Lipoxygenase: A Potential Effector Molecule for Interleukin-4

Elliott Sigal and *Douglas J. Conrad

*Syntex Discovery Research, Palo Alto, California 94304; and *Cardiovascular
Research Institute and Department of Medicine, University of California,
San Francisco, California 94143-0911*

Lipoxygenases are lipid-peroxidating enzymes implicated in the pathogenesis of a variety of inflammatory disorders (1). The 5-lipoxygenase catalyzes the first step in the biosynthesis of the potent inflammatory mediators, leukotrienes (1,2). 12- and 15-lipoxygenases are involved in the biosynthesis of other bioactive metabolites from free arachidonic acid, such as lipoxins (1). However, 15-lipoxygenase is unique among the human lipoxygenases in that it is capable of oxygenating polyenoic fatty acids esterified to membrane lipids (3) or lipoproteins, and hence it may have biologic roles distinct from its action on free arachidonic acid.

Our approach to studying the biology of human 15-lipoxygenase has been to isolate and characterize a cDNA encoding the enzyme (4,5) which, in combination with antibodies generated from the resulting expression systems, has been useful in studying tissue-specific expression in health and disease (6,7). For example, 15-lipoxygenase is expressed preferentially in the epithelial cells of human airway (6). This strategic location suggests a role in the inflammatory responses to external stimuli. Perhaps more revealing, however, is the finding that in human and rabbit atherosclerotic lesions, 15-lipoxygenase is expressed in the same location as oxidized low-density lipoprotein (LDL) (8,9). This appears relevant to the pathogenesis of atherosclerosis, in that oxidation of LDL is believed to be an essential step in foam cell formation. Furthermore, oxidized LDL exhibits many atherogenic properties in vitro.

Because 15-lipoxygenase is expressed in macrophages of human atherosclerotic lesions but not in the precursor cell, the monocyte, nor related cells such as alveolar macrophages (7,10), we searched for relevant molecules that may account for this disease-specific induction of the enzyme. Recent evidence implicates cytokines in the cellular response seen in atherosclerosis (11). We therefore examined the effect on 15-lipoxygenase expression of different cytokines produced by cells present in atherosclerotic lesions. We summarize here the studies that have identified interleukin-4 (IL-4) and interferon-$\gamma$ ($\gamma$IFN) as cytokines that potently and specifically regulate the expression of human monocyte 15-lipoxygenase. This work has been extended to airway cells and hence may have relevance to asthma. We describe a scheme that places 15-lipoxygenase in a biologic role as an effector molecule for interleukin-4 in human airway.

## MATERIALS AND METHODS

Methods for monocyte purification and culture, immunofluorescence, and RNA blots are described by Conrad et al. (12). Methods for enzymatic assays, high-pressure liquid chromatography (HPLC), and immunoblots are described by Sigal et al. (5). Methods for culturing airway epithelial cells are described by Yamaya et al. (13).

## RESULTS

We selected cytokines that were relevant to atherogenesis and monocyte/macrophage function and then incubated human monocytes (greater than 90% pure) with these cytokines for 3 days. We screened for specific immu-

**TABLE 1.** *Regulation of monocyte 15-lipoxygenase expression*[a]

| Cytokine | | Immunofluorescence | |
|---|---|---|---|
| | | Cytokine alone | With IL-4 (700 p$M$) |
| IL-1$\alpha$ | (130 p$M$) | − | + |
| IL-1$\beta$ | (110 p$M$) | − | + |
| IL-2 | (2.5 n$M$) | − | + |
| IL-3 | (1000 U/ml) | − | + |
| IL-4 | (60 p$M$) | + | |
| IL-5 | (200 p$M$) | − | + |
| IL-6 | (1000 U/ml) | − | + |
| IL-8 | (100 U/ml) | − | + |
| $\gamma$IFN | (100 p$M$) | − | − |
| GM-CSF | (30 U/ml) | − | + |
| M-CSF | (100 U/ml) | − | + |
| PDGF-BB | (3.5 n$M$) | − | + |
| TNF-$\alpha$ | (100 n$M$) | − | + |
| TGF-$\beta_1$ | (100 p$M$) | − | + |
| Oxidized LDL | (10 $\mu$g/ml) | − | + |
| PMA | (50 n$M$) | − | − |
| Hydrocortisone | (100 n$M$) | − | − |

[a] Regulation of monocyte 15-lipoxygenase by specific cytokines, oxidized low-density lipoprotein (LDL), phorbol myristate acetate (PMA), and hydrocortisone. Monocytes were cultured for 3 days and stimulated by each factor listed either alone (left column) or with interleukin-4 (right column). The doses were selected for their ability to induce relevant biologic effects in other cell systems. Cultures were assessed by indirect immunofluorescence. The results summarize at least two independent cultures per factor. (From ref. 12 with permission.)

nofluorescence using an antibody to human recombinant 15-lipoxygenase (Table 1). Monocytes cultured with IL-4 for 3 days reproducibly exhibited specific immunofluorescence, whereas freshly isolated monocytes and monocytes cultured without IL-4 exhibited no fluorescence. Dose–response studies indicated that 15-lipoxygenase was induced by IL-4 concentrations as low as 70 p$M$. Immunofluorescence was near maximal at 700 p$M$. Time course experiments revealed that 15-lipoxygenase immunofluorescence could be detected after 12 hr and was near maximal at 2 days of culture.

The IL-4 induction of 15-lipoxygenase was specific among 17 factors tested, including 14 cytokines, $Cu^{2+}$-oxidized low-density lipoprotein (LDL), hydrocortisone, and phorbol myristate acetate (PMA) (Table 1). This specificity was also demonstrated in monocytes allowed to differentiate in culture for 7 days before treatment. γIFN was the only cytokine capable of inhibiting the induction of 15-lipoxygenase (Table 1). This inhibition was dose-dependent in the range of γIFN concentrations tested (10 to 700 p$M$) and was maximal at 100 p$M$. The phorbol ester PMA (50 n$M$) and hydrocortisone (100 n$M$) also inhibited the IL-4 response.

Immunoblots of whole-cell extracts of IL-4-treated monocytes exhibited a single immunoreactive band with a molecular weight of approximately 70 kDa (Fig. 1). This band co-migrated with authentic 15-lipoxygenase prepared from human leukocytes. Furthermore, enzymatic activity of IL-4-treated monocytes confirmed the induction of 15-lipoxygenase (Fig. 2). RNA blots hybridized with a radiolabeled full-length cDNA for 15-lipoxygenase de-

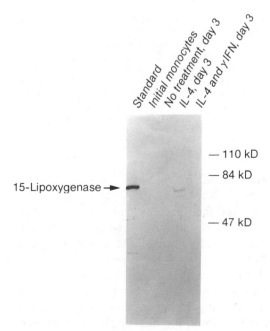

**FIG. 1.** Induction of 15-lipoxygenase in IL-4–treated human monocytes macrophages. Human monocytes were cultured for 3 days in the presence or absence of IL-4 (700 p$M$) and assayed for 15-lipoxygenase expression by immunoblot analysis. No immunoreactivity is detected in freshly isolated monocytes or in monocytes co-cultured with IL-4 (700 p$M$) and γ-interferon (100 p$M$). Partially purified human leukocyte 15-lipoxygenase was used as a standard (arrow). (From ref. 27 with permission.)

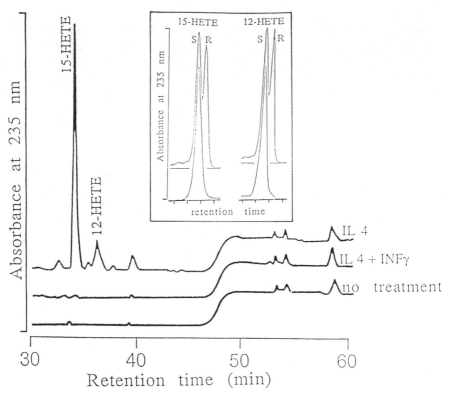

**FIG. 2.** Metabolism of exogenous arachiodonic acid by IL-4–treated monocytes. 15-Lipoxygenase activity was assessed by measuring the formation of 15-HETE from exogenous arachidonic acid (160 m*M*) by RP-HPLC. Chromatograms are shown for assays of cultured monocytes, monocytes cultured in the presence of IL-4 (700 p*M*), and monocytes cultured in the presence of both IL-4 (700 p*M*) and γIFN (100 p*M*). Each incubation contained 2 × 10⁶ cells. The IL-4–treated cells formed approximately 500 ng 15-HETE per 10⁶ cells. Retention times of authentic standards are indicated by arrows. **Inset:** Chiral-phase HPLC of the enantiomers of 12- and 15-HETE. Upper trace shows racemic standards and lower trace shows products formed by IL-4–treated monocytes. (From ref. 12 with permission.)

tected the typical RNA hybridization signal for human 15-lipoxygenase in polyadenylated RNA prepared from IL-4–treated monocytes (Fig. 3). No hybridization was seen in RNA prepared from freshly isolated monocytes, untreated monocytes, or monocytes treated with both IL-4 and γIFN. The role of transcriptional processes in the activation of the 15-lipoxygenase gene is presently under investigation.

Because IL-4 receptors are co-localized with 15-lipoxygenase in the airway epithelium (6,14) and because IL-4 may modulate airway inflammation, we investigated the role of IL-4 in regulating 15-lipoxygenase expression in cultured human airway epithelial cells. Human tracheal epithelial cells were

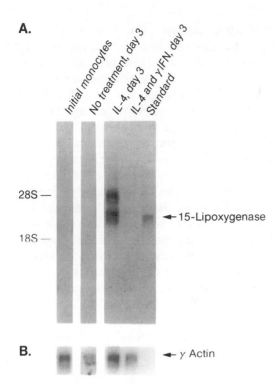

**A.**

Initial monocytes

No treatment, day 3

IL-4, day 3

IL-4 and γIFN, day 3

Standard

28S —

18S —

◄ 15-Lipoxygenase

**B.**

◄ γ Actin

**FIG. 3.** Northern blot analysis of monocyte 15-lipoxygenase induction by interleukin-4. **A:** Polyadenylated RNA was prepared from freshly isolated monocytes, cultured monocytes, monocytes cultured in the presence of IL-4 (700 pM), or monocytes cultured in the presence of both IL-4 (700 pM) and γIFN (100 pM). All lanes contained 1 μg of poly(A)$^+$ RNA except for the standard lane, which contained rabbit reticulocyte total RNA (8 μg). The positions of ribosomal RNA are indicated on the left and 15-lipoxygenase transcripts are indicated by an arrow. **B:** The same blot was probed with human γ-actin cDNA. (From ref. 12 with permission.)

isolated from postmortem specimens and cultured on Vitrogen gel-coated Cyclopore (Becton–Dickinson) filters with a lumen–air interface in medium supplemented with 2% Ultroser G. After 7 days of culture in medium supplemented with IL-4 (1.0 ng/ml), the cells were assessed for 15-lipoxygenase activity by incubation with exogenous arachidonic acid (320 μM). Analysis of the cellular lipid extracts by HPLC revealed 15-lipoxygenase metabolites in cells treated with IL-4 but not in cells cultured without IL-4 (15).

## DISCUSSION

Our results associate specific inflammatory cytokines with the regulation of 15-lipoxygenase, a lipid-peroxidating enzyme. The induction of monocyte 15-lipoxygenase by IL-4 coincides with the appearance of lipoxygenase products such as 15S-HETE in the membrane lipids (12). Because the precursor to 15-HETE is a highly reactive hydroperoxy compound, which may rapidly decompose via radical-mediated reactions, these experiments define an enzymatic pathway of radical formation with implications for host defense.

The oxidative modification of LDL has been proposed as a key event in the development of early atherosclerotic lesions (16). 15-Lipoxygenase could contribute to the oxidative modification of LDL through the production of intracellular hydroperoxy lipids, which could then initiate the extracellular oxidation of LDL. Whether IL-4 or $\gamma$IFN regulates 15-lipoxygenase expression in atherosclerosis is not known. However, activated T cells, a major cell source for IL-4, have been localized to atherosclerotic lesions. Further insights into the role of these cytokines in atherogenesis would be revealed by studies designed to detect and inhibit these factors in vivo. Such experiments could potentially identify novel therapeutic interventions.

IL-4 is a highly pleiotropic cytokine produced by the subset of T helper lymphocytes, $T_{H2}$, as well as by mast cells (17). The $T_{H2}$ cytokine response, characterized by high levels of IL-4 and low levels of $\gamma$IFN, has been increasingly associated with allergic or immediate hypersensitivity responses. Hence, IL-4 is responsible for the class switching that results in increases in serum IgE (18). In addition, IL-4 is known to increase expression of class II MHC molecules, $F_c$ receptors for IgE (19,20) and the adhesion molecules ICAM and VCAM (21,22). Importantly, transgenic mice that overexpress IL-4 develop complex inflammatory lesions characteristic of human allergic disorders (23).

Our studies suggest that the IL-4 regulation of 15-lipoxygenase may be a general mechanism and that the epithelial 15-lipoxygenase may serve an IL-4

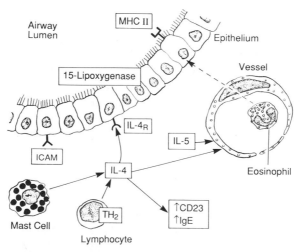

**FIG. 4.** Potential interactions of interleukin-4 and 15-lipoxygenase in human airway disease. The schematic diagram depicts a cross-section of airway epithelium expressing 15-lipoxygenase, MHC class II antigen, the adhesion molecule ICAM, and the receptor for IL-4. IL-4 and IL-5 are depicted being secreted from activated mast cells and $T_{H2}$ lymphocytes. IL-4 is known to increase IgE levels as well as the expression of CD23 (the $F_c$ receptor for IgE). IL-4 may increase eosinophil adherence through VCAM expression, and IL-5 is known to attract eosinophils to local sites of inflammation and to assist in their activation. (From ref. 27 with permission.)

function in human airway. We propose here a scheme for IL-4 and lipoxy-genase interactions in human airway (Fig. 4). In this scheme, IL-4 may be secreted along with IL-5 from activated mast cells or subset of $CD_{4+}$ lymphocytes ($T_{H2}$ cells) (24). High levels of both IL-4 and IL-5 are likely to promote eosinophil adherence and migration. These leukocytes play a prominent role in inflammatory mechanisms in asthma and contribute to epithelial shedding, hypersecretion, and bronchoconstriction. IL-4 may act further through its receptor on the epithelium to upregulate expression of ICAM, MHC class II antigens, and 15-lipoxygenase. The relationship of such coordinated events is unclear. However, the expression of 15-lipoxygenase in the airway can lead to oxygenation of cell lipids and this could affect several functions, including cellular host–defense mechanisms (i.e., production of membrane lipid peroxide radicals), intracellular signaling pathways (through the production of oxidized diacylglycerol (DAG) (25), and protein expression via oxidized lipid transcription pathways (26). It now becomes important to investigate each of these functions with specific inhibitors. Further study of these mechanisms and the effect of cytokines on the lipoxygenase reaction is expected to increase our understanding of the immune/inflammatory response in a variety of disorders, including bronchial asthma.

## ACKNOWLEDGMENT

We acknowledge the contributions of Hartmut Kühn, Mary Mulkins, and Ella Highland to the initial experiments and the help of Mitsuo Yamaya, Ella Highland, and Walter Finkbeiner in the recent extensions of the work described here. We thank Helen Guyton for assistance in manuscript preparation. This work was supported in part by National Institutes of Health Program Project Grant HL-24136 and the Council for Tobacco Research Grant 2489. E.S. is a recipient of the National Institutes for Health Clinical Investigator Award, HL-02047. D.C. is the recipient of an American Lung Association Research Fellowship.

## REFERENCES

1. Samuelsson B, Dahlén SE, Lindgren JA, Rouzer CA, Serhan CN. *Science* 1987;237: 1171–6.
2. Lewis RA, Austen KF, Soberman RJ. *N Engl J Med* 1990;323:645–55.
3. Kuhn H, Belkner J, Wiesner R, Brash AR. *J Biol Chem* 1990;265:18351–61.
4. Sigal E, Craik CS, Highland E, et al. *Biochem Biophys Res Commun* 1988;157:457–64.
5. Sigal E, Grunberger D, Highland E, Gross C, Dixon RA, Craik CS. *J Biol Chem* 1990;265: 5113–20.
6. Sigal E, Dicharry S, Highland E, Finkbeiner WE. *Am J Physiol* 1992;6:L392–8.
7. Nadel JA, Conrad DJ, Ueki IF, Schuster A, Sigal E. *J Clin Invest* 1991;87:1139–45.
8. Yla-Herttuala S, Rosenfeld ME, Parthasarathy S, et al. *Proc Natl Acad Sci USA* 1990;87:6959–63.
9. Yla-Herttuala S, Rosenfeld ME, Parthasarathy S, et al. *J Clin Invest* 1991;87:1146–52.
10. Bigby TD, Holtzman MJ. *J Immunol* 1987;138:1546–50.

11. Ross R, Masuda J, Raines EW, et al. *Science* 1990;248:1009–12.
12. Conrad DJ, Kuhn H, Mulkins M, Highland E, Sigal E. *Proc Natl Acad Sci USA* 1992;89: 217–21.
13. Yamaya M, Finkbeiner WE, Chun SY, Widdicombe JH. *Am J Physiol* 1992:L713–24.
14. Tungekar MF, Turley H, Dunnill MS, Gatter KC, Ritter MA, Harris AL. *Cancer Res* 1991;51:261–4.
15. Conrad DJ, Yamaya M, Finkbeiner WE, Widdicombe JH, Sigal E. *Am Rev Respir Dis* 1992;145:A18(abst).
16. Steinberg D, Parthasarathy S, Carew TE, Khoo JC, Witztum MD. *N Engl J Med* 1989; 320:915–24.
17. Paul WE. *Blood* 1991;77:1859–70.
18. Coffman R, Ohara J, Bond M, Carty J, Zlotnick A, Paul W. *J Immunol* 1986;136:4538–46.
19. Noelle R, Krammer PH, Ohara J, Uhr JW, Vitetta ES. *Proc Natl Acad Sci USA* 1984;81: 6149–53.
20. Kikutani H, Inui S, Sato R, et al. *Cell* 1986;47:657–61.
21. Valent P, Bevec D, Maurer D, et al. *Proc Natl Acad Sci USA* 1991;88:3339–42.
22. Schleimer RP, Sterbinsky SA, Kaiser J, et al. *J Immunol* 1992;148:1086–92.
23. Tepper RI, Levinson DA, Stanger BZ, Campos TJ, Abbas AK, Leder P. *Cell* 1990;62:457–67.
24. Robinson DS, Hamid Q, Ying S, et al. *N Engl J Med* 1992;326:298–304.
25. Legrand AB, Lawson JA, Meyrick BO, Blair IA, Oates JA. *J Biol Chem* 1991;266:7570–7.
26. Haliday EM, Ramesha CS, Ringold G. *EMBO J* 1991;10:109–15.
27. Sigal E, Sloane DL, Conrad DJ. *J Lipid Mediators* 1993;6:75–88.

*Advances in Prostaglandin, Thromboxane,*
*and Leukotriene Research,* Vol. 22, edited by
S.-E. Dahlén et al. Raven Press, Ltd., New York © 1994

# Lipoxin Recognition Sites of Human Neutrophils

## Charles N. Serhan and Stefano Fiore

*Hematology–Oncology Division, Department of Medicine, Brigham and Women's*
*Hospital and Harvard Medical School, Boston Massachusetts 02115*

Lipoxins are bioactive eicosanoids that can be generated by interactions between individual lipoxygenases and/or by cell–cell interactions (1). Lipoxin $A_4$ (LXA$_4$) displays selective actions with human polymorphonuclear leukocytes (PMN) (2–5). Exogenous addition of LXA$_4$ at submicromolar concentrations elicits PMN migration without causing aggregation (3,4), whereas prior exposure to LXA$_4$ inhibits (IC$_{50}$ $\approx$ $10^{-8}$ $M$) their subsequent chemotactic responses to either LTB$_4$ or the peptide fMLP (5). LXA$_4$ also blocks $Ca^{2+}$ mobilization and hydrolysis of phosphoinositides (6). Results from in vivo models show that LXA$_4$ inhibits LTB$_4$-induced plasma leakage and leukocyte migration (7). These findings, along with those showing blockage of both LTD$_4$- and LTC$_4$-induced responses (8,9), provide further evidence for potential counterregulatory roles of lipoxins (5–9).

Ligand-triggered signal transduction events in human PMN lend themselves to monitoring techniques with resolution of seconds (10). We have documented the initial responses of PMN on their exposure to lipoxins (2). LXA$_4$, within 5 to 15 sec, stimulates rapid lipid remodeling and release of arachidonic acid, with only a modest increment in the mobilization of intracellular $Ca^{2+}$; however, LXA$_4$ promotes neither oxygenation of arachidonic acid nor adhesion by PMN within the same temporal and concentration ranges. Release of arachidonic acid was sensitive to treatment with pertussis toxin, suggesting the involvement of G-proteins. In addition, LXA$_4$ does not block specific binding of [$^3$H]LTB$_4$ to PMN (2,6) and, unlike LTB$_4$ (11), is not rapidly further metabolized by these cells (12). This chapter describes the characteristics of [11,12-$^3$H]LXA$_4$ binding with PMN.

## METHODS

Synthetic [11,12-$^3$H]LXA$_4$ was prepared as described in (12). The specific activity was 13.5 Ci/mmol, and a higher specific activity [11,12-$^3$H] LXA$_4$ (approximately 40.5 Ci/mmol) was prepared that gave essentially identical results. Fresh peripheral blood (approximately 150 ml) was obtained from healthy volunteers, and PMN were isolated from heparinized blood directly after venipuncture by dextran sedimentation followed by Ficoll–Hypaque gradient centrifugation (13). The suspensions contained 98 ± 1% neutrophils as determined by light microscopy, and the integrity of cells was monitored by Trypan Blue exclusion (viability greater than 98% for $n = 27$ separate donors). [³H]LXA₄ and [³H]LTB₄ binding was performed as previously reported (12). PMN (1 × 10⁷ cells/0.5 ml) were layered onto a cushion of silicon oil (350 μl) in Eppendorf tubes and kept for 10 min either in an ice-water bath or at 37°C before addition of the radiolabeled eicosanoid (0.3 n$M$). Unlabeled homoligands were added in parallel samples to determine total and specific binding. Fractionation experiments also used the glass fiber filter procedure (14) and rapid centrifugation through silicon oil (15). In addition to linear regression analyses (i.e., Scatchard and Hill plots), data were processed using the Ligand program (Elsevier-Biosoft; Cambridge, U.K.). Curve fits and Boeynaems–Swillens plot (as in ref. 12) were constructed using regression fitting from Cricket Graph software (release 1.3; Computer Associates, Malvern, PA, U.S.A.).

## RESULTS

### Specific Binding of [11,12-³H]LXA₄

Total and specific binding were determined for a time course of 0 to 90 min and, for purposes of comparison, parallel incubations were carried out with [14,15-³H]LTB₄ and cells from the same donors. At 4°C, specific binding with both labels was observed within 10 to 15 sec, which increased with time to reach a plateau within 5 min (Fig. 1). At 37°C, different profiles were observed. [³H]LXA₄ binding increased for the first 60 min, whereas [³H]LTB₄ binding progressively decreased after 5 min. Nonspecific binding also increased with time. These results suggest a modest effect of tempera-

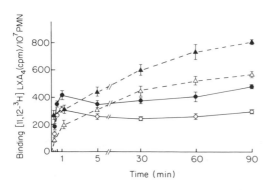

**FIG. 1.** Time course of [11,12-³H]LXA₄ binding. Human PMN (1 × 10⁷/0.5 ml) were incubated in the presence of [11,12-³H]LXA₄ (0.3 n$M$). Time course was determined at 4°C (circles) and 37°C (triangles); total (closed symbols) and specific (open symbols) binding of the radiolabels was calculated using the silicon oil cushion method and an excess of unlabeled ligand. Results are the mean ± SD of three experiments performed with duplicate determinations at each time interval.

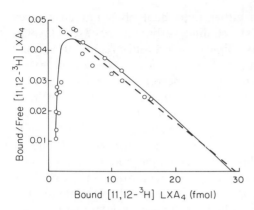

FIG. 2. Concentration dependence: binding of [11,12-³H]LXA₄ with intact PMN. Replicates containing $1 \times 10^7$ PMN per sample, were incubated in Tris buffer (pH 7.4, 4°C for 5 min) with various concentrations (0.1 to 1.6 n$M$) of [11,12-³H]LXA₄ in the presence or absence of a 3 log excess of unlabeled LXA₄. The Scatchard plot was calculated from specific binding results of the isotherms obtained from three separate experiments. For [³H]LXA₄ concentrations greater than 0.26 n$M$, a regression coefficient of $r = 0.916$ was obtained (dotted line) which resulted in a calculated $K_d$ of $0.5 \pm 0.3$ n$M$.

*Y axis: Bound/Free [11,12-³H] LXA₄*

*X axis: Bound [11,12-³H] LXA₄ (fmol)*

ture for [³H]LXA₄ binding that ranges between two and five times higher at 37°C. At 4°C (5 min), nonspecific binding was 31.6 ±7% of the maximal binding with [³H]LXA₄ compared to 12.7 ± 3.9% with [³H]LTB₄ ($n = 3$).

Binding isotherms performed with intact PMN and [11,12-³H]LXA₄ (0.1 to 1.6 n$M$) showed saturability for specific cell association (Fig. 2). For concentrations greater than 0.26 n$M$ of [³H]LXA₄, the run test analysis (seven runs) gave a $p$ value of >0.05 for a one-site binding model. Equilibrium dissociation constant ($K_d$) was $0.5 \pm 0.3 \times 10^{-9}$ $M$ and the maximal number of binding sites ($B_{max}$) was estimated to be approximately 1,830 sites/cell ($0.29 \times 10^{-13}$ mol/$1 \times 10^7$ cells or approximately $6.0 \times 10^{-10}$ $M$) for LXA₄. This value was approximately 25% of that calculated for LTB₄, which was approximately 7,351 sites/cell or $1.18 \times 10^{-13}$ mol/$1 \times 10^7$ cells determined with cells from the same donors. Construction of the Hill plot gave a Hill coefficient ($n_H$) of 1.92, suggesting positive cooperativity for LXA₄ binding. This was also supported by both Scatchard analysis and a Boeynaems–Swillens plot (12) ($r$ values of 0.97 and 0.88 were obtained for the ascendent and descendent portions of the parabolic curve, respectively).

### Recovery of [11,12-³H]LXA₄: Interactions with Cellular Components?

To determine if the observed cell association of [11,12-³H]LXA₄ was linked to either irreversible interactions with cellular components and/or further metabolism, the potential esterification or metabolism of [³H]LXA₄ was evaluated (12). For purposes of direct comparison, parallel incubations were performed with [¹⁴C]arachidonate, [³H]LXA₄, and [³H]11-*trans*-LXA₄. At 37°C, labeled AA was incorporated (esterification) into lipid classes (greater than 50% of the added label at 30 min). These findings are in sharp contrast to values obtained with either [³H]LXA₄ or [³H]11-*trans*-LXA₄.

[³H]LXs were not associated with either individual phospholipid classes (i.e., phosphatidyl-serine, -inositol(s), -choline, -ethanolamine, or phosphatidic acid), cholesterol esters, neutral lipids, or protein precipitates during the time courses. In addition, the profiles of association of labeled lipids with proteins and/or other cell components were different for labeled arachidonate (which more than doubled from 1.5% at 2 min to 3.7% at 30 min) than for both LXA₄ and its all-*trans* isomer, which remained less than 0.5% to 1% of the added labels. After addition of $A_{23187}$ (1 $\mu M$ for 3 min at 37°C), 5-min replicate samples were analyzed by ¹⁸C silica extraction and subsequent RP-HPLC of the methyl formate eluates to determine potential conversion or further metabolism. Again, the recovery of substantial amounts of the arachidonate-derived label in polar fractions and post-HPLC elution radioactive profiles (data not shown) were indicative of substantial transformation of [¹⁴C]arachidonic acid into lipoxygenase-derived products. These results were also in sharp contrast to the HPLC elution profiles obtained with both [³H]LXs that were recovered in the methyl formate eluates (94.4% for LXA₄ and 91.9% for 11-*trans*-LXA₄). RP-HPLC of the material recovered in these fractions showed that [³H]LXA₄ was essentially unaltered after exposure to intact PMN. Recovery of cell associated [11,12-³H]LXA₄ was also examined before and after competition with a 3 log excess of unlabeled LXA₄. Both the cell-associated and that displaced after competition (4°C; specifically bound [³H]LXA₄) were recovered, and evidence for further transformation or degradation was not obtained. Approximately 5% of the added [³H]LXA₄ was specifically bound to intact PMN, of which more than 99% was recovered in the methyl formate fractions. A clear reduction in nonspecific binding was obtained after competition with unlabeled LXA₄ (12). These findings indicate that [³H]LXA₄ is not metabolized or is covalently attached to either lipids or proteins of PMN during the time course of [³H]LXA₄ binding experiments.

## Structural Requirements

To assess the specificity of [11,12-³H]LXA₄ binding, we examined the abilities of structurally related compounds to displace [11,12-³H]LXA₄ from high-affinity recognition sites. The results in Fig. 3 indicate that LXA₄-Me, Mmc-LXA₄ ($IC_{50}$ 2.0 ± 0.3 n$M$) (a fluorescent derivative of LXA₄; see ref. 12), LTD₄($IC_{50}$ 56.0 ± 22.9 n$M$) and, to a lesser extent, LTC₄ ($IC_{50}$ 61.6 ± 23.4 n$M$) were able to compete for [11,12-³H]LXA₄ binding in a fashion comparable to that of the unlabeled homoligand LXA₄ ($IC_{50}$ 1.5 ± 0.7 n$M$). In contrast, LTB₄, LXB₄ (a positional isomer), 6(S)LXA₄ (an epimer at carbon-6 position of LXA₄), and 11-*trans*-LXA₄ (the all-*trans*-containing isomer) were unable to effectively displace cell-associated [³H]LXA₄ within the tested concentration range of 3 to 300 n$M$. This range encompasses a 3 log order excess from the calculated $K_d$ (see Fig. 2). SKF 104353, a potent

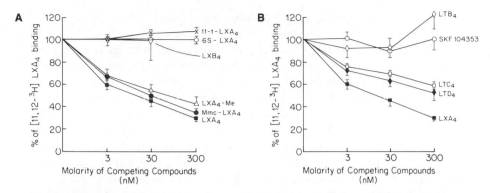

**FIG. 3. A,B:** Competition of [11,12-$^3$H]LXA$_4$ specific binding with structurally related compounds. Human PMN were incubated (5 min at 4°C) in the presence of increasing concentrations of LXA$_4$ (closed square), and related structures indicated in panels A and B. For LTB$_4$ competition, assays were performed at 4°C for 20 min to ensure equilibrium binding of LTB$_4$. Results represent the mean ± SD of three to nine separate experiments with duplicate determinations.

receptor-level antagonist of LTD$_4$ (8), did not compete for specific binding (4°C) of [$^3$H]LXA$_4$ (Fig. 3). At higher concentrations, LTB$_4$, C$_4$, and D$_4$ (greater than 300 n$M$) enhanced specific binding of [$^3$H]LXA$_4$ (not shown). In addition, treatment of PMN with proteases (chymotrypsin, pronase, and papain, 100 µg/ml each for 20 min at 25°C) led to 60% to 70% reduction in specific binding ($n = 3$).

## Subcellular Distribution

The distribution of [$^3$H]LXA$_4$ recognition sites (i.e., specific binding) was studied with nuclei-, granule-, plasma membrane-, and cytosol-enriched fractions prepared from freshly isolated PMN (12). For purposes of direct comparison, the distribution of LTB$_4$-specific binding was examined in parallel. Specific binding was obtained for both $^3$H-labeled compounds in all fractions save for the cytosol-enriched fractions. Plasma membrane- and endoplasmic reticulum-containing fractions gave the highest amount of specific binding for [11,12-$^3$H]LXA$_4$, equivalent to approximately 42.1% of the total binding capacity (expressed in fmol of ligand/mg protein). Granule-containing fractions gave 34.5% and the nuclei-containing fractions gave 23.3%. In the case of [14,15-$^3$H]LTB$_4$ specific binding with unstimulated cells, the granule fraction displayed a majority of the specific binding, with 75.7% and 16.0% of the total binding associated with membrane-enriched fractions (12). Based on analysis of the total protein content in individual fractions, there was enrichment for both LTB$_4$ receptor binding and [$^3$H]LXA$_4$ binding in the granule and membrane fractions.

### Impact of Guanosine Analogues

Specific binding of [11,12-$^3$H]LXA$_4$ was displaced with increasing concentrations of the unlabeled homoligand (Fig. 2) and was completely reduced to levels equivalent to nonspecific binding after equilibrium by addition of a 3 log order excess of unlabeled LXA$_4$ in the presence of guanosine $5^1$-[βγ/imido]triphosphate (GppNHp) at 20 μ$M$ (12). In the absence of GppNHp, the time course of [$^3$H]LXA$_4$ displacement with excess LXA$_4$ required 20 to 30 min to achieve approximately 60% reversal of specific binding. Similar results were obtained from GppNHp and [$^3$H]LTB$_4$ (0.3 n$M$) binding with intact PMN, where a reduction of 16.9 ± 3.7% was measured at 4°C for 20 min ($n$ = 2 separate donors with triplicate determinations). To define the rank order and specificity of activity for guanosine analogues, PMN membrane preparations (20 μg/250 μl) were prepared and incubated at 4°C for 20 min in the presence of [$^3$H]LXA$_4$ (0.3 n$M$) alone or added 5 min after addition of stable nucleotide analogues (50 n$M$ to 50 μ$M$). Results from these experiments showed that whereas ATPγS caused only a minimal dose-independent decrease of the specific binding, the stable guanosine analogues GDPβS, GppNHp, and GTPγS each effectively reduced [$^3$H]LXA$_4$ specific binding (12).

### DISCUSSION

Leukotrienes and prostaglandins are held to exert their actions on target tissues via interactions with plasma membrane receptors (16). In most cases, individual receptor classes that have been characterized pharmacologically display stereochemical requirements for binding with either ligands or partial antagonists. These functional assignments and binding characteristics with radiolabeled ligands have permitted the development of specific receptor level antagonists for leukotrienes (1,17). Along these lines, results show that a LTD$_4$-receptor antagonist markedly attenuates exercise-induced bronchoconstriction in human subjects with asthma (18). Therefore, this approach has provided clinically useful tools even though the individual LT receptor classes have not, to date, been isolated.

LXA$_4$ has selective actions with human PMN, in that it triggers only some specific responses (2). To elicit these responses, stereochemical requirements have been demonstrated (2–5). The present results show that [$^3$H]LXA$_4$ binding to PMN is time-dependent, saturable, specific, and reversible. [$^3$H]LXA$_4$ binding experiments performed at equilibrium saturation showed that [$^3$H]LXA$_4$ binds to intact PMN with high affinity, $K_d$ = 0.5 n$M$. In addition, Hill plot analyses suggest that [$^3$H]LXA$_4$ binds cooperatively. Positive cooperativity was also supported by Boeynaems–Swillens analysis (12). Although experiments with other $^3$H-labeled eicosanoids has not to our knowledge shown positive cooperativity in binding, glucagon binding with the hepatic adenylate cyclase system gives positive cooperativity [with a Hill coefficient ($n_H$) of approximately 1.5 calculated in ref. 19]. Competition of [³H]LXA₄ binding with related compounds provided further evidence that LXA₄ binds in a stereoselective fashion to sites not shared by either LTB₄ or LXB₄ (Fig. 3).

LTB₄ receptors of human PMN can exist in high- and low-affinity states (17,20). The range reported for high affinity includes $K_d$ = 0.08 to 10 n$M$ and low-affinity from 50 to 500 nM (21; see ref. 17 for review). A portion of the LTB₄ receptors in the high-affinity state can be converted by guanine nucleotide analogs to lower affinity (21). Whether PMN LTB₄ receptors exist as two distinct and separate classes (20) or as one interconverting population (21) that undergoes altered binding properties in cycling from granule to plasma membrane must await structural elucidation of the LTB₄ recognition sites. Nevertheless, clear differences were noted between the characteristics of [³H]LTB₄ binding and those observed with [11,12-³H]LXA₄ (12). First, LTB₄ cell association at 37°C decreased with time, unlike LXA₄ (Fig. 1). This difference may be explained by rapid ω-oxidation of LTB₄ (11) to ω-OH-LTB₄ and ω-COOH-LTB₄, which are known to bind less avidly with LTB₄ receptors (17). [³H]LXA₄ was not further metabolized by the ω-oxidation pathway in isolated PMN and was recovered after binding. These results indicate that [³H]LXA₄, unlike LTB₄, is not transformed or modified by PMN during the time course of these binding experiments. Neither irreversible association to cellular components (covalent linkage) nor further metabolism of the labeled compound complicated binding analyses of [³H]LXA₄ (see Results). Second, binding isotherms of [³H]LXA₄ performed with equilibrium binding conditions at 4°C (Fig. 2). showed that the $K_d$ of LXA₄ was approximately three times less than that of LTB₄, specifically compared in parallel using PMN from the same donors. LXA₄ recognition sites (approximately 1,830 sites/PMN; Fig. 2) were three to five times fewer than those for LTB₄. Although low in number, the density of [³H]LXA₄ sites (approximately 1,830/PMN) appears to be relevant when compared to 100 to 500 receptors/PMN demonstrated for GM-CSF, which displays potent actions on PMN (22). Third, subcellular distribution of specific binding sites for [³H]LTB₄ and [³H]LXA₄ gave different profiles. Taken together, these results indicate that LXA₄ binds to specific recognition sites with human PMN that are distinct from LTB₄ sites.

In general, both prostaglandin and leukotriene receptors show strict requirements for binding, which are evident in the rank order of specific binding activity with radioligands (17). Human PMN responses to LXA₄ also show strict stereochemical requirements to elicit both stimulatory (early responses) (2–4) and inhibitory actions (5–7). 6S-LXA₄ and 11-*trans*-LXA₄ were found to be less effective (5–9), and in the present experiments neither LTB₄, 6S-LXA₄, 11-*trans*-LXA₄, nor LXB₄ competed for [³H]LXA₄ specific binding (Fig. 3). $LXB_4$ can also induce rapid activation of PMN lipid remodeling (2) but appears not to inhibit these PMN responses (5). It therefore appears that $LXB_4$ and $LXA_4$ do not share a common site of action with human PMN.

Rapid lipid remodeling, the generation of phosphatidate, and the release of $[1-^{14}C]C20:4$ elicited by $LXA_4$ were pertussis toxin-sensitive (2). Additional evidence for the involvement of G-proteins in $LXA_4$ interactions with PMN comes from the finding that guanosine $5'-[\beta\gamma$-imido]triphosphate, a known modulator of $LTB_4$-receptor binding (17), altered the time course of $[^3H]LXA_4$ displacement (12). A rank order of guanosine analogue reactivity, i.e., $GTP\gamma S > GppNHp >>> ATP\gamma S$, was obtained with membrane preparations, which provides strong evidence for a structurally specific impact of these analogs in the specific binding of $[^3H]LXA_4$. Therefore, the recognition sites for $[^3H]LXA_4$ observed in membrane-enriched fractions (12) may be involved in $LXA_4$ signal transduction events that are sensitive to pertussis toxin treatment (2). Whether the specific recognition sites located in granule and nuclei-enriched fractions prove to be identical structures, as well as their biologic significance, remains to be elucidated. Nevertheless, the present results with guanosine analogs indicate that $[^3H]LXA_4$ specific binding to PMN membrane is regulated and altered by putative G-proteins.

$LXA_4$ can block the action of $LTC_4$ on guinea pig ileum, and the contractile actions of $LXA_4$ on human bronchi are blocked by the cysteinyl leukotriene receptor antagonist L-648,051 (reviewed in refs. 1 and 9). $LXA_4$ also stimulates vasodilatation and can block the vasoconstrictor actions of $LTD_4$ both in vivo in rats and in $[^3H]LTD_4$ binding to intact mesangial cells in vitro, responses that can be inhibited by the $LTD_4$-receptor antagonist SKF 104353 (8). These observations lead to the concept that $LXA_4$ and cysteinyl LTs may share binding domains at the receptor level, particularly since both molecules contain polar groups at carbons 5 and 6 in the 5S and 6R configurations, which have been shown to be critical for eliciting biologic activity (8,9). SKF 104353 did not block specific binding of $[^3H]LXA_4$ to intact PMN, although $LTC_4$ and $LTD_4$ partially compete for $LXA_4$ binding (Fig. 3). $LTC_4$ binding sites have been documented with intact PMN (14); however, their functional role with human PMN is not clear. Taken together, these (2,6,12) and the present results suggest that $LXA_4$ interacts with specific recognition sites with human PMN that are distinct from those described for $LTB_4$ and may be distinct from $LTC_4$ on human PMN or $LTD_4$, as defined by the absence of an effect with SKF 104353 in blocking $[^3H]LXA_4$ binding with these cells (Fig. 3B). Therefore, the sensitivity of $LXA_4$ to SKF 104353 may reflect species or subclass differences in recognition sites.

Results from competition experiments with $[^3H]LXA_4$ also provide evidence suggesting that the carbon 11 position and the chirality of the alcohol group at the carbon 6 position of $LXA_4$ are relevant determinants for $LXA_4$ interaction with PMN. Along these lines, the *cis* double bond at carbon 11

($\Delta$11) is required for $LXA_4$ to assume its globular conformation (23). Recent results show that $LXA_4$ ($10^{-10}$ $M$) stimulates colony formation with human marrow, whereas higher concentrations (greater than $10^{-8}$ $M$) were without agonist effects but displayed antagonist effects (24). The range and specificity of this bioactivity are in agreement with the $K_d$ for $LXA_4$ binding determined in the present study ($K_d$ 0.5 n$M$). These results provide the first evidence that the actions of $LXA_4$ may be mediated by interaction with specific functional receptors and that G-protein regulatory units might be critical components involved in their regulation.

## ACKNOWLEDGMENT

The authors thank Mary Halm Small for skillful preparation of the manuscript. These studies were supported in part by National Institutes of Health grant GM38765. C.N.S. is an Established Investigator of the American Heart Association. S.F. is the recipient of an Arthritis Foundation Postdoctoral Fellowship.

## REFERENCES

 1. Dahlén S-E, Serhan CN. In: Crooke ST, Wong A, eds. *Lipoxygenases and their products.* San Diego: Academic Press; 1991;235–76.
 2. Nigam S, Fiore S, Luscinskas FW, Serhan CN. *J Cell Physiol* 1990;143:512–23.
 3. Palmblad J, Gyllenhammar H, Ringertz B. In: Wong PY-K, Serhan CN, eds. *Advances in experimental medicine and biology,* Vol. 229. New York: Plenum Press; 1988;137–45.
 4. Serhan CN, Hamberg M, Samuelsson B. *Proc Natl Acad Sci USA* 1984;81:5335–9.
 5. Lee TH, Horton CE, Kyan-Aung U, Haskard D, Crea AEG, Spur BW. *Clin Sci* 1989;77: 195–203.
 6. Grandordy BM, Lacrois H, Mavoungou E, et al. *Biochem Biophys Res Commun* 1990;167: 1022–9.
 7. Hedqvist P, Raud J, Palmertz U, Haeggström J, Nicolaou KC, Dahlén S-E. *Acta Physiol Scand* 1989;137:571–2.
 8. Badr KF, DeBoer DK, Schwartzberg M, Serhan CN. *Proc Natl Acad Sci USA* 1989;86: 3438–42.
 9. Dahlén S-E, Franzén L, Raud J, et al. In: Wong PY-K, Serhan CN, eds. *Advances in experimental medicine and biology,* Vol. 229. New York: Plenum Press; 1988;107–30.
10. Weissmann G, Smolen JE, Korchak HM. *N Engl J Med* 1980;303:27–34.
11. Shak S, Goldstein IM. *J Clin Invest* 1985;76:1218–28.
12. Fiore S, Ryeom SW, Weller PF, Serhan CN. *J Biol Chem* 1992;267:16168–76.
13. Böyum A. *Scand J Clin Lab Invest* 1986;21(suppl 97):77–89.
14. Baud L, Koo CH, Goetzl EJ. *Immunology* 1987;62:53–9.
15. Yamazaki M, Gomez-Cambronero J, Durstin M, Molski TFP, Becker EL, Sha'afi RI. *Proc Natl Acad Sci USA* 1989;86:5791–4.
16. Munson PJ, Rodbard D. *Anal Biochem* 1980;107:220–39.
17. Mong S. In: Crooke ST, Wong A, eds. *Lipoxygenases and their products.* San Diego: Academic Press; 1991;185–206.
18. Manning PJ, Watson RM, Margolskee DJ, Williams VC, Schwartz JI, O'Byrne PM. *N Engl J Med* 1990;323:1736–9.
19. Rodbell M, Lin MC, Solomon Y. *J Biol Chem* 1974;249:59–65.
20. Goldman DW, Gifford LA, Marotti T, Koo CH, Goetzl EJ. *Fed Proc* 1987;46:200–3.
21. Votta B, Mong S. *Biochem J* 1990;265:841–7.

22. Cannistra SA, Koenigsmann M, DiCarlo J, Groshek P, Griffin JD. *J Biol Chem* 1990;265: 12656–63.
23. Brasseur R, Deleers M, Ruysschaert J-M, Samuelsson B, Serhan CN. *Biochem Biophys Acta* 1988;960;245–52.
24. Stenke L, Mansour M, Edenius C, Reizenstein P, Lindgren JA. *Biochem Biophys Res Commun* 1991;180:255–61.

*Advances in Prostaglandin, Thromboxane,*
*and Leukotriene Research,* Vol. 22, edited by
S.-E. Dahlén et al. Raven Press, Ltd., New York © 1994

# Regulation of Leukotriene Production
# by Cytokines

## Clemens A. Dahinden

*Institute of Clinical Immunology, University Hospital, Inselspital,*
*CH-3010 Bern, Switzerland*

Inflammatory reactions are somewhat redundant and stereotypical, albeit very complex, responses of the macroorganism to tissue damage of different causes (e.g., infections with microorganisms, trauma, physical and chemical insults, immunologic and neurogenic triggers) and play an important role in the pathogenesis of diseases of almost any etiology. Inflammatory responses of different etiologies probably display more common features than dissimilarities, because all leukocyte types, humoral effector systems, and even tissue cells participate, to various degrees, in a complex network of cellular interactions. These cellular interactions are controlled by a redundant system of a very large number of humoral and cell-derived factors, with partially distinct and partially overlapping biologic activities. Inflammation usually begins with a vascular response involving plasma exudation and edema caused by activation of resident tissue cells, either directly or through humoral systems such as complement. This vascular phase is usually followed by infiltration of the affected tissue with blood leukocytes (cellular exudate, tumor) and, finally, by tissue repair, remodeling, or fibrosis. Clinically, the cellular phase of inflammation is of particular importance to the severity of the disease because activation of the infiltrating leukocytes can in itself lead to further tissue damage owing to the release of secondary inflammatory mediators and cytotoxic products, thus leading to a vicious cycle and further amplification of the inflammatory reaction. Lipid mediators, particularly leukotrienes and platelet-activating factor (PAF), are formed in both the vascular and the cellular phase of inflammation and may therefore play an important part in the evolution of different inflammatory diseases.

Despite the redundant nature of inflammatory reactions, the relative importance of a particular effector cell, the profile of the mediators formed, and the composition of the different leukocyte types that infiltrate the site of the insult differ in diseases of distinct etiologies. For example, in most acute inflammatory reactions the neutrophil is the predominant leukocyte, whereas in many chronic processes activated monocytes/macrophages prevail. However, parasitic infections, certain autoimmune diseases and, in particular, immediate-type hypersensitivity diseases are characterized by the predominant infiltration and activation of eosinophils and basophils, often in association with activated lymphocyte subsets (1). In allergic IgE-mediated reactions such as asthma, the immediate (vascular) phase is particularly prominent owing to the activation of mast cells bearing high-affinity IgE receptors. However, even in allergic diseases, the severity of the clinical manifestations is determined primarily by the degree of cellular infiltration with leukocytes such as eosinophils, the so-called late-phase reaction, which does not strongly correlate with the amount of antigen-specific IgE. Leukotriene $C_4$ ($LTC_4$) is formed in the immediate reaction by antigen-activated mast cells, but even higher levels are found in allergic late-phase reactions. Therefore, leukotrienes may also be of particular importance in both the mast cell-mediated response and the clinically more pertinent cellular phase of allergic inflammation, and they represent an interesting target for therapeutic intervention. Under experimental challenge conditions in human subjects, the profile of mediators in allergic late-phase reactions corresponds to that formed by basophils (histamine, $LTC_4$) and by eosinophils (eosinophilic cationic proteins, $LTC_4$), but not by mast cells (no prostaglandin $D_2$, no tryptase), indicating that the $LTC_4$ formed must derive from infiltrating leukocytes rather than from resident mast cells. Because allergic late-phase reactions occur hours after allergen challenge, leukocytes must be capable of producing leukotrienes in an antigen-independent manner in response to activation by endogenous humoral and/or cell-derived factors. This conclusion is further supported by the fact that, in "intrinsic" forms of asthma, no exogenous antigen triggers are involved at all. Finally, many inflammatory processes in which other leukocyte types, such as neutrophils and monocytes, are the major effector cells are also antigen-independent but are nevertheless accompanied by the generation of leukotrienes.

The definition of endogenous soluble factors capable of promoting leukotriene synthesis in leukocytes therefore appears critical to our understanding of the pathogenesis of inflammatory processes in general and of allergic disease in particular. Here we present the concept that two signals are required for the induction of lipid mediator synthesis in leukocytes. Our studies indicate that the combined and sequential actions of certain cytokines and cell agonists are critical for the regulation of mediator release in effector cells. Furthermore, the profile of cytokines present may also determine the distinct features of inflammatory processes of different etiologies.

## DIRECT AGONIST PROMOTION OF LEUKOTRIENE SYNTHESIS

Leukocytes of the myeloid lineage are clearly the most important source of leukotrienes and PAF. Depending on the $LTA_4$ metabolizing enzyme they express, $LTC_4$ (mast cells, basophils, eosinophils, monocytes) and/or $LTB_4$ (neutrophils, monocytes) is produced, which mediate plasma exudation and smooth muscle contraction or chemotaxis and activation of granulocytes, respectively. The different lipoxygenase products have been primarily characterized from supernatants of leukocytes stimulated with calcium ionophore, which induces the production of large amounts of lipid mediators. Crosslinking of immunoglobulin receptors by antigen and, in particular, activation of the high-affinity IgE receptor on mast cells and basophils, can directly induce leukotriene generation. Small amounts of leukotrienes are also formed in response to particulate phagocytic stimuli by neutrophils and monocytes. However, years after the discovery and structural elucidation of the arachidonate products of the 5-lipoxygenase pathway, the only soluble agents identified as weak agonists of LT formation were exogenous bacterial products (pore-forming toxins, fMLP for basophils and eosinophils). Clearly, neither particulate triggers nor bacterial products can explain why leukotrienes are formed by leukocytes in pathologic exudates of allergic late-phase reactions and in many other inflammatory processes. To date, no soluble endogenous bioactive molecules have yet been found capable of directly promoting the formation of leukotrienes in any leukocyte type, despite the fact that a large number of novel cell agonists are being discovered at an increasing pace. In the case of neutrophils, the intriguing observation that these cells do not generate leukotrienes in response to diverse agonists, although they possess the machinery to produce them, has been termed "the leukotriene $B_4$ paradox" by Weissmann's group (2).

## LEUKOTRIENE PRODUCTION FROM EXOGENOUS ARACHIDONIC ACID

Resting neutrophils (PMN) do not produce leukotrienes when exposed to arachidonic acid complexed to albumin. On stimulation with C5a and fMLP, however, PMN rapidly and transiently metabolize exogenous arachidonic acid (AA) into leukotrienes (3). Probably all agonists interacting with G-protein-coupled receptors that induce an increase in cytosolic free calcium concentration have this effect, since similar observations have been made for interleukin 8 (IL-8) (4) and even for $LTB_4$ itself (unpublished observation). These observations indicate that the 5-lipoxygenase is inactive in resting PMN as the formation of leukotrienes does not solely depend on the availability of free AA which largely controls prostaglandin generation. The second messengers formed in response to chemotactic cell agonists are sufficient to activate the 5-lipoxygenase, and the activity of the 5-lipoxygenase and of the phospholipase(s) (e.g., $PLA_2$) are separately regulated, as no leukotrienes are formed from endogenous AA pools on stimulation with these neutrophil agonists alone.

Although the level of free AA is tightly controlled in vivo, the ability of these myeloid cell agonists to promote leukotriene generation from exogenous AA could nevertheless play a local role at inflammatory sites, where AA may be released by necrotic tissues or by the action of extracellular $PLA_2$, which is indeed present in different inflammatory processes.

## EFFECTOR CELL PRIMING FOR LEUKOTRIENE SYNTHESIS BY CYTOKINES

Cytokines are defined as cell-derived protein mediators. They have been primarily characterized on the basis of their growth-promoting and/or cell-differentiating properties for leukocytes of the myeloid and lymphoid lineage, and are therefore important regulators of the function of the adaptive immune system. However, more recent studies have clearly established that several cytokines, most of which have been initially identified as hematopoietic growth factors, not only regulate the growth and differentiation of immature leukocyte precursors but also modulate and amplify inflammatory reactions by their action on mature effector leukocytes. These "priming" cytokines, which we also termed "cell response modifiers," do not directly trigger effector cell functions but rather enhance the responsiveness of different leukocyte types toward stimulation by all triggering molecules examined thus far. All the effector functions that have been tested are strongly potentiated (i.e., chemotaxis, release of preformed and de novo synthesized mediators or cytotoxic products, cell adhesiveness, cytotoxicity). This priming phenomenon has been observed in all myeloid cell types (neutrophils, eosinophils, basophils, monocytes) and even in tissue mast cells. However, the target cell profile is distinct for the different modulatory cytokines. In addition to these rapid effects on cell function, prolonged exposure of mature effector cells to appropriate priming cytokines can lead to increased cell survival and to further functional and phenotypic alterations by de novo gene expression and protein synthesis (5; and unpublished observations).

Several studies from our laboratory, first performed with neutrophils and, more recently, with mature human basophils and eosinophils, showed that these cytokines are also critical regulators of lipid mediator formation ($LTB_4$ and PAF in neutrophils; $LTC_4$ in basophils; $LTC_4$ and PAF in eosinophils) (6). In fact, cytokine-primed inflammatory effector cells produce considerable amounts of lipid mediators in response to most soluble chemotactic cell agonists, which are by themselves ineffective in promoting lipid mediator formation (Fig. 1) We therefore propose that the presence of priming cytokines determines whether or not mature effector cells produce lipid mediators, whereas the target-cell profile of the cytokines present largely determines which cell types respond.

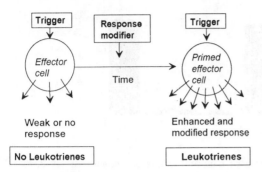

**FIG. 1.** Priming of effector cells by cytokines.

### Priming of Basophils and Mast Cells by Cytokines

Basophils and mast cells are particularly potent sources of $LTC_4$. In fact, basophils produce 10 to 1,000 times more $LTC_4$ than eosinophils when sequentially stimulated with a priming cytokine and different cell agonists, at least in vitro. Therefore, basophils should be considered as important effector cells of allergic late-phase reactions, even if their number compared to eosinophils is lower in an allergic exudate. In basophils, three related cytokines, IL-3, IL-5, and GM-CSF, enhance the releasability of the cells (7–12). More recently, a neurotrophic cytokine, nerve growth factor (NGF), has been added to the list of potent basophil-priming cytokines, suggesting a modulation of allergic inflammation by the nervous system (13). In contrast, a large number of other cytokines were inactive in modulating basophil function. Exposure of basophils to IL-3, IL-5, GM-CSF, or NGF for 5 to 10 min augments the release of preformed (e.g., histamine) and de novo-generated lipid mediators in response to IgE receptor or fMLP stimulation. More importantly, primed basophils produce large amounts of $LTC_4$ in response to C5a (7,11) and the monocyte chemotactic peptide 1 (MCP-1) (14), two potent endogenous basophil agonists that by themselves induce degranulation only. Furthermore, a large number of cell-derived (PAF, IL-8/NAP-1), and other intercrines/chemokines; see below) or humoral (C3a) cell agonists, which do not induce any mediator release in unprimed basophils, promote degranulation as well as $LTC_4$ formation by basophils exposed to either IL-3, IL-5, GM-CSF, or NGF (8–10,12). Therefore, these priming cytokines not only enhance the cellular responsiveness but lead to a qualitative alteration in the behavior of the cells (Fig. 2).

Human mucosal lung mast cells do not appear to release mediators in response to the many IgE-independent agonists, including those that trigger human basophils. C-KIT ligand (KL), a hematopoietic stem cell growth factor that can be produced by tissue cells in either a transmembrane or a soluble form, was found to be a unique potentiator of mediator release by

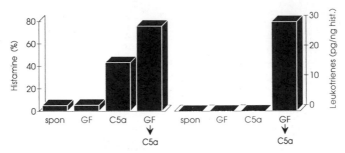

**FIG. 2.** Growth factors (GF) as mediators of basophil mediator release; GF: IL-3, IL-5, GM–CSF, or NGF.

lung mast cells in response to IgE-receptor stimulation (15). KL increases the sensitivity of mast cells to IgE receptor cross-linking and also increases the amount of mediators formed in response to maximal IgE-receptor stimulation. It is still unclear whether KL acts mainly as a priming agent or also as a direct agonist, because, depending on the experimental conditions, KL can by itself induce the release of considerable amounts of mast-cell mediators, including $LTC_4$ (unpublished observations). In rodents, and probably in human subjects as well, KL is also an important mast-cell growth and differentiating factor. Therfore, the extent of expression of KL by tissue cells may regulate both the number and the function of mucosal mast cells. By contrast, a large number of cytokines, including basophil-priming cytokines and the mast-cell growth factors/agonists in rodents (i.e., IL-3, IL-4, IL-9, NGF) neither modulate nor induce mediator release by lung mast cells, indicating that observations made in rodents cannot be easily extrapolated to the human system and that mouse mucosal mast cells functionally resemble more the human basophils than the human mucosal lung mast cells (15; and references therein).

### Priming of Eosinophils by Cytokines

Eosinophils and basophils are developmentally and functionally closely related cell types, both with regard to the cytokine profile that enhances their responsiveness and to the cell agonists to which they respond (16). There are a few exceptions: NGF does not prime eosinophil function, and tumor necrosis factor (TNF), which does not affect basophils, increases $LTC_4$ formation by eosinophils (17). It is interesting that a particular set of cytokines, IL-3, IL-5, and GM-CSF, primes both cell types in a similar manner, indicating that these cytokines are of particular importance in allergic late-phase reactions. The similarity of action of IL-3, IL-5, and GM-CSF can now be explained in molecular terms, since the different ligand α-chain receptor complexes of these three cytokines interact with a common β-chain, which is necessary for high-affinity binding and signal transduction. Our recent observation that the priming effect of IL-3, IL-5, and GM-CSF can be inhibited by small peptide analogue of a consensus sequence of the cytokine receptor family indicates that it may become feasible to design β-chain antagonists that will inhibit an entire group of cytokines (18).

In contrast to basophils, the regulation of degranulation and lipid mediator formation in eosinophils is still poorly defined. Even after priming with IL-3, IL-5, or GM-CSF, eosinophils produce relatively little $LTC_4$ in response to C5a or PAF (16,17), and other recently identified eosinophil agonists, such as C3a, RANTES, and MIP-1a, do not promote the formation of detectable amounts of $LTC_4$ (19). It has been reported that $LTC_4$ production in response to fMLP is further enhanced by prolonged culture in the presence of GM-CSF and fibroblasts, indicating that unknown factors from tissue cells may also regulate lipid mediator formation. However, it is not yet known whether the response to endogenous agonists is affected in a similar way.

### Priming of Neutrophils by Cytokines

Neutrophils are the principal effector cells of acute inflammation and defense against bacterial infection. In contract to basophils and eosinophils, only GM-CSF, but not IL-3 and IL-5, primes neutrophils to produce $LTB_4$ in response to the chemotactic agonists C5a or fMLP (20). IL-1 and TNF enhance other cell functions, such as oxygen radical release and degranulation, but do not prime neutrophils for C5a-induced $LTB_4$ synthesis. PAF formation through the phospholipase $A_2$/acetyltransferase pathway is regulated in an identical manner, further indicating the cytokine priming is particularly important for activation of cytoplasmic $PLA_2$ (21,22). Interestingly, however, IL-8/NAP-1, a potent chemotactic cytokine that activates neutrophils through G-protein–coupled receptors in a manner identical to that of C5a or fMLP with regard to chemotaxis and cell activation (respiratory burst and granule release), does not induce lipid mediator formation even by GM-CSF–primed neutrophils, indicating that the signal-transducing pathways for the different chemotactic cell agonists are not entirely identical (23).

### CYTOKINES ACTING AS CHEMOTACTIC CELL AGONISTS (CHEMOKINES)

In recent years, a large superfamily of homologous cytokines (platelet factor-4/intercrine/chemokine superfamily) has been gradually identified, and other members of this family may still be discovered. In bioactivity they resemble other cell-derived or humoral inflammatory mediators, such as C5a, fMLP or PAF, but with a more restricted target-cell profile (24).

Members of the C-X-C branch (according to the position of the first two cysteines in the conserved motif), also termed the IL-8 or α-chemokine family, attract and activate mainly neutrophils and are therefore important mediators of acute inflammatory processes. IL-8 receptors are also expressed on basophils and eosinophils; however, these cell types must be primed by appropriate response-modifying cytokines to appreciably respond to IL-8 stimulation. The biologic activities of the members of the C–C branch or β-chemokine family of cytokines are less well defined. They do not appear to activate neutrophils, but rather attract certain mononuclear cells, and may therefore be important mediators of chronic inflammatory processes. RANTES, macrophage inflammatory protein MIP-1α, and MIP-1β are chemotactic for distinct lymphocyte subpopulations and MCP-1 is a particularly potent monocyte chemotactic factor (24).

Work from our laboratory and other groups has revealed that distinct members of the β-chemokines are potent agonists for basophils and eosinophils, indicating that this group of cytokines may be particularly important mediators of allergic inflammation. MCP-1 is the most potent cell-derived basophil agonist identified thus far, inducing the release of histamine by itself and promoting the generation of large amounts of $LTC_4$ by cytokine-primed basophils (Fig. 2) (14). MCP-1 does not activate or attract eosinophils, thus representing the first recognized basophil trigger incapable of activating eosinophils (18). RANTES and MIP-1α, however, activate both cell types in an identical manner, in contrast to MIP-1β, which is inactive (18,25). All of these agonists activate basophils and eosinophils by a similar mechanism that induces pertussis toxin-sensitive changes in intracellular calcium concentrations of identical kinetics, similar to the chemotaxin C5a (14,18). Despite these similarities in signal transduction, the fine specificities for activating the different effector functions are distinct, even in the same cell type. For example, RANTES attracts basophils with higher efficacy than MCP-1, despite a much lower mediator-releasing capacity that is similar to that of IL-8/NAP-1.

The distinct and relatively restricted target cell profiles of the members of the β-chemokine family of cytokines, and the fact that they preferentially promote distinct cellular functions even in the same cell type, indicate that these cytokines regulate the fine tuning of chronic inflammatory processes of diverse etiologies. In allergic inflammation, MCP-1 may be particularly important for activating basophil mediator release. RANTES is a potent chemotactic factor for T-helper memory cells, eosinophils, and basophils (but not neutrophils), and may therefore mediate the selective attraction of these effector cells in allergic late phase reactions.

Therefore, the specificity of allergic inflammation may be determined not only by the profile of cytokines enhancing the cellular responsiveness of particular effector cells to pleiotophic cell agonists, as suggested earlier, but also by the profile of the members of the chemokine family that act as relatively oligotrophic chemotactic agonists.

## MECHANISMS OF PRIMING AND CELL ACTIVATION IN BASOPHILS

The mechanisms of priming for leukotriene production has been most extensively studied in basophils, because in these cell types priming occurs within minutes, making interpretations of pharmacologic interventions easier. In neutrophils and eosinophils, however, priming for lipid mediator formation by hematopoietic growth factors requires 90 to 120 min and is partially dependent on gene expression and de novo synthesis of proteins (22). Therefore, despite obvious analogies, the mechanism of priming may not be completely identical for the different effector leukocyte types.

Only the sequential action of a response modifier and a cell agonist leads to an enhancement of cellular functions such as degranulation and can induce leukotriene generation. No other combination is able to induce leukotriene formation (Fig. 3) (26,27). These observations not only indicate that the time of appearance of a cytokine or agonist is of equal importance for the outcome of inflammatory reactions as the profile of the factors produced, but also suggest that the mechanism of action of cell response modifiers must be completely different from that of cell agonists. This fundamental difference in the mode of action between response modifiers and triggers is paralleled by the different classes of receptors with which they interact (cytokine receptor or tyrosine kinase receptor superfamilies, and G-protein–

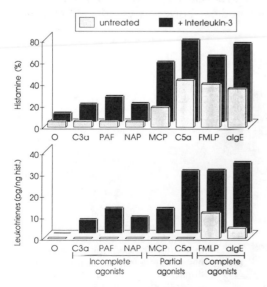

**FIG. 3.** Basophils were exposed to IL-3 (10 ng/ml) for 10 min or to buffer (untreated) and then stimulated with the agonists indicated. Histamine release and leukotriene generation are shown.

coupled receptor superfamily, respectively), and by different intracellular signaling pathways utilized by these ligands. All basophil triggers promote a transient rise in cytoplasmic free calcium $[Ca^{2++}]_i$. This response is independent on cytokine priming even for incomplete agonists and is similar for MCP-1, IL-8, and other chemokines, although only MCP-1, in contrast to IL-8, efficiently induces degranulation in unprimed basophils. IgE-independent histamine release, but not basophil priming by growth factors, is dependent on extracellular calcium and pertussis toxin-sensitive G-proteins, and both cellular responses are independent of PKC activation. Therefore, basophil histamine release requires calcium and a second yet unknown signal. The IL-3 signal and IL-3-dependent $LTC_4$ synthesis are independent of PKC activation, independent of pertussis toxin-sensitive G-proteins, dependent on tyrosine phosphorylation, and are antagonized by PKC activation. These studies indicate that lipid mediator generation and cytokine priming of basophils are regulated by tyrosine and serine/threonine phosphorylation events in an antagonistic manner (28,29) (Figs. 4 and 5).

Our studies are consistent with the hypothesis that the priming effect is due to activation of a tyrosine kinase, which is a necessary but not sufficient step for leukotriene production. The second signal is provided, at least in part, by activation of a phospholipase C, either through G-protein–coupled receptors or directly by the phosphorylation of PLC-$\gamma$1 by IgE receptor crosslinking or activation of the C-KIT receptor in mast cells, in which case a second signal is not needed (full agonists). Much more work is needed, however, to better define the intracellular signals for leukotriene production. It has been postulated that PKC activation is involved in the induction of leukotriene formation because of a synergism of calcium ionophore and phorbol esters in neutrophils. Our studies, however, clearly showed that

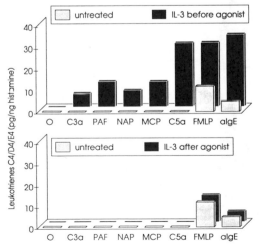

**FIG. 4.** Basophils were exposed to IL-3 either 10 min before **(above)** or 10 min after **(below)** the different agonists. Otherwise, experimental conditions were as in Fig. 3. Leukotriene generation is shown.

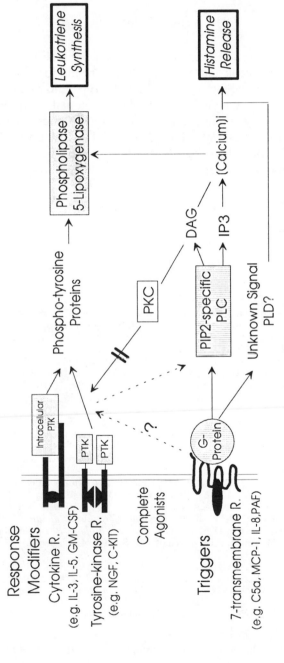

**FIG. 5.** Regulation of mediator release by human basophils.

leukotrienes can be generated without PKC activation, indicating that interpretations based on the effects of xenobiotics are difficult.

## CONCLUSIONS

The capacity of certain cytokines to enhance the responsiveness of inflammatory effector cells and, in particular, to prime for lipid mediator formation may be a critical factor controlling the type and extent of inflammatory processes. Pharmacologic interventions aimed at interfering with leukocyte priming by inhibiting the production of these cytokines or by blocking their effect either at the receptor level or by interference with the signal-transducing pathways, could provide novel approaches to anti-allergic and anti-inflammatory therapy.

## ACKNOWLEDGMENT

This work was supported by the Swiss National Science Foundation Grant 31 36033.92.

## REFERENCES

1. Robinson DR, Hamid Q, Yin S, et al. *N Engl J Med* 1992;326:298–304.
2. Haines KA, Giedd KN, Rich AM, Korchak HM, Weissmann G. *Biochem J* 1987;241:55–62.
3. Clancy RM, Dahinden CA, Hugli TE. *Proc Natl Acad Sci USA* 1989;80:7200–4.
4. Schröder JM. *J Exp Med* 1989;170:847–63.
5. Lopez AF, Eglinton JM, Lyons AB, et al. *J Cell Physiol* 1990;145:69.
6. de Weck AL, Stadler BM, Dahinden CA. *Int Arch Allergy Appl Immunol* 1989;90:17–21.
7. Kurimoto Y, de Weck AL, Dahinden CA. *J Exp Med* 1989;170:476–79.
8. Dahinden CA, Kurimoto Y, de Weck AL, Lindley I, Dewald B, Baggiolini M. *J Exp Med* 1989;170:1787–92.
9. Bischoff SC, Brunner Th, de Weck, AL, Dahinden CA. *J Exp Med* 1990;172:1577–82.
10. Bischoff SC, de Weck AL, Dahinden CA. *Proc Natl Acad Sci USA* 1990;87:6813–7.
11. Kurimoto Y, de Weck AL, Dahinden CA. *Eur J Immunol* 1991;21:361–8.
12. Brunner Th, de Weck AL, Dahinden CA. *J Immunol* 1991;147:237–42.
13. Bischoff SC, Dahinden CA. *Blood* 1992;79:2662–9.
14. Bischoff SC, Krieger M, Brunner Th, Dahinden CA. *J Exp Med* 1992;175:1271–5.
15. Bischoff SC, Dahinden CA. *J Exp Med* 1992;175:237–44.
16. Takafuji S, Bischoff SC, de Weck AL, Dahinden CA. *J Immunol* 1991;147:3855–61.
17. Takafuji S, Bischoff SC, de Weck AL, Dahinden CA. *Eur J Immunol* 1992;22:969–74.
18. Bischoff SC, de Weck AL, Dahinden CA. *Biochem Biophys Res Commun* 1992;11:33–7.
19. Rot A, Krieger M, Brunner Th, Bischoff SC, Shall T, Dahinden CA. *J Exp Med* 1992:1489–95.
20. Dahinden CA, Zingg J, Maly FE, de Weck AL. *J Exp Med* 1988;167:1281–95.
21. Wirthmüller U, de Weck AL, Dahinden CA. *J Immunol* 1989;142:3213–8.
22. Wirthmüller U, de Weck AL, Dahinden CA. *Biochem Biophys Res Commun* 1990;170:556–62.
23. Wirthmüller U, Baggiolini M, de Weck AL, Dahinden Ca. *Biochem Biophys Res Commun* 1991;176:972–8.
24. Schall TJ. *Cytokine* 1991;3:165–83.
25. Kameyoshi Y, Dörscher A, Mallet AJ, Christophers E, Schröder JM. *J Exp Med* 1992;176:587–92.

26. Dahinden CA, Bischoff SC, Brunner Th, Krieger M, Takafuji S, de Weck AL. *Int Arch Allergy Appl Immunol* 1991;94:161–4.
27. Bischoff SC, Baggiolini M, de Weck AL, Dahinden CA. *Biochem Biophys Res Commun* 1991;179:628–33.
28. Krieger M, von Tscharner V, Dahinden CA. *Eur J Immunol* 1992:2907–13.
29. Krieger M, Brunner Th, Bischoff SC, et al. *J Immunol* 1992:2662–7.

*Advances in Prostaglandin, Thromboxane,*
*and Leukotriene Research*, Vol. 22, edited by
S.-E. Dahlén et al. Raven Press, Ltd., New York © 1994

# Current Approaches to Estimation of Eicosanoid Formation In Vivo

## Robert C. Murphy and *Garret A. FitzGerald

*Department of Pediatrics, National Jewish Center for Immunology and Respiratory Medicine, Denver, Colorado 80206; and *Center for Experimental Therapeutics, University of Pennsylvania, Philadelphia, Pennsylvania 19104*

The potent biologic activities of eicosanoids suggest that these metabolites of arachidonic acid play an important role in pathophysiology if not normal physiology. However, direct assessment of the involvement of eicosanoids in any particular disease of normal biologic function has been a difficult task. This is in large part because these molecules are lipid mediators and, as such, exert their effects only a short distance from the site of biosynthesis. These molecules are not pre-stored in specific intracellular granules like the neurotransmitters, and biosynthesis results only after cell stimulation. Furthermore, these molecules do not circulate in the blood as hormones, and therefore the measurement of blood levels is meaningless if not misleading because those eicosanoids found in blood samples are probably due to immediate biosynthesis during the blood collection process. The strategy that has proven most useful in the evaluation of in vivo eicosanoid biosynthesis is the measurement of secondary metabolites in a physiologic fluid, particularly in urine.

Recent clinical studies testing 5-lipoxygenase inhibitors have relied on the measurement of $LTE_4$ as a metabolite of cysteinyl leukotrienes to assess drug efficacy. However, events involved in the metabolic transformations taking place with this arachidonic acid derivative are an important facet, implied by the hypothesis that measurement of a urinary metabolite is a valid index of in vivo eicosanoid production.

## PROSTAGLANDIN METABOLISM

A great deal is known about the metabolism of the prostanoids as well as the specific enzymes that mediate the variety of chemical reactions leading to the final urinary metabolites. An example is the metabolism of $PGE_2$, which is known to undergo oxidation as well as reduction reactions to form a predominant metabolite 13,14-dihydro-15-keto-$PGE_2$ (Fig. 1.). This metab-

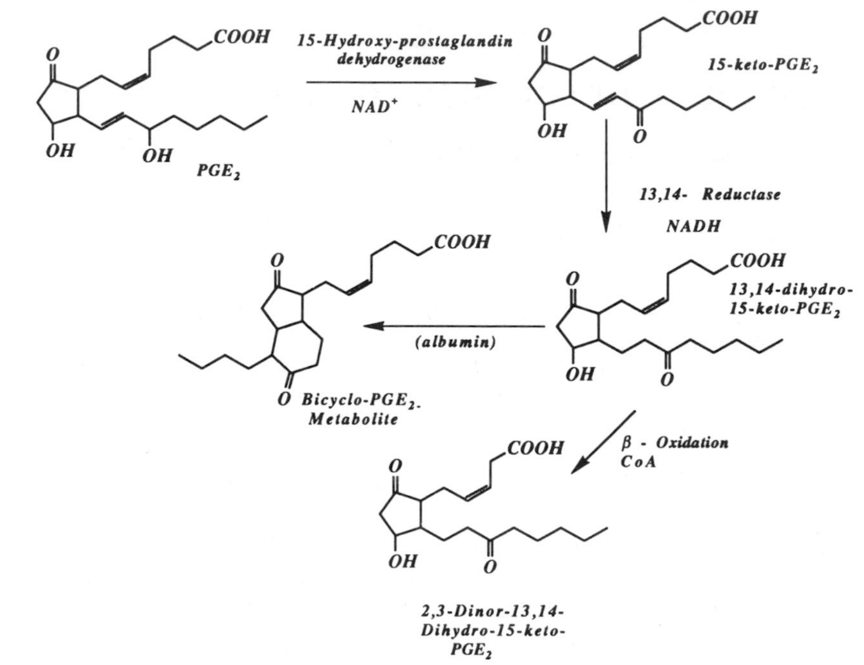

**FIG. 1.** Prostaglandin metabolism: the bicyclo-PGE$_2$ metabolite.

olite can be cyclized in vitro or in vivo to yield the bicyclo-PGE$_2$ metabolite. The bicyclo-PGE$_2$ metabolite has been measured in urine as an index of production of PGE$_2$ in vivo (1). The enzyme 15-hydroxy prostaglandin dehydrogenase is widely distributed and mediates the oxidation of the 15-hydroxyl group to the 15-keto group, the first step in this metabolic transformation. The α/β unsaturated ketone is then reduced by prostaglandin 13,14-reductase using either NAD$^+$ or NADP$^+$ as co-factor. This results in saturation of the 13,14 double bond. Another pathway of PGE$_2$ is metabolism through β-oxidation from the carboxy terminus (C$_1$) followed by one and two rounds of β-oxidation. This route of metabolism results in the dinor and tetranor series of prostaglandins. As this process probably takes place in the peroxisome (2), formation of the CoA ester is required as a necessary first step. The importance of the unsaturated group at $\Delta^{5,6}$ has been suggested as critical to the occurrence of the tetranor series, which may involve prior saturation of this double bond (3).

## THROMBOXANE

The biologically active thromboxane (thromboxane A$_2$) is nonenzymatically hydrated to form thromboxane B$_2$. Although one can readily measure

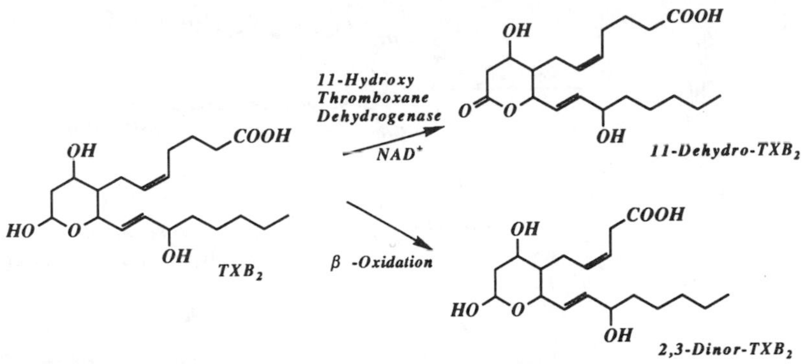

**FIG. 2.** Oxidation of thromboxane $B_2$ by 11-hydroxy thromboxane dehydrogenase: 11-dehydro-TxB$_2$.

the presence of thromboxane $B_2$ in blood or urine, its presence is largely either an artifact of platelet activation occurring during blood collection or of direct kidney production, respectively (4). Therefore, the measurement of a metabolite that is thought to be formed within the liver and eliminated by the kidney has been considered to be a better indicator of in vivo thromboxane $A_2$ production. Thromboxane $B_2$ can be metabolized by two different pathways, both leading to measurable urinary metabolites. The first pathway is through direct oxidation of thromboxane $B_2$ by 11-hydroxy thromboxane dehydrogenase, leading to 11-dehydro-TxB$_2$ (Fig. 2). The fallacy in measurement of plasma levels of TxB$_2$ as a quantitative index of in vivo thromboxane $A_2$ formation was nicely revealed in a study carried out with coincident measurement of plasma TxB$_2$ and 11-dehydro-TxB$_2$ from sequential samples collected through a catheter. Compared with samples drawn from separate venipuncture collections, the concentration of 11-dehydro-TxB$_2$ did not change significantly compared with concentrations of TxB$_2$, which increased in magnitude as well as variance with time (5).

A second pathway, β-oxidation, occurs from the carboxy terminus ($C_1$) and results in 2,3-dinor-TxB$_2$. As neither of these metabolites can be made directly in blood or by the kidney, they serve as excellent indicators of TxA$_2$ production in vivo.

The measurement of these metabolites was performed in a carefully controlled infusion study to assess the normal entry rate of thromboxane into the circulation. The results of these studies have revealed that 0.11 ng/kg/min TxA$_2$ is formed in vivo (6).

## PROSTACYCLIN

Prostacyclin is another important biologically active prostaglandin that is rapidly metabolized in vivo to relatively stable metabolites. The most com-

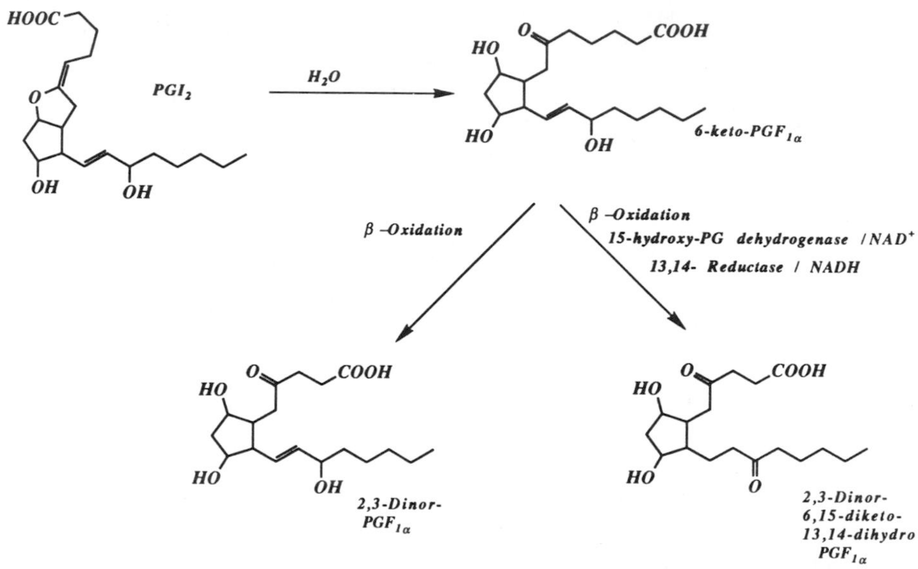

**FIG. 3.** Prostacyclin: measurement of two separate metabolites.

monly measured metabolite is 6-keto-PGF$_{1\alpha}$. Detection of 6-keto-PGF$_{1\alpha}$ in the urine, however, is not believed to reflect in vivo prostacyclin production per se. In a study to test the hypothesis that because PGI$_1$ is not extensively metabolized by the lung it may act as an antiplatelet hormone circulating in vivo, measurement of two separate metabolites was carried out (Fig. 3). The results of these studies indicated that the entry rate of prostacyclin into the circulatory system was approximately 0.1 ng/kg/min, a concentration that was unlikely to exert a physiologic effect and was therefore not supportive of the hypothesis that PGI$_2$ acts as a circulating antiplatelet agent (7).

## CYSTEINYL LEUKOTRIENES

Shortly after the elucidation of the structure of slow-reacting substance as LTC$_4$, the other sulfur-containing leukotrienes possessing biologic activity were structurally characterized as LTD$_4$ and LTE$_4$. It was found that LTC$_4$ was rapidly converted to LTD$_4$ by $\gamma$-glutamyl transpeptidase and LTD$_4$ to LTE$_4$ through various dipeptidases found in most cells, even in plasma. LTE$_4$ was also found to be a urinary metabolite of LTC$_4$ or LTD$_4$ infused into human subjects. The entry rate of LTC$_4$ into the circulation has been estimated to be 0.026 ng/kg/min; yet other metabolites were discovered to predominate and to follow an initial $\omega$-oxidation of LTE$_4$ and two and three rounds of $\beta$-oxidation (8). It is interesting that the sulfur-containing leukotrienes differ substantially from the metabolism of prostaglandins and throm-

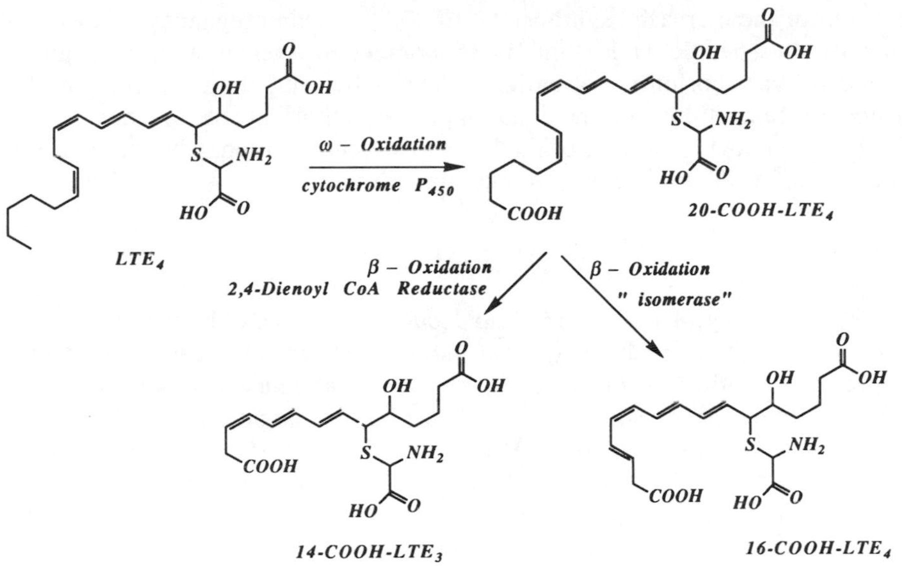

**FIG. 4.** Cysteinyl leukotrienes.

boxane in that β-oxidation is not observed from the carboxyl ($C_1$) terminus, but rather only after ω-oxidation does β-oxidation from the methyl ($C_{20}$) terminus proceed (Fig. 4). In careful infusion studies it was found that these latter ω/β-oxidized metabolites of $LTC_4$ are excreted over a long period of time (8). $LTE_4$ appears only in urine collected immediately after infusion of $LTC_4$, suggesting that only an initial extraction from the blood by the kidney may be taking place. If a continual synthesis of $LTC_4$ is taking place in human subjects, the measurement of $LTE_4$ in urine would be an appropriate index of cysteinyl leukotriene biosynthesis. However, if periodic synthesis of $LTC_4$ is taking place, the measurement of urinary $LTE_4$ may not precisely correlate with the initiation of 5-lipoxygenase activation. Rather, the ω/β-oxidized metabolites might be more appropriate measurements of cysteinyl leukotriene synthesis in these subjects. Unfortunately, little is known about the time course of leukotriene biosynthesis in vivo.

## CYTOCHROME P450 METABOLITES

One of the more recently discovered pathways of arachidonic acid metabolism is by cytochrome P450. This pathway leads to a variety of metabolites, including epoxyeicosatrienoic acids (EET) and their dihydroxy metabolites (DHET). Recent observations revealed an increased elimination of 8,9-, 11,12-, and 14,15-DHET in urine of healthy pregnant women and of patients who have demonstrated pregnancy-induced hypertension (9). The reason for the increased synthesis of EETs in human pregnancy and formation of the specific 11,12- and 14,15-isomers in women with pregnancy-induced hypertension is not entirely clear. However, the discovery of elevated concentrations in urine does suggest an important role for these EETs in the physiologic response of the human subject to pregnancy and possibly the pathophysiology of pregnancy-induced hypertension.

## ISOPROSTANES

The discovery of the isoprostanoid class of eicosanoids in the urine of animals challenged with agents that induce free radical events in vivo (10) represents another example of eicosanoid metabolites observed in urine. The identification of isoprostanes led to pharmacologic studies of biologic activity and discovery of the potent action of at least one member, 8-epi $PGF_{2\alpha}$ on the renal vascular system (11). It is likely that measurement of these compounds may be a measure of noncyclooxygenase/free radical-catalyzed metabolism of arachidonic acid probably occurring at the level of tissue phospholipids (12).

## 15-LIPOXYGENASE

The work of Sigal and co-workers (13) has been provocative in suggesting an important role of 15-lipoxygenase in various diseases. The expression of 15-lipoxygenase in the human epithelial airway places it in a strategic location for metabolites to affect airway responses (13). As with the prostaglandins, thromboxanes, and leukotrienes, evaluation of the in vivo involvement of 15-lipoxygenase is a challenging undertaking.

We know little about the in vivo secondary metabolism of 15-lipoxygenase products, including lipoxins, which have been studied extensively in the laboratories of Serhan and Samuelsson (14). One future area of investigation would be to assess the production of lipoxins through measurement of urinary metabolites. The precise role these interesting metabolites of arachidonic acid play through their myriad biologic activities, as well as specific receptors (15), could be expanded.

One class of 15-lipoxygenase metabolites is rather unique in that this enzyme can work directly on arachidonate esterified in cellular phospholipids. Such metabolites might serve as a specific indicator of 15-lipoxygenase activity in mediating specific disease processes.

## SUMMARY AND CAUTIONARY COMMENTS

The measurement of urinary metabolites of prostaglandins, thromboxanes, leukotrienes, and other eicosanoids has served as an important means by which to assess lipid mediator production in vivo. Furthermore, the measurement of specific metabolites serves as a positive means that can directly assess pharmacologic inhibition of a target enzyme such as cyclooxygenase or, more recently, 5-lipoxygenase. However, an understanding of the formation of these metabolites is important to the general hypothesis that assessment of urinary metabolites is a valid tool by which one can evaluate in vivo eicosanoid biosynthesis. Although the collection of urine is a noninvasive process, the measurement of urinary eicosanoid metabolites precludes an understanding of the precise tissue contribution in the biosynthesis of the parent active eicosanoid. In other words, a urinary metabolite that is largely the result of biosynthesis in one tissue (e.g., the skin) reflects little in terms of the biosynthetic events that may be occurring in the organ of interest (e.g., the lung).

Finally, there are methodologic considerations as to how one quantitatively assesses the level of a urinary metabolite. The problems are largely due to the fact that hundreds if not thousands of molecules are present in urine at the trace concentrations encountered for eicosanoid metabolites. This results in several problems, such as antibody crossreactivity with closely related or even quite structurally diverse molecules. Immunoassays in urine must be carefully validated. Mass spectrometry is also not without its problems, as it relies on a powerful chromatographic step such as gas chromatography or, more recently, high-pressure liquid chromatography, to separate all endogenous or dietary substances found in the urine from the compound of interest. Interfering compounds can influence detection of an otherwise specific ion. As with all analytical techniques employed in microanalysis, great care must be exercised in data interpretation from any assay.

## ACKNOWLEDGMENT

This work was supported in part by grants from the National Institutes of Health (HL25785 and HL30400) and a program grant from the Wellcare Trust.

## REFERENCES

1. Bothwell WM, Verburg MT, Wynalda MA, Daniels EG, Fitzpatrick FA. *J Pharmacol Exp Ther* 1982;220:229–35.
2. Schepers L, Casteels M, Vamecq J, Parmentier G, Van Veldhoven PP, Mannaerts GP. *J Biol Chem.* 1988;263:2724–31.
3. Tserng K-Y, Jin S-J. *J Biol Chem* 1991;266:11614–20.
4. Samuelsson B, Granstrom E, Green K, Hamberg M, Hammarstrom S. *Annu Rev Biochem* 1975;44:669–95.
5. Catella F, Healy D, Lawson JA, FitzGerald GA. *Proc Natl Acad Sci USA* 1986;83:5861–5.
6. Patrono C, Ciabattoni G, Pugliese F, Pierucci A, Blair IA, FitzGerald GA. *J Clin Invest* 1986;77:590–4.
7. FitzGerald GA, Brash AR, Falardeau P, Oates JA. *J Clin Invest* 1981;68:1272–6.
8. Maclouf J, Antoine C, De Caterina R, et al. *Am J Physiol* 1992;263:H244–9.

9. Catella F, Lawson JA, Fitzgerald DJ, FitzGerald GA. *Proc Natl Acad Sci USA* 1990;87: 5893–7.
10. Morrow JD, Hill KE, Burk RF, Nammour TM, Badr KF, Roberts LJ. *Proc Natl Acad Sci USA* 1990;87:9383–7.
11. Takahashi K, Nammour TM, Fukunaga M, et al. *J Clin Invest* 1992;90:136–41.
12. Carella F, Reilly MP, Meaghes EA, et al. *Adv Prostaglandin Thromboxane Leukot Res* [*in press*].
13. Sigal E, Dicharry S, Highland E, Finkbeiner WE. *Am J Physiol* 1992;6:L392–8.
14. Serhan CN, Hamberg M, Samuelsson B. *Proc Natl Acad Sci USA* 1984;81:5335–9.
15. Fiore S, Ryeom SW, Weller PF, Serhan CN. *J Biol Chem* 1992;267:16168–76.

# Subject Index